AF328007

Emerging Cancer Therapeutics

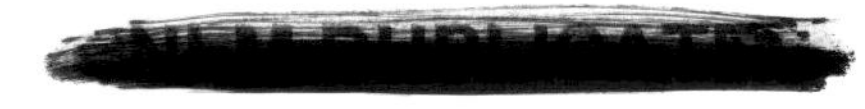

Jame Abraham, MD, FACP

Editor-in-Chief

Bonnie Wells Wilson Distinguished Professor and Eminent Scholar
Chief, Section of Hematology-Oncology
Medical Director, Mary Babb Randolph Cancer Center
West Virginia University
Morgantown, West Virginia

Editorial Board

Ross Donehower, MD
Virginia and D. K. Ludwig Professor in Clinical
   Investigation of Cancer
Director
Division of Medical Oncology
The Johns Hopkins University School of Medicine
Baltimore, Maryland

Ramaswamy Govindan, MD
Associate Professor of Medicine
Division of Oncology
Washington University School of Medicine
St. Louis, Missouri

James L. Gulley, MD, PhD, FACP
Director
Clinical Immunotherapy Group
Laboratory of Tumor Immunology and Biology
National Cancer Institute
National Institutes of Health
Bethesda, Maryland

Scott Howard, MD, MS
Director of Clinical Trials
International Outreach Program
St. Jude Children's Research Hospital
Associate Professor
University of Tennessee College of Medicine
Memphis, Tennessee

Robert Lowsky, MD
Associate Professor of Medicine
Blood and Marrow Transplantation
Stanford School of Medicine
Stanford, California

Joyce O'Shaughnessy, MD
Director
Breast Cancer Research
U. S. Oncology
Dallas, Texas

Shreyaskumar Patel, MD
Professor and Deputy Chair
Sarcoma Medical Oncology
MD Anderson Cancer Center
Houston, Texas

Edith Perez, MD
Professor of Medicine
Mayo Clinic
Jacksonville, Florida

Stephen P. Povoski, MD
Associate Professor of Surgery
Director
High Risk and Breast Cancer Prevention Program
Division of Surgical Oncology
Arthur G. James Cancer Hospital
Richard J. Solove Research Institute
Columbus, Ohio

Kanti Rai, MD
Professor of Medicine
Long Island Jewish Medical Center
New York, New York

Scot C. Remick, MD
Director and Professor of Medicine
The Laurence and Jean DeLynn Chair of Oncology
Mary Babb Randolph Cancer Center
West Virginia University
Morgantown, West Virginia

Stuart Schnitt, MD
Professor
Department of Pathology
Harvard Medical School
Director, Division of Anatomic Pathology
Beth Israel Deaconess Medical Center
Boston, Massachusetts

Forthcoming Issue

Breast Cancer
Antoinette R. Tan, MD, Guest Editor

Emerging Cancer Therapeutics

VOLUME 1, ISSUE 2

Multiple Myeloma

Shaji Kumar, MD
Guest Editor

Associate Professor of Medicine
Hematology and Internal Medicine
Mayo Clinic
Rochester, Minnesota

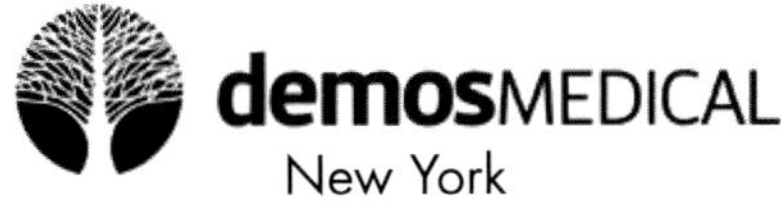

demosMEDICAL
New York

Acquisitions Editor: Richard Winters
Cover Design: Joe Tenerelli
Compositor: NewGen Imaging
Printer: Hamilton Printing

Visit our website at www.demosmedpub.com

Emerging Cancer Therapeutics is published three times a year by Demos Medical Publishing.

Business Office. All business correspondence including subscriptions, renewals, and address changes should be sent to Demos Medical Publishing, 11 West 42nd Street, 15th Floor, New York, NY, 10036.

Copyright © 2010 Demos Medical Publishing. All rights reserved. No part of this publication may be reproduced, stored in a retrieval system, or transmitted in any form or by any means, electronic, mechanical, photocopying, recording, or otherwise, without the prior permission of Demos Medical Publishing, or authorization through payment of the appropriate fees to the Copyright Clearance Center, Inc., 222 Rosewood Drive, Danvers, MA 01923, 978-750-8400, fax 978-646-8600, info@copyright.com or on the web at www.copyright.com.

The ideas and opinions expressed in *Emerging Cancer Therapeutics* do not necessarily reflect those of the Publisher. The Publisher does not assume any responsibility for any injury and/or damage to persons or property arising out of or related to any use of the material contained in this periodical. The reader is advised to check the appropriate medical literature and the product information currently provided by the manufacturer of each drug to be administered to verify the dosage, the method and duration of administration, or contraindications. It is the responsibility of the treating physician or other health care professional relying on independent experience and knowledge of the patient, to determine drug dosages and the best treatment for the patient. Mention of any product in this issue should not be construed as endorsement by the contributors, editors, or the Publisher of the product or manufacturer's claims.

ISSN: 2151-4194
ISBN: 978-1-933864-91-4

Library of Congress Cataloging-in-Publication Data

Multiple myeloma / guest editor, Shaji Kumar.
     p. ; cm. — (Emerging cancer therapeutics, ISSN 2151-4194 ; v. 1, issue 2)
  Includes bibliographical references and index.
  ISBN 978-1-933864-91-4
  1. Multiple myeloma. I. Kumar, Shaji. II. Series: Emerging cancer therapeutics ; v. 1, issue 2. 2151-4194
    [DNLM: 1. Multiple Myeloma. WH 540 M9606 2010]

RC280.B6M847 2010
616.99'418—dc22

2010018635

Reprints. For copies of 100 or more of articles in this publication, please contact Reina Santana, Special Sales Manager.

Special discounts on bulk quantities of Demos Medical Publishing books are available to corporations, professional associations, pharmaceutical companies, health care organizations, and other qualifying groups. For details, please contact:

Reina Santana, Special Sales Manager
Demos Medical Publishing
11 W. 42nd Street
New York, NY 10036
Phone: 800–532–8663 or 212–683–0072
Fax: 212–941–7842
E-mail: rsantana@demosmedpub.com

Made in the United States of America
10 11 12 13 14   5 4 3 2 1

Contents

Foreword

Cancer treatment is one of the fastest growing specialties in modern medicine, with better understanding of the disease, improved diagnostic tools, better prognostic information, and ever-changing management options. The most important tool a clinician can have in the fight against cancer is access to current information.

The *Emerging Cancer Therapeutics (ECAT)* periodicals provide a thorough analysis of key clinical research related to cancer therapeutics, including a discussion and assessment of current evidence, current clinical best practice, and likely near future developments. The content is in the form of review articles, but the volume format will allow for much more in-depth discussion than the typical journal review article. As a periodical, the content can be dynamic and updated more frequently and regularly than the typical static textbook discussion. The goal is to provide for the practicing clinician a source of thorough ongoing analysis and translational assessment of "hot topics" and areas of rapidly emerging new data in cancer therapeutics with significant implications for clinical care.

Each *ECAT* issue is a valuable tool for practicing cancer specialists of all disciplines. It provides the most comprehensive evidence-based review of pathology, radiology, pharmacology, surgical oncology, radiation oncology, and medical oncology of the topic.

Multiple Myeloma provides a comprehensive approach in the pathophysiology, epidemiology, clinical features, diagnostic modalities, and current and future treatment options. Experts from Mayo Clinic and around the world contributed to this issue. This will be a valuable tool for any clinician, researcher, or student of oncology.

Jame Abraham, MD, FACP
Editor-in-Chief

Bonnie Wells Wilson Distinguished Professor and Eminent Scholar
Chief, Section of Hematology-Oncology
Medical Director, Mary Babb Randolph Cancer Center
West Virginia University
Morgantown, WV

Preface

Multiple myeloma represents a malignant proliferation of plasma cells that predominantly affects older patients, with a median age of 65 to 70 years at diagnosis. Multiple myeloma is the second most common hematological malignancy after non-Hodgkin lymphoma and is a part of the spectrum of monoclonal gammopathies, of which monoclonal gammopathy of undetermined significance (MGUS) constitutes the majority. While it has become clear in recent years that MGUS always precedes development of myeloma, the risk remains fairly small with less than 1% of patients progressing to myeloma annually. Myeloma is characterized pathologically by accumulation of clonal plasma cells in the marrow and clinically by development of anemia, renal insufficiency, hypercalcemia or bone destruction, and pathological fractures. Even though myeloma appears to be incurable with current approaches, the past decade has witnessed a paradigm shift in understanding the disease as well as the treatment options available to the patient with myeloma. We have made great strides in understanding the underlying biology of myeloma, particularly the genetic underpinnings of the disease. This has helped to shed light on the underlying heterogeneity of the disease, especially in terms of the genetic groups that have allowed us to better risk stratify patients with myeloma. The therapies have improved with the introduction of the immunomodulatory drugs (thalidomide and lenalidomide) and the proteasome inhibitor bortezomib, improving the outcome of patient, both short term and long term. The overall survival of patients with myeloma has nearly doubled in the past decade, a testament to improved therapies as well as supportive care.

During this time there have been significant changes in the clinical approach to the patient with myeloma regarding diagnosis, risk stratification, and the treatment and monitoring of patients. The explosion of information has made it difficult to obtain a clear view of the practical approach to patients with myeloma. This issue of *Emerging Cancer Therapeutics* is focused on summarizing the state of the art in myeloma, with an emphasis on the practical approach to management of patients with myeloma. The articles cover the entire spectrum, from the diagnosis, risk stratification and treatment, with the treatment sections covering every aspect in great detail. *Multiple Myeloma* brings together experts from several countries, to provide a succinct yet comprehensive description of the state of the art in myeloma. This issue will serve as an up-to-date book for anyone needing to study the entire topic in detail as well as a great reference for someone seeking information about any particular aspect of the disease. I would like to thank all the authors who have contributed to this volume, which will undoubtedly be a great resource for everyone in the field. I hope you will find this book of great value in improving your knowledge and allowing excellent care for patients with myeloma.

Shaji Kumar, MD

Contributors

Melissa Alsina, MD
Associate Professor
Department of Blood and Marrow
  Transplantation
H. Lee Moffitt Cancer Center and Research
  Institute
Department of Oncological Sciences
University of South Florida
Tampa, Florida

Kenneth Andersonm, MD
Professor
Department of Medicine
Harvard Medical School
Boston, Massachusetts

Francis Buadi, MB. ChB
Assistant Professor of Medicine
Division of Hematology
Department of Medicine
Mayo Clinic
Rochester, Minnesota

Wee J. Chng, MB. ChB
Associate Professor of Medicine
Department of Haematology-Oncology
National University Cancer Institute of
  Singapore
National University Health System
National University of Singapore
Singapore

Kathleen A. Donovan, PhD
Professional Associate in Research
Division of Hematology
Mayo Clinic
Rochester, Minnesota

Francesca Gay, MD
Myeloma Unit, Division of Hematology,
  University of Torino
A.O.U. San Giovanni Battista
Torino, Italy

Myo Htut, MD
Clinical Instructor
Hematology and Hematopoietic Cell
  Transplantation
City of Hope Medical Center
Duarte, California

Prashant Kapoor, MD
Fellow, Hematology Oncology
Department of Oncology
Mayo Clinic
Rochester, Minnesota

Amrita Krishnan, MD
Director, Multiple Myeloma Program
Hematology and Hematopoietic Cell
  Transplantation
City of Hope Medical Center
Duarte, California

Shaji Kumar, MD
Associate Professor of Medicine
Hematology and Internal Medicine
Mayo Clinic
Rochester, Minnesota

Jacob Laubach, MD
Instructor
Department of Medicine
Harvard Medical School
Boston, Massachusetts

John A. Lust, MD, PhD
Associate Professor of Medicine
Division of Hematology
Mayo Clinic
Rochester, Minnesota

Sumit Madan, MD
Postdoctoral research fellow
Division of Hematology
Mayo Clinic
Rochester, Minnesota

Constantine Mitsiades, MD, PhD
Instructor
Department of Medicine
Harvard Medical School
Boston, Massachusetts

Taiga Nishihori, MD
BMT Fellow
Department of Blood and Marrow
    Transplantation
H. Lee Moffitt Cancer Center and Research
    Institute
Department of Oncological Sciences
University of South Florida
Tampa, Florida

Stefania Oliva, MD
Myeloma Unit, Division of Hematology,
    University of Torino
A.O.U. San Giovanni Battista
Torino, Italy

Antonio Palumbo, MD
Myeloma Unit, Division of Hematology,
    University of Torino
A.O.U. San Giovanni Battista
Torino, Italy

Hari Parameswaran, MD, MRCP, MS
Center for International Blood and Marrow
    Transplant Research
Division of Neoplastic Diseases and Related
    Disorders
Medical College of Wisconsin
Milwaukee, Wisconsin

Noopur Raje, MD
Director
Center for Multiple Myeloma
Division of Hematology/Oncology
Massachusetts General Hospital
Boston, Massachusetts

Vincent Rajkumar, MD
Professor of Medicine
Division of Hematology
Mayo Clinic
Rochester, Minnesota

Paul Richardson, MD
Associate Professor
Department of Medicine
Harvard Medical School
Clinical Director
Jerome Lipper Center for Multiple Myeloma
Boston, Massachusetts

Ayman Saad, MD
Division of Neoplastic Diseases and Related
    Disorders
Medical College of Wisconsin
Milwaukee, Wisconsin

Loredana Santo, MD
Research Associate
Division of Hematology/Oncology
Massachusetts General Hospital
Boston, Massachusetts

Robert Schlossman, MD
Assistant Professor
Department of Medicine
Harvard Medical School
Boston, Massachusetts

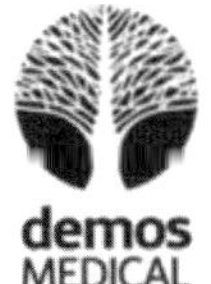

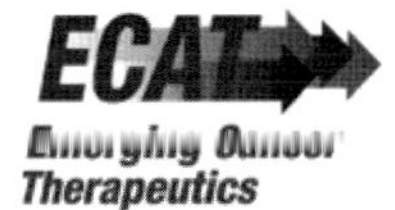

The Etiology and Pathophysiology of Multiple Myeloma

Loredana Santo and Noopur Raje*

*Massachusetts General Hospital Cancer Center and the
Dana Farber Cancer Institute, Harvard Medical School, Boston, MA*

■ ABSTRACT

Although the introduction of novel agents has changed the landscape of multiple myeloma (MM) outcomes, it remains an incurable malignancy of plasma cells. Its development is associated with dysregulated expression and function of multiple cellular genes controlling apoptosis, proliferation, and cell growth. Understanding the etiology and pathogenesis of MM may provide the framework for identification of novel therapeutic targets. Here, we provide a comprehensive review of the latest advances in the study of MM pathogenesis, including the evolution of MM from monoclonal gammopathy of unclear significance. Bone marrow microenvironmental interactions are highlighted in the context of promoting proliferation, survival, drug resistance, and migration of MM cells, with a focus on signaling cascades and cytokines mediating this interaction.

■ INTRODUCTION

Multiple myeloma (MM) is an incurable plasma cell disorder originating in the bone marrow (BM). An understanding of its pathogenesis has been critical to newer insights into the biology of the disease and consequent development of several novel therapies. Here, we will review the pathogenesis of MM, with a focus on novel targets identified and their potential as therapeutic targets.

■ PATHOGENESIS

Etiology

The many studies focused on the etiology of MM have not pinned down a single major causative agent for the disease but rather diverse risk factors including genetic components, lifestyle, and

*Corresponding author, POB 216, MGH Cancer Center, Massachusetts General Hospital, 55 Fruit St, Boston, MA 02114

E-mail address: nraje@partners.org

Emerging Cancer Therapeutics 1:2 (2010) 197–214.
© 2010 Demos Medical Publishing LLC. All rights reserved.
DOI: 10.5003/2151–4194.1.2.197

dietary behavior as well as exposure to external agents. Cohort analyses have identified exposure to high doses of radiation or petroleum products as possible risk factors for MM development. These epidemiological observations are consistent with the property of these agents to induce chromosome abnormalities, oncogenic deregulation, and cellular malignant transformation (1).

A genetic predisposition in MM development has been confirmed in case-control studies that show an increased risk of MM in families with a history of breast, lung, and genitourinary cancer in two or more individuals (2). An association between increased risk of MM and obesity has been reported in a 1994 study. In this study, a positive correlation between body mass index (BMI) and the incidence of MM in white men independent of the presence of diabetes mellitus has been shown (3). Most recent studies (4) confirm that high BMI and alterations in glucose metabolism are correlated with higher MM incidence, and high BMI correlates with particular genotype that increases interleukin-6 (IL-6) production (5). Other factors as hypothesized in other cancers, such as fresh fish intake in the diet, could decrease the MM risk (6).

Although monoclonal gammopathy of unclear significance (MGUS) has been considered a premalignant condition, the rate of conversion to MM remains low and often associated with additional genetic changes (7,8). Repeated infections or antigenic stimulation of the plasma cell compartments has also been suggested as a possible precondition for myeloma. A proposed correlation between MM and infectious or autoimmune diseases, in particular with the presence of human herpesvirus 8 (HHV-8) and Kaposi sarcoma, had been previously made. However, this association, observed in some studies, was not confirmed by other studies (9–11).

MM Evolution from MGUS

MM is preceded by asymptomatic MGUS in 1% of individuals older than 50 years. MGUS can progress to MM with a 1% annual risk and a 25% cumulative probability of progression over 20 years (8). Understanding the evolution of myeloma from MGUS has provided a background for a multistep process involving alterations in various oncogenes and tumor suppressor genes. A multistep development model suggests that MGUS might progress first to smoldering (asymptomatic) MM, next to symptomatic (intramedullary) MM, and finally to extramedullary MM/plasma cell leukemia (PCL). Smoldering MM is considered an intermediate entity between MGUS and active MM without MM-related symptoms, but it can often progress to symptomatic MM. In advanced disease, malignant plasma cells can form extramedullary lesions (e.g., soft tissue plasmacytomas) and can be detected in the circulation as PCL.

Molecular Pathogenesis of MM

MM development is associated with dysregulated expression and function of multiple cellular genes controlling apoptosis, cell growth, and proliferation. Under normal physiological conditions, immature B lymphocytes differentiate after rearrangement of heavy-chain (IgH) and light-chain immunoglobulin (IgL) genes in the BM. The cells with functional expression of IgM migrate to secondary lymphatic tissues, where antigenic stimulation leads to proliferation and differentiation of B lymphocyte in two different types of plasmablasts depending on their passage through the germinal center: (a) cells that have not gone through the germinal center (pregerminal center plasmablasts) and can produce IgM or switch immunoglobulin production (these cells are short-lived plasma cells that do not undergo hypermutation of heavy chain [IgH]) and (b) cells that have gone through the germinal center (postgerminal center plasmablasts). In the germinal center, cells undergo active hypermutation of IgH and IgL gene sequences and antigenic stimulation. Somatically mutated IgM-positive B cells migrate into the blood as memory cells. The postgerminal center plasmablasts that switch immunoglobulin production from IgM to

IgG or IgA and sometimes to IgD or IgE migrate to the BM and differentiate to form long-lived plasma cells (12). In MM, the postgerminal B cells have a phenotype similar to long-lived BM plasma cells.

During the different stages of lymphopoiesis, the postgerminal center plasma cells undergo specific DNA modification like the other B cells that have passed through the germinal center. These DNA modification processes involve VDJ recombination, somatic hypermutation, and IgH switch recombination. Some errors may occur in these DNA modifications of B cells, eventually leading to chromosome translocations, deletions, insertions, and mutations. Because MM is almost exclusively a tumor of plasma cells that have undergone the processes of somatic hypermutation and isotype switch recombination in germinal centers, errors during these physiological processes may occur, leading to chromosome translocations involving the immunoglobulin genes. Almost all cases of MM are characterized by chromosomal abnormalities as demonstrated by cytogenetic and molecular investigations. By interphase fluorescent in situ hybridization (FISH) analysis, two studies have reported that at least one chromosome is trisomic in nearly 90% of MM tumor samples (13,14). By FISH analysis, the incidence of trisomy for at least one chromosome was reported in more than 40% of MGUS cells (13,15). The characteristic numerical abnormalities are monosomy 13 and trisomies of chromosome 3, 5, 7, 9, 11, 15, and 19.

Abnormalities of 14q (the location of IgH) are most common in MM. In addition, chromosomal translocations that involve one of the IgL loci can be present in MM (16). The consequence of Ig translocations is dysregulation or increased expression of an oncogene located near one or more strong Ig enhancers. For MM, most translocations involve five recurrent translocation partners (4p16 [multiple myeloma set domain, *MMSET*, and usually fibroblast growth factor receptor 3, *FGFR3*]; 6p21 [*cyclin* D3]; 11q13 [*cyclin* D1]; 16q23 [c-*MAF*]; 20q12 [*MAFB*]) and appear to be primary translocations that occurred from errors in IgH switch recombination (less often errors in somatic hypermutation) during B-cell development in germinal centers.

Primary translocations occur very early, perhaps initiating events during tumor pathogenesis, whereas secondary translocations occur at the time of progression (17). Secondary translocations are usually complex, unbalanced translocations or insertions, often involving three different chromosomes and sometimes with associated inversions, deletions, duplications, or amplifications (18,19). Conventional karyotypic analyses show that translocations involving 14q32 are present in 20% to 40% of patients with MM with abnormal karyotype. Conventional cytogenetics have failed to identify recurrent IgH translocations in MM because of the low proliferative index of MM cells, the complexity of karyotypes, and the telomeric location of both IgH locus and the partner loci involved. By molecular and FISH techniques, 14q32 region has been found to be involved in translocations in 50% of MGUS and 90% of advanced myeloma. The demonstration of this abnormality in MGUS suggests its involvement in the initial step of the transformation (20–22). The partner chromosomal locus is 11q13 (*cyclin* D1) and is seen in about 30% of these translocations (23). t(11;14)(q13;q32) and t(6;14)(p21;q32) increase the expression of cyclins. t(11;14)(q13;q32), present in 15% to 20% of patients with MM, induces cyclin D1 overexpression (24). t(6;14)(p21;q32), present in 2% to 3% of MM cases, increases the expression of cyclin D3 (25). Another translocation, t(4;14)(p16.3;q32), is present in approximately 15% of patients. It dysregulates the expression of both the MMSET and the receptor tyrosine kinase FGFR3 (26,27). Finally, the t(14;16)(q32;q23) dysregulates the oncogene *MAF*, a basic leucine zipper transcription factor, in 5% to 10% of patients (28); and the t(14;20) affects another member of this family, *MAFB*, in 2% to 5% of cases (29). Although 14q32 is one of the common translocations, its role in MM pathogenesis remains unclear because of the variety of partner chromosomes involved and lack of its prognostic significance. Other recurrent partner loci have been identified infrequently, including 8q24 (*c-myc*) in less than 5%, 18q21 (*bcl2*), 11q23 (*mcl-1*), and 6p21.1 (12).

By interphase FISH analyses, it has been observed that the c-myc locus is rearranged in 3% of MGUS/smoldering myeloma tumors, 10% of MM tumors with a low tumor mass, and 19% of MM tumors with high tumor mass (β2 microglobulin > 3), and it is frequently heterogeneous within a tumor (30). Translocation (14;18) occurs at a low frequency (0–15%) in MM; however, an overexpression of *bcl-2* is observed in numerous myeloma cell lines as well as primary cells express high levels of *bcl-2* (31,32). High levels of Bcl-2 protein are likely to mediate the resistance of MM cells to apoptosis induced by IL-6 deprivation, staurosporine, or other drugs (33). *Mcl-1* is another antiapoptotic gene that is overexpressed in MM and is upregulated by IL-6. Its overexpression mediates potent resistance to apoptosis. t(6;14)(p21;q32) is a rare translocation present in 1 of 30 MM cell lines and in about 4% of primary MM specimens (34). The translocation results in overexpression of cyclin D3. *Ras* mutations are identified in about 39% of patients with newly diagnosed MM and are more frequently observed with disease progression (35,36). Mutually exclusive activating mutations of *K-* or *N-Ras* are rare or absent in MGUS, whereas *Ras* mutations are present in 30% to 40% of early MM (37). *p53* mutations are infrequent in MM. They occur in 5% of inactive MM and in 20% to 40% of acute PCL. *p53* abnormalities represent an important late event associated with progression to an aggressive form of the disease. *p53* mutations may cause a block of plasmablastic apoptosis and differentiation at the final stages of plasma cell maturation (37,38).

In the past decades, different models have been proposed to clarify the molecular evolution and progression of MM. A common pathogenic model hypothesizes that the immortalizing event occurs in the GC and correlates to a primary IgH translocation occurring at the time of switch recombination and somatic hypermutation. Primary IgH translocation causes the ectopic expression of an oncogene that drives proliferation of the long-lived plasmablast/plasma cell. It has been postulated that karyotypic instability is the initiating oncogenic event in MM, independent of the presence of IgH translocations. Secondary translocations that dysregulate *c-myc* and *p53* mutations contribute to subsequent progression and increased proliferation (18).

Cellular Origin of MM

In physiological conditions, pre-B cells (immature B-cell precursors) are CD10+ CD19– CD22– CD34+ during the B-cell development. Their Ig genes remain germline or affect only D-JH joining. At the next stage, pre-pre-B and early pre-B cells express CD19 and present a rearrangement of IgH genes. The pre-B cells express the µ-chain in their cytoplasm, CD34 is no longer present, and CD22 is expressed. IgL genes are rearranged in late pre-B cells, and production of IgL causes the expression of the surface µ-chain typical of B cells (39). Unique idiotypic determinants can identify clones of peripheral blood lymphocytes in patients with macroglobulinemia, MM, MGUS, and chronic lymphocytic leukemia, as demonstrated by studies using antiidiotypic antibodies (40). The presence of idiotypic determinants on cytoplasmic µ-containing pre-B cells in MM BM has suggested that the oncogenic event may occur at the pre-B cell stage. Aneuploid marrow MM cells can express mRNA for cell surface proteins characteristic of myeloid, erythroid, and platelet lineages. This observation strengthens the evidence that the malignant clone can extend from an early stage of differentiation (41).

B and T cells characterized by the presence of identical idiotypic determinants have been identified, suggesting that target cells for oncogenic transformation could be precursor cells for both B- and T-cell clones (42). The cells that accumulate in the BM of patients with MM have plasma cell or plasmablast morphology. It has been shown that monoclonal B lineage cells in peripheral blood of patients with MM, which are late-stage B cells (low CD19 and CD20, moderate CALLA and PCA-1, with strong CD45RO antigen expression), are in continuous progression toward the plasma cell stage (43). However, it has not been identified yet which cell within the malignant clone is "clonogenic" and capable of self-renewal.

■ ROLE OF MICROENVIRONMENT IN MM PATHOGENESIS

Adhesion of MM Cells to the BM

Gene expression in tumor cells and bone marrow stromal cells (BMSCs) is affected by adhesion of MM cells to BM. This interaction influences tumor growth, survival, drug resistance, and migration in the BM environment. Complex and dynamic interplay of MM cells with their local bone microenvironment strongly determines the biological behavior of MM cells (44).

Adhesion of MM cells to extracellular matrix (ECM) proteins or BMSCs is regulated by several adhesion molecules involved in the pathogenesis of disease progression. After switching class in the LN, adhesion molecules (e.g., CD44, VLA-4, VLA-5, LFA-1, CD56, syndecan-1, intercellular adhesion molecule [ICAM1], and MPC-1) help MM homing to the BM (45–47) (Figure 1). Subsequently, binding of MM cells occurs to BMSCs; for example, VLA4 expressed on MM cells mediates both binding to the ECM and to BMSCs, through fibronectin and VCAM1,

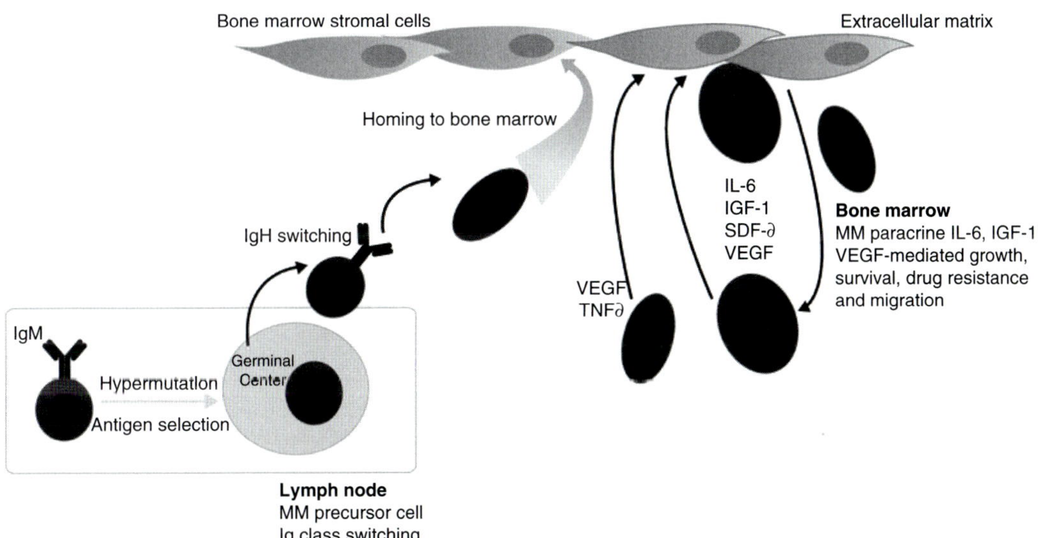

FIGURE 1

Maturation and homing of plasma cells in multiple myeloma (MM) progression: In the germinal center, cells undergo active hypermutation of IgH and IgL gene sequences and antigenic stimulation. The postgerminal center plasmablasts that switch immunoglobulin production from IgM to IgG or IgA and sometimes to IgD or IgE migrate to the bone marrow (BM) and differentiate to form long-lived plasma cells. Myeloma cells interact with different cell types within the BM microenvironment promoting direct adhesion-mediated signaling and triggering the secretion of growth and/or anti-apoptotic factors, including interleukin (IL)-6, insulin-like growth factor (IGF)-1, vascular endothelial growth factor (VEGF), B-cell activating factor (BAFF), fibroblast growth factor (FGF), stromal cell-derived factor (SDF) 1α, and tumor necrosis factor (TNF)-α.

respectively. Binding to fibronectin upregulates p27 (encoded by CDKN1B) and induces nuclear factor κB (NF-κB) activation in MM cells (48), which provides cell adhesion-mediated drug resistance (CAMDR) to conventional chemotherapy (49,50). Moreover, such binding not only localizes tumor cells in the BM microenvironment but also stimulates IL-6 transcription and secretion from BMSCs with related paracrine growth of MM cells (51–53). Other cytokines, like tumor necrosis factor (TNF)-α, upregulate adhesion molecules on MM cells and BMSCs, thereby increasing binding and CAMDR (54).

Syndecan 1, a transmembrane heparan sulphate-bearing proteoglycan, is expressed in most MM cells. The adhesion of MM cells to the ECM through the binding of syndecan 1 to type I collagen induces the expression of matrix metalloproteinase 1 (MMP1), which favors bone resorption and tumor invasion (55). Increased serum soluble syndecan 1 correlates with increased tumor cell mass, decreased MMP9 activity, and poor prognosis. The adhesion of MM cells to the ECM through the binding of syndecan 1 to type I collagen induces the expression of MMP1, which favors bone resorption and tumor invasion. Soluble syndecan 1 promotes the growth of MM cells in vivo. It also mediates decreased osteoclast (OC) and increased osteoblast (OB) differentiation (56,57).

As the disease progresses, the development of PCL is characterized by decreased expression of certain adhesion molecules (e.g., CD56, VLA-5, MPC-1, and syndecan-1), which, in turn, facilitates tumor cell mobilization; extramedullary spread of MM cells is facilitated by the reappearance of CD56, VLA-5, MPC-1, and syndecan-1. Because adhesion molecules play a central role in the pathogenesis of MM, therapeutic strategies targeting these molecules have been developed and tested in animal models; for example, anti-ICAM-1 antibodies have been shown to inhibit tumor development in severe combined immunodeficient (SCID) mice (58). Moreover, the introduction of fetal human bone into SCID mice (SCID-hu) has enabled studying the importance of stromal cell/

MM cell interactions, the biological sequence of binding, and testing novel treatments based on interruption of this process (59,60). Novel agents, including thalidomide (Thal) and its immunomodulatory derivatives (IMiDs), as well as the proteasome inhibitor, bortezomib, can target both tumor cells and the BM microenvironment; as a consequence, they overcome CAMDR (37,61).

Role of BM Microenvironmental Components

Homing of MM cells to BM is a complex process; however, its detailed understanding can reveal crucial information regarding disease progression and drug resistance. Studies of the homing mechanism have enabled promising therapies aimed at both the MM and BM microenvironment in a direct or an indirect fashion. Myeloma cells strongly interact with many different cell types in the BM microenvironment, such as BMSCs, endothelial cells, OC, OB, and immune cells. This interaction is central to MM pathogenesis promoting direct adhesion-mediated signaling and triggering the secretion of growth and/or antiapoptotic factors, including IL-6, insulin-like growth factor (IGF)-1, vascular endothelial growth factor (VEGF), B-cell activating factor (BAFF), fibroblast growth factor (FGF), stromal cell-derived factor (SDF)-1α, and TNF-α. In turn, these secreted agents not only mediate tumor cell growth, proliferation, survival, drug resistance, and migration but are also involved in osteoclastogenesis and angiogenesis. Many proliferative/antiapoptotic signaling pathways in MM cells are determined by these physical interactions, either through cell adhesion molecule-mediated interactions of MM cells with BMSCs, OCs, other BM cellular compartments or the ECM or, indirectly, through other cytokines/growth factors released by MM cells and/or BMSCs (48).

When MM cells bind to BMSCs, NF-κB is stimulated and upregulates adhesion molecules and cytokine secretion, which further increase MM cell growth, survival, drug resistance, and migration.

In addition, NF-κB also mediates the expression of many adhesion molecules expressed in both MM and BM microenvironment. Moreover, activation of NF-κB by cell adhesion and cytokines (such as TNF-α) augments the binding of MM cells to BMSCs, which, in turn, induces IL-6 transcription and secretion in BMSCs (54,62).

In addition to NF-κB, several pathways are involved in the BM microenvironment–MM cells interaction. Adhesion and cytokines activate p42/44 mitogen-activated protein kinase (MAPK), which mediates proliferation of MM cells, Janus kinase (JAK)/signal transducer, and activator of transcription 3 (STAT3), which along with upregulation of Bcl-X$_L$ and Mcl-1 regulates survival and/ or phosphatidylinositol 3-kinase (PI3K)/Akt and their downstream pathways. Specifically, PI3K/ Akt mediates antiapoptosis through downstream activation of BAD and NF-κB and/or inactivation of caspase-9. NF-κB and forkhead in rhabdomyosarcoma (FKHR) modulate cyclin D and KIP1, thus regulating cell-cycle progression. Signaling through PI3K induces downstream protein kinase C (PKC) activity and MM cell migration (37,63,64) (Figure 2).

Osteolytic lesions are a crucial clinical signature of MM and a major cause of morbidity and mortality (44). The defining property of patients with osteolytic bone lesions is an unbalanced bone remodeling usually due to accumulations of MM cells within the BM that increase bone turnover rates. In physiological conditions, the skeleton optimizes the stress-bearing capacity of bones by constant structural remodeling. This remodeling is made of two coordinated processes of old bone resorption mediated by OCs and compensatory new bone formation by OBs. In MM, the concomitant strengthening of many positive regulators of OC formation and function together with the suppression of negative regulators of osteoclastogenesis and/or positive regulators of bone formation tend to decouple these two processes (65,66). BMSCs and OBs regulate osteoclastogenesis through the production of receptor activator of NF-κB ligand (RANKL) and osteoprotegerin (OPG) (67,68), a

soluble decoy receptor for RANKL. RANK is a TNF-receptor superfamily member expressed on OCs and their precursors. RANKL is expressed on BMSCs and OBs and secreted by activated lymphocytes. RANKL binds to RANK receptor on OC precursors, thereby triggering OC differentiation and resorptive activity. OPG, produced by OBs as well as other cell types, blocks the interactions of RANKL with RANK, thereby limiting osteoclastogenesis.

Expression of RANKL by BMSCs is drastically increased upon contact with MM cells, whereas OPG is suppressed and inactivated by syndecan-mediated internalization in myeloma cells. Moreover, MM cells potentiate OC activity by triggering the upregulation of multiple pro-osteoclastogenic cytokines (e.g., IL-6, IL-1α, IL-1β, IL-11, MIP-1α, M-CSF, TNF-α, PTHrP, VEGF), which are either produced by MM cells or by host BM cells (e.g., BMSCs) following paracrine/ juxtacrine stimulation by MM cells (65,69,70) (Figure 3). MIP-1α is a chemokine that strongly induces OC formation independently of RANKL and promotes both RANKL- and IL-6-stimulated OC formation. Moreover, MIP-1α increases adhesive interactions between MM cells and BMSCs by increasing the expression of β1 integrins on MM cells. This leads to increased production of RANKL, IL-6, VEGF, and TNF-α by the marrow stromal compartment, which further triggers MM cell growth, angiogenesis, and bone destruction (71). Although the role of IL-6 as a proliferative factor for plasma cells is well known, its precise role in MM bone disease is not fully determined yet. IL-6 production by OCs can increase tumor burden, leading to enhanced bone destruction as well as act as an autocrine/paracrine factor to increase OC formation (72). In addition to RANKL and MIP-1α, IL-3 is also significantly elevated in BM plasma of patients with MM compared with normal controls. IL-3 indirectly influences osteoclastogenesis by triggering the effects of RANKL and MIP-1α on the growth and development of OCs (73). IL-3 also inhibits OB formation through a factor produced by macrophages

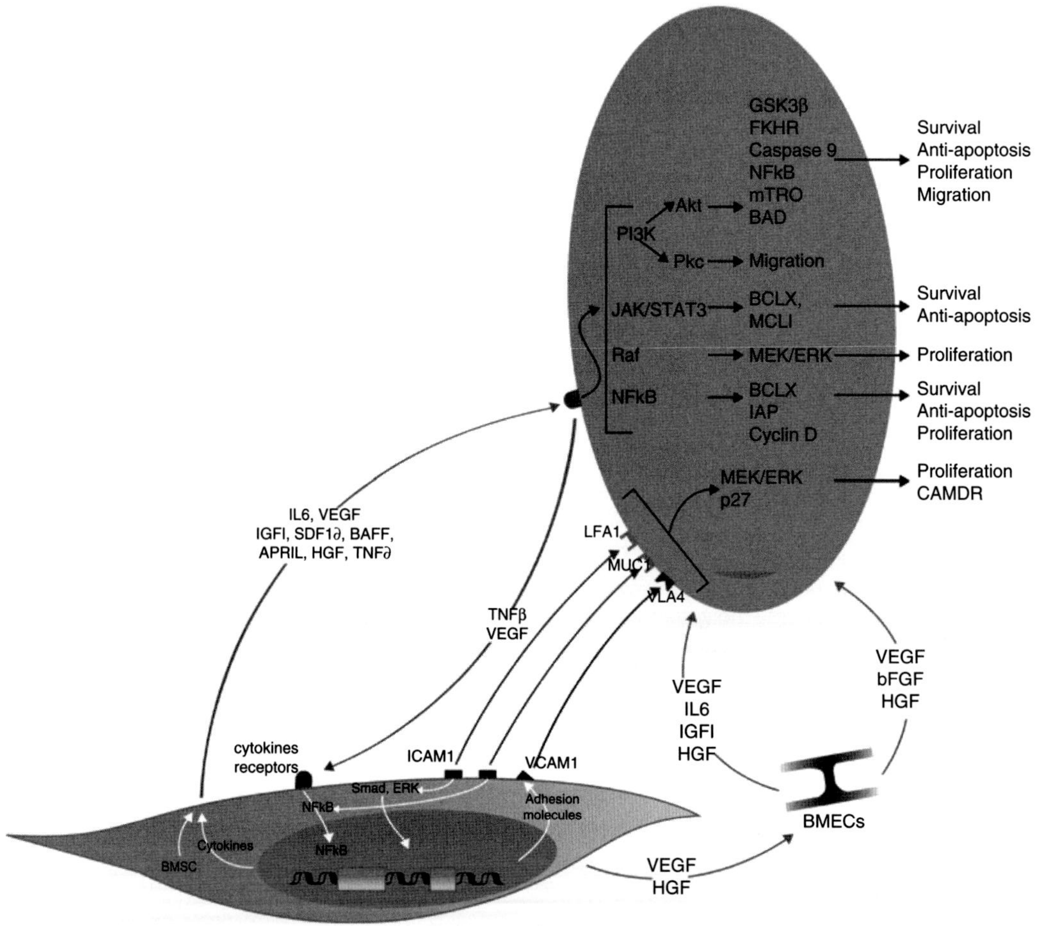

FIGURE 2

Role of the bone marrow (BM) microenvironment in myeloma pathogenesis: Adhesion of multiple myeloma (MM) cells to BMSCs is regulated by several adhesion molecules (e.g., CD44, VLA-4, VLA-5, LFA-1, CD56, syndecan-1, intercellular adhesion molecule [ICAM1], and MPC-1) resulting in MM homing to the BM. Binding of MM cells to BMSCs via, for example, VLA4 expressed on MM cells through fibronectin and VCAM1 on BMSCs upregulates p27 and induces nuclear factor-κB (NF-κB) activation in MM cells, which induces cell adhesion-mediated drug resistance (CAMDR) to conventional chemotherapy. This interaction leads to NF-κB activation and induction of adhesion molecules and cytokine secretion, which further induce signaling cascades and augment MM cell growth, survival, drug resistance, and migration. Modified from Ref. 37.

in the marrow microenvironment (74). Moreover, OB activity is significantly suppressed in MM. The formation and differentiation of OBs from mesenchymal cells require the activity and function of the transcription factor Runx2/Cbfal (75). Increased Runx2/Cbfal activity without change in Runx2 protein levels leads to human OB differentiation, even though Runx2/Cbfal overexpression can impair bone formation. In MM bone disease, the inhibition of Runx2/Cbfal activity has been

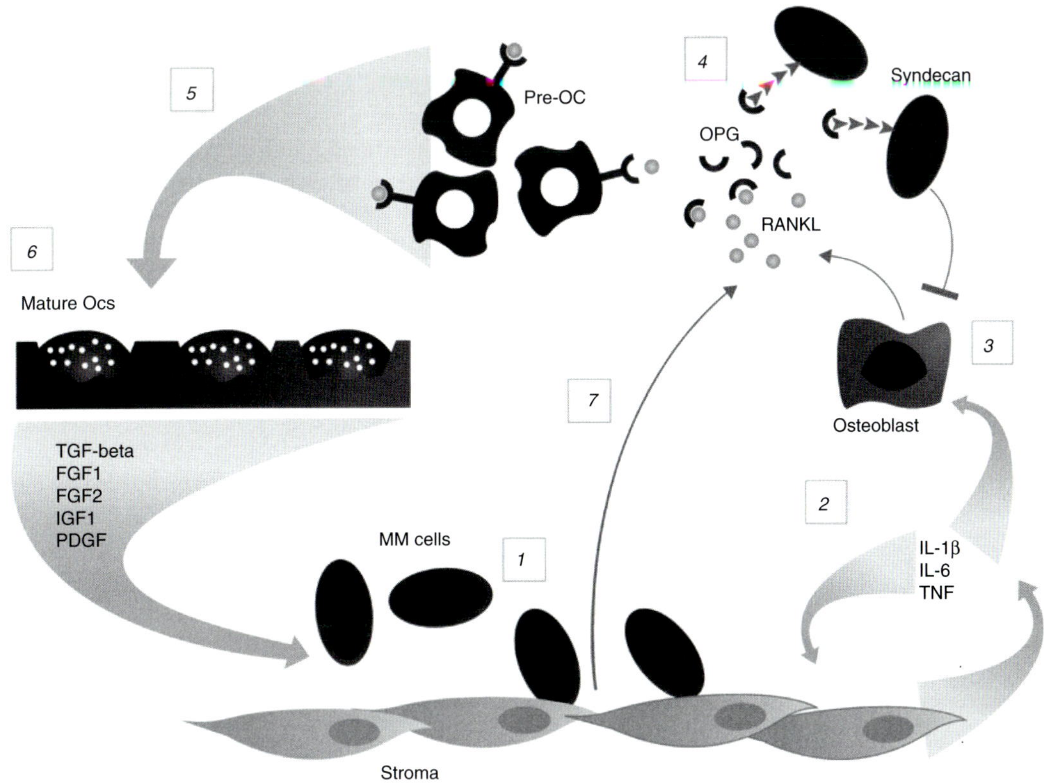

FIGURE 3

Role of osteoclasts and osteoblasts and the cytokine regulatory loop in myeloma bone disease: Adhesion of multiple myeloma (MM) cells to stroma (1) results in secretion of osteoclast activating factors (OAFs) from stroma (2). OAFs induce stroma and osteoblasts to secrete RANKL (3), which is blocked by OPG; syndecan secreted by MM cells binds OPG and reduces OPG concentration (4). Excess RANKL stimulates osteoclasts (5) leading to increased osteoclast activity (6) resulting in cytokines released from bone matrix stimulating MM cell growth. These cytokines cause release of PTHrP from MM cells (7), which activate stromal cells to secrete RANKL.

observed. IL-3, besides its role in OC formation and bone resorption, can indirectly inhibit OB formation (74). Similarly, IL-7 can also inhibit OBs in MM. IL-7 levels are increased in marrow plasma samples from patients with MM (76). IL-7 is a potent inhibitor of OB differentiation and can affect OB formation in several ways including via interference of Runx2 activity (77).

Other factors such as Dickoppf-1 (DKK1), expressed and secreted by MM cells, interfere with Wnt signaling, thereby inhibiting OB differentiation and maturation and aggravating bone destruction (78). Recombinant human DKK1 or BM plasma with increased levels of DKK1 inhibit the differentiation of OB precursor cells and bone formation in vitro (79) through a DKK1-mediated attenuation of Wnt3a-induced stabilization of β-catenin (80). Elevated DKK1 levels can also enhance osteoclastogenesis. DKK1 suppression of Wnt in BMSC/OB leads to increased production of RANKL and IL-6 and decreased production of OPG. Immature OBs produce a significant amount of IL-6; however, upon differentiation, IL-6 production decreases substantially (81,82).

Multiple stimulators of OC activity and suppressors of OB differentiation are present in MM and together result in the devastating bone disease (77) pathognomic of MM. Understanding the pathophysiology of MM bone disease has fostered the creation of novel pharmacological approaches targeting both MM cell proliferation and the complex interaction between MM cells and BM microenvironment. Activin A, a transforming growth factor β (TGF-β) superfamily member, is involved in bone remodeling, where it promotes osteoclastogenesis. Activin, usually synthesized and secreted by BMSCs, directs an autocrine regulatory loop of stromal differentiation into OB (83,84). Although OB differentiation effects have not been clearly identified yet, exogenous activin has been reported to both inhibit and promote OB differentiation in vitro (85,86). However, in vivo, activin A seems to perform an inhibitory role on OB. Enhanced bone formation rate and bone mass has been observed in vivo as a result of treatment with a soluble receptor for activin, RAP-011 (87,88). Increased activin A levels have been associated with high lytic burden in patients with MM independently of the disease stage (89). In addition, activin A is used by MM cells to modify their niche; conversely, this niche modification supports MM growth, which creates a microenvironmental positive feedback loop. A novel strategy to treat MM is aimed at disrupting this loop by targeting activin A (89).

Role of Cytokines and Growth Factors

Myeloma cells and BMSCs produce various cytokines that play a crucial role in tumor growth, survival, migration, and drug resistance: IL-6 (90), IGF-1 (91), VEGF (92), SDF-1 (93), TNF (54), TGF-β (94), BAFF (95), IL-21 (96), and others.

Interleukin-6

IL-6 is a critical growth and survival factor for MM cells. IL-6 binds to gp80 (IL-6R) inducing gp130 phosphorylation and homodimerization (97). When IL-6 interacts with its receptor, it triggers the MAPK, PI3K/Akt, and JAK/STAT signaling cascades, which mediates growth, survival, and drug resistance (64). IL-6 is mostly produced by BMSCs, following binding of myeloma cells; it mediates MM cell growth and prevents apoptotic cell death. Importantly, both autocrine and paracrine growth of myeloma cells is mediated by IL-6. Autocrine production of IL-6 corresponds to a highly malignant phenotype, high proliferative index, and significant resistance to drug-induced apoptosis (98).

In addition, IL-6 confers resistance to dexamethasone (Dex). MM apoptosis induced by Dex is regulated by the release of second mitochondria activator of caspase (Smac) from mitochondria (but not by cytochrome c release), followed by caspase 9 and 3 cleavage activation. IL-6 blocks caspase 9 activation, thus preventing cell death induced by Dex (99).

Dex-induced apoptosis is also mediated by the activation of related adhesion focal tyrosine kinase (RAFTK) (100). IL-6 prevents Dex-induced apoptosis via PI3-K/Akt signaling (64) and specific activation of src homology 2-domain containing tyrosine phosphatase 2 (SHP2); in this way, the activation of RAFTK is blocked (101).

The importance of IL-6 has also been demonstrated in the growth of MM in vivo. Elevated IL-6 serum levels correlate to poor prognosis and higher tumor cell mass (102,103). Moreover, patients with MGUS and indolent or smoldering MM have relatively normal IL-6 serum levels, whereas patients with advanced MM or PCL have the highest IL-6 levels. IL-6 and soluble IL-6Rα are involved in bone resorption by OCs. In therapy, specific antibodies for IL-6 or its receptor and IL-6 superantagonists, which compete for IL-6R binding but do not activate downstream signaling (104), have been used; nevertheless, these treatments have only triggered transient responses in patients with MM (105,106). Newer classes of neutralizing antibodies are currently being investigated.

Insulin-Like Growth Factor-1

The multifunctional peptide IGF-1 is mostly produced and secreted by the BMSCs. IGF-1 induces proliferation and survival in MM cells (107,108).

IGF-1 activates ERK and PI3-K/Akt signaling pathways (109) without an effect on JAK2/STAT signaling pathway. Specifically, IGF-1 activates PI3-K/Akt and NF-κB (62); induces phosphorylation of FKHR (forkhead) transcription factor; upregulates antiapoptotic proteins including FLIP, survivin, cIAP-2, A1/Bfl-1, and XIAP; strengthens telomerase activity via induction of PI3-K/Akt/NF-κB (110); and lowers drug sensitivity of MM cells (62).

IGFs and their receptors are considered attractive therapeutic targets given their high levels in serum and in the BM environment due to paracrine release by OBs and BMSCs. IGF-1-driven therapies targeting IGF-1, for example, involving inhibitors of IGF-1 receptor, have shown preclinical anti-MM activity (111).

Vascular Endothelial Growth Factor

VEGF, crucially involved in tumor cell migration and angiogenesis (92,112), is produced both by MM cells and BMSCs. VEGF secretion is upregulated by IL-6, and CD40 activation induces p53-dependent VEGF production in human MM cells (113).

VEGF triggers the phosphorylation and activation of VEGF receptor Flt-1, highly expressed in MM cell lines and patient cells. Moreover, VEGF activates MEK/ERK and PI-3K/PKCα signaling pathway inducing MM cell proliferation and migration (92). The aforementioned effects of VEGF on tumor cells, together with the VEGF-induced BM angiogenesis, suggest VEGF as a therapeutic target. The VEGF receptor tyrosine kinase PTK787 and anti-VEGF antibody have shown promising antimyeloma activity (114). Increased angiogenesis enhances microvessel density in BM of patients with MM compared with individuals with MGUS (115–117). Moreover, increased microvascular density correlates with disease progression and poor prognosis (118,119).

B-Cell Activating Factor

BAFF (also known as BlyS or B lymphocyte stimulator, TALL1, zTNF-4, THANK, and TNFSF13B) is a member of TNF family involved in B-cell maturation and survival and T-cell activation (95,120). Moreover, BAFF costimulates B-cell proliferation and immunoglobulin secretion. It has been shown that B cells isolated from BAFF transgenic mice have elevated Bcl-2 levels and prolonged survival (121,122), demonstrating a role for BAFF in attenuating apoptosis.

APRIL, a proliferation-inducing ligand, is another member of TNF family, which shares two receptors with BAFF, transmembrane activator and calcium-modulator and cyclophilin ligand interactor, and B-cell maturation antigen. BAFF also specifically binds to a third receptor, BAFF receptor (BAFF-R), that seems to be the primary BAFF-binding receptor responsible for B-cell development and survival (123). In fact, mice with a mutation in the BAFF-R have a loss of follicular and marginal zone B cells in secondary lymphoid organs, a phenotype similar to BAFF-deficient mice (121,122). BAFF and APRIL play an important role in MM pathogenesis and in multiple-drug resistance and disease relapse of MM. It has been shown that both BAFF and APRIL contribute to the survival of human myeloma cell lines and primary MM cells and can protect MM cell apoptosis induced by IL-6 deprivation and Dex (124). In addition, BAFF and APRIL have been found to be elevated in the serum of patients with MM (125,126). Anti-BAFF antibodies have demonstrated direct anti-MM activity in an SCID model of human MM with a reduction in radiologically evident lytic lesions in anti-BAFF-treated animals underscoring the role of BAFF in the BM microenvironment (125).

BAFF and APRIL modulate NF-κB (127), making these cytokines interesting in the context of MM because increased NF-κB activity is associated with enhanced tumor cell survival. A recent study showed that different MM cell lines and primary MM cells express BAFF, APRIL, and their three receptors. Treatment with bortezomib decreases the concentration of BAFF and APRIL by lowering their autocrine secretion and reduces MM cell proliferation by inhibiting the noncanonical NF-κB pathway transduced by BAFF and APRIL (128). Importantly, specific neutralizing antibodies to BAFF are currently undergoing clinical testing.

Fibroblast Growth Factor

FGF is expressed and secreted by MM cells. In progressive MM, FGF increases the angiogenic potential of BMSCs (115,129). Stimulation of BMSCs by FGF triggers time- and dose-dependent increase in IL-6 secretion; conversely, stimulation with IL-6 enhanced FGF triggers expression and secretion by MM cell lines as well as MM patient cells (130). This suggests paracrine interaction of IL-6 and FGF between MM and BMSCs. This interaction plays a pivotal role in MM cell growth and survival in the BM microenvironment (131).

Wnt

Wnts are a family of 19 secreted glycoproteins that are critically involved in stem cell maintenance and development (132) and MM pathogenesis (133). Wnt proteins bind to frizzled receptors alone or complexed with low-density lipoprotein receptor-related proteins 5/6. Many effects of Wnts are mediated through β-catenin, essential in the canonical Wnt pathway.

Intracellularly, the Wnt-signaling cascade blocks degradation of β-catenin in proteasomes, thereby leading to accumulation of β-catenin in the cytoplasm. In MM, a canonical Wnt-signaling pathway is activated after treatment with Wnt-3a, associated with accumulation of β-catenin. In addition, Wnt-3a treatment leads to significant morphological changes in MM cells, accompanied by rearrangement of the actin cytoskeleton (134). However, the activation of canonical Wnt signaling by Wnt3a or by LiCl has no effect on the proliferation of MM cells or on the antiapoptotic signals conferred on MM cells (133,134). In contrast to these data, other studies have reported that the activation of the Wnt/β-catenin pathway

by sFRP1, a Wnt antagonist, inhibits cell growth (135,136). Potential reasons behind these apparently contradictory results could be the inhibition of both canonical and noncanonical Wnt signaling, by sFRP1, as a soluble decoy receptor (137).

Canonical Wnt signaling is essential for osteoblastogenesis and normal bone metabolism. The secretion of Wnt-signaling antagonists by MM cells contributes to the bone-destructive process as well as disease progression (138). MM plasma cells secrete the Wnt-signaling inhibitor DKK1 as previously described and using a neutralizing antibody results in inhibition of bone destruction and tumor progression in a xenograft mouse model of human MM (139).

Other Cytokines

SDF-1α is expressed by BMSCs, and its receptor CXCR4 is expressed by myeloma cells. Higher expression of CXCR4 has been reported in patient-derived cells and MM cell lines (140). SDF-1α helps internalization of CXCR4 and induces cytoskeletal rearrangement of MM cells. On the other hand, specific inhibitors of CXCR4 anti-CXCR4 antibodies prevent migration of MM cells in vitro, which indicates that the SDF1α–CXCR4 interaction is an important regulator of MM homing (93,141). SDF-1α regulates the migration of normal hematopoietic stem cells (142), promotes proliferation, induces migration, and protects against Dex-induced apoptosis in MM cells (93). Although SDF-1α plays a role in the pathophysiology of MM, its effects are modest compared with other cytokines.

TNF-α is secreted by myeloma cells. TNF-α strongly activates NF-κB, thus upregulating adhesion molecules, with resultant binding of myeloma cells to BM and related CAMDR (48). TNF-α induces only modest activation of MAPK/ERK in MM cells, without any significant direct effect on myeloma cell growth and survival. Specific antibody inhibitors of TNF-α have not shown clinical response; nonetheless, Thal and its IMiD analogs have potent anti-TNF-α activity and can overcome CAMDR (61,143). IL-21 induces proliferation and prevents apoptosis independent of IL-6 signaling. It triggers phosphorylation of Jak1, Stat3, and Erk1/2 (p44/42 MAPK). TNF-α upregulates expression of both IL-21 and IL-21 receptors (IL-21R).

TGF-α is produced by MM cells and induces secretion of IL-6 by BMSCs; it also contributes to immunosuppression characteristic of myeloma. Osteoclast-activating factors, such as IL-6, IL-1α, IL-1β, IL-11, MIP-1α, M-CSF, TNF-α, PTHrP, and VEGF, are secreted by stromal cells as a consequence of adhesion of MM cells have been previously discussed.

The enormous research effort aimed at studying MM biology is tightly linked to present improvements and future innovations in the clinical management of MM. For example, we now have a clearer understanding of the pathogenesis of MM, which has highlighted specific pathways important in the multistep transformation process of normal plasma cells to MM. In addition, the in-depth knowledge of the molecular pathogenesis of MM as well as the role of BM in MM development have allowed and continue to allow the identification of critical molecules and pathways potentially useful as novel therapeutic targets for improved MM patients outcome.

■ REFERENCES

1. Riedel DA, Pottern LM. The epidemiology of multiple myeloma. *Hematol Oncol Clin North Am* 1992;6(2):225–247.
2. Bourguet CC, Grufferman S, Delzell E, et al. Multiple-myeloma and family history of cancer—a case control study. *Cancer* 1985;56(8):2133–2139.
3. Friedman GD, Herrinton LJ. Obesity and multiple-myeloma. *Cancer Causes Control* 1994;5(5):479–483.
4. Renehan AG, Tyson M, Egger M, Heller RF, Zwahlen M. Body-mass index and incidence of cancer: a systematic review and meta-analysis of prospective observational studies. *Lancet* 2008;371(9612):569–578.
5. Cozen W, Gebregziabher M, Conti DV, et al. Interleukin-6-related genotypes, body mass index, and risk of multiple myeloma and plasmacytoma. *Cancer Epidemiol Biomarkers Prev* 2006;15(11):2285–2291.
6. Fritschi L, Ambrosini GL, Kliewer EV, Johnson KC; Canadian Cancer Registries Epidemiologic Research Group. Dietary fish intake and risk of leukaemia, multiple myeloma and non-Hodgkin lymphoma. *Cancer Epidemiol Biomarkers Prev* 2004;13(4):532–537.
7. Avet-Loiseau H, Facon T, Daviet A, et al. 14q32 translocations and monosomy 13 observed in monoclonal gammopathy of undetermined significance delineate a multistep process for the oncogenesis of multiple myeloma. *Cancer Res* 1999;59(18):4546–4550.
8. Kyle RA, Therneau TM, Rajkumar SV, et al. A long-term study of prognosis in monoclonal gammopathy of undetermined significance. *N Engl J Med* 2002;346(8):564–569.
9. Goedert JJ, Coté TR, Virgo P, et al. Spectrum of AIDS-associated malignant disorders. *Lancet* 1998;351(9119):1833–1839.
10. Rettig MB, Ma HJ, Vescio RA, et al. Kaposi's sarcoma-associated herpesvirus infection of bone marrow dendritic cells from multiple myeloma patients. *Science* 1997;276(5320):1851–1854.
11. Schalling M, Ekman M, Kaaya EE, Linde A, Biberfeld P. A role for a new herpes-virus (KSHV) in different forms of kaposis-sarcoma. *Nat Med* 1995; 1(7):707–708.
12. Seidl S, Kaufmann H, Drach J. New insights into the pathophysiology of multiple myeloma. *Lancet Oncol* 2003;4(9):557–564.
13. Drach J, Angerler J, Schuster J, et al. Interphase fluorescence in-situ hybridization identifies chromosomal-abnormalities in plasma-cells from patients with monoclonal gammopathy of undetermined significance. *Blood* 1995;86(10):3915–3921.
14. Flactif M, Zandecki M, Laï JL, et al. Interphase fluorescence in situ hybridization (FISH) as a powerful tool for the detection of aneuploidy in multiple myeloma. *Leukemia* 1995;9(12):2109–2114.
15. Zandecki M, Obein V, Bernardi F, et al. Monoclonal gammopathy of undetermined significance—chromosome changes are a common finding within bone-marrow plasma-cells. *Br J Haematol* 1995;90(3):693–696.
16. Gabrea A, Berysagel PL, Kuehl WM. Distinguishing primary and secondary translocations in multiple myeloma. *DNA Repair* 2006;5(9–10):1225–1233.
17. Bergsagel PL, Kuehl WM. Chromosome translocations in multiple myeloma. *Oncogene* 2001;20(40): 5611–5622.
18. Kuehl WM, Bergsagel PL. Multiple myeloma: evolving genetic events and host interactions. *Nat Rev Cancer* 2002;2(3):175–187.

19. Sawyer JR, Lukacs JL, Munshi N, et al. Identification of new nonrandom translocations in multiple myeloma with multicolor spectral karyotyping. *Blood* 1998;92(11):4269–4278.

20. Dewald GW, Kyle RA, Hicks GA, Greipp PR. The clinical-significance of cytogenetic studies in 100 patients with multiple-myeloma, plasma-cell leukemia, or amyloidosis. *Blood* 1985;66(2):380–390.

21. Hallek M, Bergsagel PL, Anderson KC. Multiple myeloma: increasing evidence for a multistep transformation process. *Blood* 1998;91(1):3–21.

22. Hayman SR, Bailey RJ, Jalal SM, et al. Translocations involving the immunoglobulin heavy-chain locus are possible early genetic events in patients with primary systemic amyloidosis. *Blood* 2001;98(7):2266–2268.

23. Fonseca R, Bailey RJ, Ahmann GJ, et al. Genomic abnormalities in monoclonal gammopathy of undetermined significance. *Blood* 2002;100(4):1417–1424.

24. Chesi M, Bergsagel PL, Brents LA, et al. Dysregulation of cyclin D1 by translocation into an IgH gamma switch region in two multiple myeloma cell lines. *Blood* 1996;88(2):674–681.

25. Shaughnessy J, Gabrea A, Qi Y, et al. Cyclin D3 at 6p21 is dysregulated by recurrent chromosomal translocations to immunoglobulin loci in multiple myeloma. *Blood* 2001;98(1):217–223.

26. Chesi M, Nardini E, Lim RS, et al. The t(4;14) translocation in myeloma dysregulates both FGFR3 and a novel gene, MMSET, resulting in IgH/MMSET hybrid transcripts. *Blood* 1998;92(9):3025–3034.

27. Richelda R, Ronchetti D, Baldini L, et al. A novel chromosomal translocation t(4;14)(p16.3;q32) in multiple myeloma involves the fibroblast growth-factor receptor 3 gene. *Blood* 1997;90(10):4062–4070.

28. Chesi M, Bergsagel PL, Shonukan OO, et al. Frequent dysregulation of the c-maf proto-oncogene at 16q23 by translocation to an Ig locus in multiple myeloma. *Blood* 1998;91(12):4457–4463.

29. Hanamura I, Iida S, Akano Y, et al. Ectopic expression of MAFB gene in human myeloma cells carrying (14;20)(q32;q11) chromosomal translocations. *Jpn J Cancer Res* 2001;92(6):638–644.

30. Avet-Loiseau H, Gerson F, Magrangeas F, et al. Rearrangements of the c-myc oncogene are present in 15% of primary human multiple myeloma tumors. *Blood* 2001;98(10):3082–3086.

31. Ong F, van Nieuwkoop JA, de Groot-Swings GM, et al. Bcl-2 protein expression is not related to short survival in multiple myeloma. *Leukemia* 1995;9(7):1282–1284.

32. Pettersson M, Jernberg-Wiklund H, Larsson LG, et al. Expression of the bcl-2 gene in human multiple-myeloma cell-lines and normal plasma-cells. *Blood* 1992;79(2):495–502.

33. Tian EM, Gazitt Y. The role of p53, bcl-2 and bax network in dexamethasone induced apoptosis in multiple myeloma cell lines. *Int J Oncol* 1996;8(4):719–726.

34. Grogan TM, Durie BG, Lomen C, et al. Delineation of a novel pre-B cell component in plasma-cell myeloma—immunochemical, immunophenotypic, genotypic, cytologic, cell-culture, and kinetic features. *Blood* 1987;70(4):932–942.

35. Corradini P, Ladetto M, Voena C, et al. Mutational activation of n-ras and k-ras oncogenes in plasma-cell dyscrasias. *Blood* 1993;81(10):2708–2713.

36. Neri A, Murphy JP, Cro L, et al. RAS oncogene mutation in multiple-myeloma. *J Exp Med* 1989;170(5):1715–1725.

37. Hideshima T, Bergsagel PL, Kuehl WM, Anderson KC. Advances in biology of multiple myeloma: clinical applications. *Blood* 2004;104(3):607–618.

38. Portier M, Molès JP, Mazars GR, et al. P53 and ras gene-mutations in multiple-myeloma. *Oncogene* 1992;7(12):2539–2543.

39. Kiyoi H, Naoe T. Immunoglobulin variable region structure and B-cell malignancies. *Int J Hematol* 2001;73(1):47–53.

40. Kubagawa H, Vogler LB, Capra JD, et al. Studies on the clonal origin of multiple-myeloma—use of individually specific (idiotype) antibodies to trace the oncogenic event to its earliest point of expression in B-cell differentiation. *J Exp Med* 1979;150(4):792–807.

41. Epstein J, Xiao HQ, He XY. Markers of multiple hematopoietic-cell lineages in multiple-myeloma. *N Engl J Med* 1990;322(10):664–668.

42. Preud'homme JL, Klein M, Labaume S, Seligmann M. Idiotype-bearing and antigen-binding receptors produced by blood T lymphocytes in a case of human myeloma. *Eur J Immunol* 1977;7(12):840–846.

43. Jensen GS, Mant MJ, Belch AJ, Berenson JR, Ruether BA, Pilarski LM. Selective expression of CD45 isoforms defines CALLA+ monoclonal B-lineage cells in peripheral-blood from myeloma patients as late stage B-cells. *Blood* 1991;78(3):711–719.

44. Mitsiades CS, Mitsiades N, Munshi NC, Anderson KC. Mitsiades N, Munshi NC. Focus on multiple myeloma. *Cancer Cell* 2004;6(5):439–444.

45. Teoh G, Anderson KC. Interaction of tumor and host cells with adhesion and extracellular matrix molecules in the development of multiple myeloma. *Hematol Oncol Clin North Am* 1997;11(1):27–42.

46. Ahsmann EJ, Lokhorst HM, Dekker AW, Bloem AC. Lymphocyte function-associated antigen-1 expression on plasma-cells correlates with tumor-growth in multiple-myeloma. *Blood* 1992;79(8):2068–2075.

47. Ridley RC, Xiao H, Hata H, et al. Expression of syndecan regulates human myeloma plasma-cell adhesion to type-I collagen. *Blood* 1993;81(3):767–774.

48. Landowski TH, Olashaw NE, Agrawal D, Dalton WS. Olashaw NE, Agrawal D. Cell adhesion-mediated drug resistance (CAM-DR) is associated with activation of NF-kappa B (RelB/p50) in myeloma cells. *Oncogene* 2003;22(16):2417–2421.

49. Damiano JS, Cress AE, Hazlehurst LA, Shtil AA, Dalton WS. Cell adhesion mediated drug resistance (CAM-DR): role of integrins and resistance to apoptosis in human myeloma cell lines. *Blood* 1999;93(5):1658–1667.

50. Damiano JS, Dalton WS. Integrin-mediated drug resistance in multiple myeloma. *Leuk Lymphoma* 2000;38(1–2):71–81.

51. Chauhan D, Uchiyama H, Akbarali Y, et al. Multiple myeloma cell adhesion-induced interleukin-6 expression in bone marrow stromal cells involves activation of NF-kappa B. *Blood* 1996;87(3):1104–1112.

52. Lokhorst HM, Lamme T, de Smet M, et al. Primary tumor-cells of myeloma patients induce interleukin-6 secretion in long-term bone-marrow cultures. *Blood* 1994;84(7):2269–2277.

53. Uchiyama H, Barut BA, Mohrbacher AF, Chauhan D, Anderson KC. Adhesion of human myeloma-derived cell-lines to bone-marrow stromal cells stimulates interleukin-6 secretion. *Blood* 1993;82(12):3712–3720.

54. Hideshima T, Chauhan D, Schlossman R, Richardson P, Anderson KC. The role of tumor necrosis factor alpha in the pathophysiology of human multiple myeloma: therapeutic applications. *Oncogene* 2001;20(33):4519–4527.

55. Sanderson RD, Turnbull, JE, Gallagher, JT, Lander, AD. Fine structure of heparan-sulfate regulates syndecan-1 function and cell behavior. *J Biol Chem* 1994;269(18):13100–13106.

56. Yang Y, Macleod V, Miao HQ, et al. Heparanase enhances syndecan-1 shedding—a novel mechanism for stimulation of tumor growth and metastasis. *J Biol Chem* 2007;282(18):13326–13333.

57. Yang Y, Yaccoby S, Liu W, et al. Soluble syndecan-1 promotes growth of myeloma tumors in vivo. *Blood* 2002;100(2):610–617.

58. Huang YW, Richardson JA, Vitetta ES. Anti-CD54 (icam-1) has antitumor-activity in scid mice with human myeloma cells. *Cancer Res* 1995;55(3):610–616.

59. Yaccoby S, Barlogie B, Epstein J. Primary myeloma cells growing in SCID-hu mice: a model for studying the biology and treatment of myeloma and its manifestations. *Blood* 1998;92(8):2908–2913.

60. Urashima M, Chen BP, Chen S, et al. The development of a model for the homing of multiple myeloma cells to human bone marrow. *Blood* 1997;90(2):754–765.

61. Hideshima T, Chauhan D, Shima Y, et al. Thalidomide and its analogs overcome drug resistance of human multiple myeloma cells to conventional therapy. *Blood* 2000;96(9):2943–2950.

62. Mitsiades CS, Mitsiades N, Poulaki V, et al. Activation of NF-kappa B and upregulation of intracellular anti-apoptotic proteins via the IGF-1/Akt signaling in human multiple myeloma cells: therapeutic implications. *Oncogene* 2002;21(37):5673–5683.

63. Hideshima T, Mitsiades C, Tonon G, Richardson PG, Anderson KC. Understanding multiple myeloma pathogenesis in the bone marrow to identify new therapeutic targets. *Nat Rev Cancer* 2007;7(8):585–598.

64. Hideshima T, Noriaki N, Dharminder C, Kenneth AC. Biologic sequelae of interleukin-6 induced P13-K/Akt signaling in multiple myeloma. *Oncogene* 2001;20(42):5991–6000.

65. Ashcroft AJ, Davies FE, Morgan GJ. Aetiology of bone disease and the role of bisphosphonates in multiple myeloma. *Lancet Oncol* 2003;4(5):284–292.

66. Roodman GD. Pathogenesis of myeloma bone disease. *Leukemia* 2009;23(3):435–441.

67. Gori F, Hofbauer LC, Dunstan CR, Spelsberg TC, Khosla S, Riggs BL The expression of osteoprotegerin and RANK ligand and the support of osteoclast formation by stromal-osteoblast lineage cells is developmentally regulated. *Endocrinology* 2000;141(12):4768–4776.

68. Giuliani N, Colla S, Rizzoli V. New insight in the mechanism of osteoclast activation and formation in multiple myeloma: focus on the receptor activator of NF-kappa B ligand (RANKL). *Exp Hematol* 2004;32(8):685–691.

69. Bataille R, Chappard D, Marcelli C, et al. Mechanisms of bone destruction in multiple myeloma: the importance of an unbalanced process in determining the severity of lytic bone disease. *J Clin Oncol* 1989;7(12):1909–1914.

70. Han JH, Choi SJ, Kurihara N, Koide M, Oba Y, Roodman GD. Macrophage inflammatory protein-1-alpha is an osteoclastogenic factor in myeloma that

is independent of receptor activator of nuclear factor kappaB ligand. *Blood* 2001;97(11):3349–3353.

71. Oba Y, Lee JW, Ehrlich LA, et al. MIP-1 alpha utilizes both CCR1 and CCR5 to induce osteoclast formation and increase adhesion of myeloma cells to marrow stromal cells. *Exp Hematol* 2005;33(3):272–278.

72. Abe M, Hiura K, Wilde J, et al. Osteoclasts enhance myeloma cell growth and survival via cell-cell contact: a vicious cycle between bone destruction and myeloma expansion. *Blood* 2004;104(8):2484–2491.

73. Lee JW, Chung HY, Ehrlich LA, et al. IL-3 expression by myeloma cells increases both osteoclast formation and growth of myeloma cells. *Blood* 2004;103(6):2308–2315.

74. Ehrlich LA, Chung HY, Ghobrial I, et al. IL-3 is a potential inhibitor of osteoblast differentiation in multiple myeloma. *Blood* 2005;106(4):1407–1414.

75. Kobayashi T, Kronenberg H. Minireview: transcriptional regulation in development of bone. *Endocrinology* 2005;146(3):1012–1017.

76. Giuliani N, Colla S, Morandi F, et al. Myeloma cells block RUNX2/CBFA1 activity in human bone marrow osteoblast progenitors and inhibit osteoblast formation and differentiation. *Blood* 2005;106(7):2472–2483.

77. Roodman GD. Pathogenesis of myeloma bone disease. *Blood Cells Mol Dis* 2004;32(2):290–292.

78. Sen M. Wnt signalling in rheumatoid arthritis. *Rheumatology* 2005;44(6):708–713.

79. Giuliani N, Morandi F, Tagliaferri S, et al. Production of Wnt inhibitors by myeloma cells: potential effects on canonical Wnt pathway in the bone microenvironment. *Cancer Res* 2007;67(16):7665–7674.

80. Qiang YW, Barlogie B, Rudikoff S, Shaughnessy JD. Dkk1-induced inhibition of Wnt signaling in osteoblast differentiation is an underlying mechanism of bone loss in multiple myeloma. *Bone* 2008;42(4):669–680.

81. Gregory CA, Singh H, Perry AS, Prockop DJ. The Wnt signaling inhibitor dickkopf-1 is required for reentry into the cell cycle of human adult stem cells from bone marrow. *J Biol Chem* 2003;278(30):28067–28078.

82. Gunn WG, Conley A, Deininger L, Olson SD, Prockop DJ, Gregory CA. A crosstalk between myeloma cells and marrow stromal cells stimulates production of Dkk1 and interleukin-6: a potential role in the development of lytic bone disease and tumor progression in multiple myeloma. *Stem Cells* 2006;24(4):986–991.

83. Shao LE, Frigon NL Jr, Yu A, Palyash J, Yu J. Contrasting effects of inflammatory cytokines and glucocorticoids on the production of activin A in human marrow stromal cells and their implications. *Cytokine* 1998;10(3):227–235.

84. Shav-Tal Y, Zipori D. The role of activin a in regulation of hemopoiesis. *Stem Cells* 2002;20(6):493–500.

85. Ikenoue T, Jingushi S, Urabe K, Okazaki K, Iwamoto Y. Inhibitory effects of activin-A on osteoblast differentiation during cultures of fetal rat calvarial cells. *J Cell Biochem* 1999;75(2):206–214.

86. Eijken M, Swagemakers S, Koedam M, et al. The activin A-follistatin system: potent regulator of human extracellular matrix mineralization. *FASEB J* 2007;21(11):2949–2960.

87. Pearsall RS, Canalis E, Cornwall-Brady M, et al. A soluble activin type IIA receptor induces bone formation and improves skeletal integrity. *Proc Natl Acad Sci U S A* 2008;105(19):7082–7087.

88. Perrien DS, Akel NS, Edwards PK, et al. Inhibin A is an endocrine stimulator of bone mass and strength. *Endocrinology* 2007;148(4):1654–1665.

89. Vallet S, Mukherjee S, Vaghela N, et al. Targeting myeloma bone disease via activin A inhibition. *Clin Lymphoma Myeloma* 2009;9:S126–S127.

90. Chauhan D, Uchiyama H, Urashima M, Yamamoto K, Anderson KC. Regulation of interleukin 6 in multiple myeloma and bone marrow stromal cells. *Stem Cells* 1995;13(suppl 2):35–39.

91. Tai YT, Podar K, Catley L, et al. Insulin-like growth factor-1 induces adhesion and migration in human multiple myeloma cells via activation of beta1-integrin and phosphatidylinositol 3'-kinase/AKT signaling. *Cancer Res* 2003;63(18):5850–5858.

92. Podar K, Tai YT, Davies FE, et al. Vascular endothelial growth factor triggers signaling cascades mediating multiple myeloma cell growth and migration. *Blood* 2001;98(2):428–435.

93. Hideshima T, Chauhan D, Hayashi T, et al. The biological sequelae of stromal cell-derived factor-1 alpha in multiple myeloma. *Mol Cancer Ther* 2002;1(7):539–544.

94. Urashima M, Ogata A, Chauhan D, et al. Transforming growth factor-beta1: differential effects on multiple myeloma versus normal B cells. *Blood* 1996;87(5):1928–1938.

95. Schneider P, MacKay F, Steiner V, et al. BAFF, a novel ligand of the tumor necrosis factor family, stimulates B cell growth. *J Exp Med* 1999;189(11):1747–1756.

96. Brenne AT, Ro TB, Waage A, Sundan A, Borset M, Hjorth-Hansen H. Interleukin-21 is a growth and survival factor for human myeloma cells. *Blood* 2002;99(10):3756–3762.

97. Kurth I, Horsten U, Pflanz S, et al. Activation of the signal transducer glycoprotein 130 by both IL-6 and IL-11 requires two distinct binding epitopes. *J Immunol* 1999;162(3):1480–1487.

98. Frassanito MA, Cusmai A, Iodice G, Dammacco F. Autocrine interleukin-6 production and highly malignant multiple myeloma: relation with resistance to drug-induced apoptosis. *Blood* 2001;97(2):483–489.

99. Chauhan D, Hideshima T, Rosen S, et al. Apaf-1/cytochrome c-independent and Smac-dependent induction of apoptosis in multiple myeloma (MM) cells. *J Biol Chem* 2001;276(27):24453–24456.

100. Chauhan D, Hideshima T, Pandey P, et al. RAFTK/PYK2-dependent and independent apoptosis in multiple myeloma cells. *Oncogene* 1999;18(48):6733–6740.

101. Chauhan D, Pandey P, Hideshima T, et al. SHP2 mediates the protective effect of interleukin-6 against dexamethasone-induced apoptosis in multiple myeloma cells. *J Biol Chem* 2000;275(36):27845–27850.

102. Ludwig H, Nachbaur DM, Fritz E, et al. Interleukin-6 is a prognostic factor in multiple-myeloma. *Blood* 1991;77(12):2794–2795.

103. Bataille R, Jourdan M, Zhang XG, Klein B. Serum levels of interleukin-6, a potent myeloma cell-growth factor, as a reflect of disease severity in plasma-cell dyscrasias. *J Clin Invest* 1989;84(6):2008–2011.

104. Demartis A, Bernassola F, Savino R, Melino G, Ciliberto G. Interleukin 6 receptor superantagonists are potent inducers of human multiple myeloma cell death. *Cancer Res* 1996;56(18):4213–4218.

105. Barille S, Collette M, Bataille R, Amiot M. Myeloma cells up-regulate interleukin-6 secretion in osteoblastic cells through cell-to-cell contact but down-regulate osteocalcin. *Blood* 1995;86(8):3151–3159.

106. Bataille R, Barlogie B, Lu ZY, et al. Biologic effects of anti-interleukin-6 murine monoclonal-antibody in advanced multiple-myeloma. *Blood* 1995;86(2):685–691.

107. Jelinek DF, Witzig TE, Arendt BK. A role for insulin-like growth factor in the regulation of IL-6-responsive human myeloma cell line growth. *J Immunol* 1997;159(1):487–496.

108. Ge NL, Rudikoff S. Insulin-like growth factor I is a dual effector of multiple myeloma cell growth. *Blood* 2000;96(8):2856–2861.

109. Qiang YW, Kopantzev E, Rudikoff S. Insulin like growth factor-I signaling in multiple myeloma: downstream elements, functional correlates, and pathway cross-talk. *Blood* 2002;99(11):4138–4146.

110. Akiyama M, Hideshima T, Hayashi T, et al. Cytokines modulate telomerase activity in a human multiple myeloma cell line. *Cancer Res* 2002;62(13):3876–3882.

111. Mitsiades CS, Mitsiades NS, McMullan CJ, et al. Inhibition of the insulin-like growth factor receptor-1 tyrosine kinase activity as a therapeutic strategy for multiple myeloma, other hematologic malignancies, and solid tumors. *Cancer Cell* 2004;5(3):221–230.

112. Podar K, Tai YT, Lin BK, et al. Vascular endothelial growth factor-induced migration of multiple myeloma cells is associated with beta(1) integrin and phosphatidylinositol 3-kinase-dependent PKC alpha activation. *J Biol Chem* 2002;277(10):7875–7881.

113. Tai YT, Podar K, Gupta D, et al. CD40 activation induces p53-dependent vascular endothelial growth factor (VEGF) secretion in human multiple myeloma (MM) cells. *Blood* 2001;98(11):2674.

114. Lin B, Podar K, Gupta D, et al. The vascular endothelial growth factor receptor tyrosine kinase inhibitor PTK787/ZK222584 inhibits growth and migration of multiple myeloma cells in the bone marrow microenvironment. *Cancer Res* 2002;62(17):5019–5026.

115. Vacca A, Ribatti D, Presta M, et al. Bone marrow neovascularization, plasma cell angiogenic potential, and matrix metalloproteinase-2 secretion parallel progression of human multiple myeloma. *Blood* 1999;93(9):3064–3073.

116. Rajkumar SV, Fonseca R, Witzig TE, Gertz MA, Greipp PR. Bone marrow angiogenesis in patients achieving complete response after stem cell transplantation for multiple myeloma. *Leukemia* 1999;13(3):469–472.

117. Rajkumar SV, Mesa RA, Fonseca, et al. Bone marrow angiogenesis in 400 patients with monoclonal gammopathy of undetermined significance, multiple myeloma, and primary amyloidosis. *Clin Cancer Res* 2002;8(7):2210–2216.

118. Munshi NC, Wilson C. Increased bone marrow microvessel density in newly diagnosed multiple myeloma carries a poor prognosis. *Semin Oncol* 2001;28(6):565–569.

119. Kumar S, Fonseca R, Dispenzieri A, et al. Bone marrow angiogenesis in multiple myeloma: effect of therapy. *Br J Haematol* 2002;119(3):665–671.

120. Moore PA, Belvedere O, Orr A, et al. BLyS: member of the tumor necrosis factor family and B lymphocyte stimulator. *Science* 1999;285(5425):260–263.

121. Gross JA, Johnston J, Mudri S, et al. TACI and BCMA are receptors for a TNF homologue implicated in B-cell autoimmune disease. *Nature* 2000;404(6781):995–999.

122. Mackay F, Woodcock, SA, Lawton. P, et al. Mice transgenic for BAFF develop lymphocytic disorders along with autoimmune manifestations. *J Exp Med* 1999;190(11):1697–1710.

123. Bossen C, Schneider P. BAFF, APRIL and their receptors: structure, function and signaling. *Semin Immunol* 2006;18(5):263–275.

124. Moreaux J, Legouffe E, Jourdan E, et al. BAFF and APRIL protect myeloma cells from apoptosis induced by interleukin 6 deprivation and dexamethasone. *Blood* 2004;103(8):3148–3157.

125. Neri P, Kumar S, Fulciniti MT, et al. Neutralizing B-cell-activating factor antibody improves survival and inhibits osteoclastogenesis in a severe combined immunodeficient human multiple myeloma model. *Clin Cancer Res* 2007;13(19):5903–5909.

126. Tai YT, Li XF, Breitkreutz I, et al. Role of B-cell-activating factor in adhesion and growth of human multiple myeloma cells in the bone marrow microenvironment. *Cancer Res* 2006;66(13): 6675–6682.

127. Endo T, Nishio M, Enzler T, et al. BAFF and APRIL support chronic lymphocytic leukemia B-cell survival through activation of the canonical NF-kappa B pathway. *Blood* 2007;109(2):703–710.

128. Li W, Li J, Su C, Zou WY, Luo S. New targets of PS-341: BAFF and APRIL. *Med Oncol* 2009.

129. Otsuki T, Yamada O, Yata K, et al. Expression of fibroblast growth factor and FGF-receptor family genes in human myeloma cells, including lines possessing t(4;14)(q16.3;q32.3) and FGFR3 translocation. *Int J Oncol* 1999;15(6):1205–1212.

130. Bisping G, Leo R, Wenning D, et al. Paracrine interactions of basic fibroblast growth factor and interleukin-6 in multiple myeloma. *Blood* 2003;101(7):2775–2783.

131. Chesi M, Brents LA, Ely SA, et al. Activated fibroblast growth factor receptor 3 is an oncogene that contributes to tumor progression in multiple myeloma. *Blood* 2001;97(3):729–736.

132. Nusse R. Wnt signaling in disease and in development. *Cell Res.* 2005;15(1):28–32.

133. Qiang YW, Endo Y, Rubin JS, Rudikoff S. Wnt signaling in B-cell neoplasia. *Oncogene* 2003;22(10): 1536–1545.

134. Qiang YW, Walsh K, Yao L, et al. Wnts induce migration and invasion of rnyeloma plasma cells. *Blood* 2005;106(5):1786–1793.

135. Sukhdeo K, Mani M, Zhang Y, et al. Targeting the beta-catenin/TCF transcriptional complex in the treatment of multiple myeloma. *Proc Natl Acad Sci U S A* 2007;104(18):7516–7521.

136. Derksen PWB, Tjin E, Meijer HP, et al. Illegitimate Wnt signaling promotes proliferation of multiple myeloma cells. *Proc Natl Acad Sci U S A* 2004;101(16):6122–6127.

137. Uren A, Reichsman F, Anest V, et al. Secreted frizzled-related protein-1 binds directly to wingless and is a biphasic modulator of Wnt signaling. *J Biol Chem* 2000;275(6):4374–4382.

138. Tian E, Zhan F, Walker R, et al. The role of the Wnt-signaling antagonist DKK1 in the development of osteolytic lesions in multiple myeloma. *N Engl J Med* 2003;349(26):2483–2494.

139. Yaccoby S, Ling W, Zhan F, Walker R, Barlogie B, Shaughnessy JD Jr. Antibody-based inhibition of DKK1 suppresses tumor-induced bone resorption and multiple myeloma growth in vivo. *Blood* 2007;109(5):2106–2111.

140. Möller C, Strömberg T, Juremalm M, Nilsson K, Nilsson G. Expression and function of chemokine receptors in human multiple myeloma. *Leukemia* 2003;17(1):203–210.

141. Alsayed Y, Ngo H, Runnels J, et al. Mechanisms of regulation of CXCR4/SDF-1 (CXCL12)-dependent migration and homing in multiple myeloma. *Blood* 2007;109(7):2708–2717.

142. Wang JF, Liu ZY, Groopman JE. The alpha-chemokine receptor CXCR4 is expressed on the megakaryocytic lineage from progenitor to platelets and modulates migration and adhesion. *Blood* 1998;92(3):756–764.

143. Gupta D, Treon SP, Shima Y, et al. Adherence of multiple myeloma cells to bone marrow stromal cells upregulates vascular endothelial growth factor secretion: therapeutic applications. *Leukemia* 2001;15(12):1950–1961.

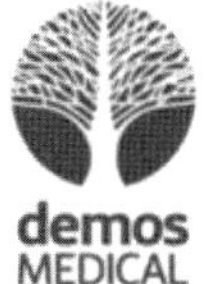

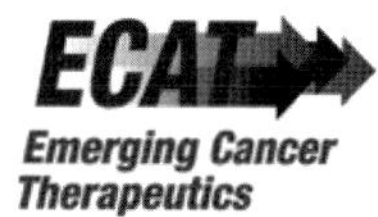

Genetic Abnormalities in Multiple Myeloma

Wee J. Chng*

*National University Cancer Institute of Singapore, National University
Health System, National University of Singapore, Singapore*

■ ABSTRACT

Multiple myeloma (MM) is the second most common hematological malignancy. Over the last decade, tremendous progress has been made in understanding the genetics and molecular biology of the disease, from disease initiation and transformation to clonal evolution and progression. As a result, progress has been made in risk stratification, development of novel therapeutics, and rationale therapeutic strategies.

■ INTRODUCTION

In recent years, significant progress in the understanding of multiple myeloma (MM) at the genetic and molecular level has led to better understanding of disease heterogeneity, pathogenesis, and biology. This coupled with the current expansion in our treatment armamentarium and the differential response of tumors with different underlying genetic abnormalities to different therapeutic agents mean that risk-stratified treatment of myeloma is now feasible. This is a step toward individualized therapy.

■ GENETIC TECHNIQUES

G-Banding Karyotype

Study of cytogenetics in MM using conventional G-banding karyotyping is limited by the poor yield of karyotypic abnormalities from MM bone marrow (BM) samples (1). In 50% to 70% of cases, the karyotype reveals normal metaphases that originate from more proliferative myeloid cells (1–9). Furthermore, some important genetic abnormalities such as t(4;14)(p16.3;q32) and t(14;16)(q32;q23) are cytogenetically cryptic as they involve telomeric sequences (10–12). A further limitation is that it cannot describe possible heterogeneity within a population of clonal cells. However, karyotyping can efficiently identify numerical chromosomal abnormalities and, in fact, is the gold standard in assigning ploidy categories

*Corresponding author, Department of Haematology-Oncology, National University Cancer Institute of Singapore, National University Health System, National University of Singapore, 5 Lower Kent Ridge Rd, Singapore 119074

E-mail address: mdccwj@nus.edu.sg

Emerging Cancer Therapeutics 1:2 (2010) 215–236.
© 2010 Demos Medical Publishing LLC. All rights reserved.
DOI: 10.5003/2151–4194.1.2.215

demosmedpub.com/ecat

that may have important prognostic implications. It is recommended that all patients have conventional cytogenetics performed at diagnosis as the test is available from most clinical laboratories and, in patients with informative karyotype, the results carry useful prognostic information.

Fluorescence In Situ Hybridization

Fluorescence in situ hybridization (FISH) utilizes fluorescent-labeled DNA sequence to probe for complementary DNA sequences in the cell of interest. This can be used to detect copy number gains and losses as well as gene fusion/translocations and gene rearrangement. It has the advantage of detecting genetic abnormalities in nondividing cells (interphase FISH), which is a distinct advantage in a low proliferative malignant condition such as myeloma (13–19). Interphase FISH is best done on purified cells or using simultaneous immunofluorescence (14,16–25). This is of paramount importance in conditions where there is a low percentage of plasmacytosis such as monoclonal gammopathy of undetermined significance (MGUS) and smoldering multiple myeloma (SMM) (20,26–28).

Metaphase Spectral Karyotype Imaging/ Multicolor-FISH and Comparative Genomic Hybridization

In an effort to improve on the accuracy of conventional karyotype analysis, other methods of investigation have been attempted. Multicolor metaphase FISH has been used to provide greater details of complex karyotypes (12,29,30). This technique is still limited by the need for the cell to undergo mitosis. Another interphase technique is comparative genomic hybridization (CGH). However, CGH allows only for the detection of net DNA gain or loss and cannot detect balanced structural abnormalities, and it needs to be done on purified cell populations. CGH has been used to study MM, and several recurrent areas of abnormalities have been identified including 6q and 13q loss as well as gains of 9q and 11q (31–35).

Microarray aCGH, SNP Arrays, GEP

Microarray technology allows the spotting of small probes onto an inert surface such as a glass slide. Many probes can be "arrayed," allowing the study of a large number of genetic elements in a highly paralleled fashion. The input material is usually labeled with a dye and hybridized onto the chip. The presence of complementary sequences in the input material to the immobilized probes will lead to binding. The relative quantity of each sequence in the input material can then be detected based on the amount of fluorescence emitted for each spot. This information is acquired by scanning the chip after hybridization and processing the scanned data using algorithms that can subtract background signals to give a relatively accurate quantification of signals arising from each probe. In some ways, the number of probes or features that can be arrayed is limited by the resolution of the scanner. With technological advancement, the number of features that can be arrayed has increased by about 50-fold and typically at least a million features can be arrayed on the latest generation of chips. In terms of genomic spacing between probes and fine resolution of aberrations, this has improved to about 10 kb. At this resolution, one can detect intragenic rearrangements.

The type of assay that microarray technology can be used for is dependent on the probe design and input material. The improvements in array manufacturing and probe design have made these tests much more robust, and there are now different companies offering these assays using different manufacturing technologies. The most common platforms used in myeloma are gene expression arrays, array CGH (aCGH), and single-nucleotide polymorphism (SNP) arrays.

In gene expression profiling (GEP), the input material is tumor RNA, and the output is the relative expression level of large number of transcripts on the microarray. A number of gene expression studies in myeloma have been published (36–52). Significantly, molecular classification (39,43,51) and powerful prognostic signatures (42,44) have been derived.

In aCGH, the input material is tumor DNA, and this is usually cohybridized with normal reference DNA in equal amounts onto the microarray. Because of the much higher resolution, new abnormalities previously undetectable by conventional G-banding, or even metaphase aCGH, are now identified, including deletions and rearrangement of genes involved in the nuclear factor (NF)-κB signaling (53,54) and *CDKN2C* (55).

SNP-based arrays consist of sets of oligonucleotides specific for polymorphisms in the genome. In simplistic terms, each SNP has two different oligonucleotide sets, one for each allele, when hybridized with sample DNA gives a signal intensity relating to copy number and an SNP call referring to allele in the sample, which can be homozygous AA, BB, or heterozygous AB. SNP-based techniques have the advantage of not only identifying copy number changes but also copy number neutral loss of heterozygosity, such as uniparental disomy (56).

■ ANEUPLOIDY

Aneuploidy is almost universal in MM. The main exception appears to be a subset of MM with t(11;14)(q13;q32), which tends to be diploid. The most common trisomies involve those of chromosomes 3, 5, 7, 9, 11, 15, 19, and 21, whereas the most common monosomies involve chromosomes 13, 14, 16, and 22. Patients can be segregated into the following categories based on ploidy category alone: hypodiploid, pseudodiploid, near-tetraploid, constituting nonhyperdiploid (NHRD) MM, and hyperdiploid (HRD) (3,4,9). When ploidy was studied using conventional karyotyping, the determined cutoff values for the different categories are as follows: hypodiploid up to 44 chromosomes, pseudodiploid 45 to 47 chromosomes, hyperdiploid greater than 47 but less than 75 chromosomes and near-tetraploid 76 or more chromosomes (3,4,9). An alternative method is measuring the DNA content using propidium iodide by flow cytometry. The cutoff values used for this method is hypodiploid <0.95, pseudodiploid 0.95 to 1.05, hyperdiploid >1.05 and <1.75, and near-tetraploid 1.75 or greater (57,58). We and others have also recently developed FISH-based methods that are highly predictive of HRD state in PC tumors (59,60).

■ DELETIONS/AMPLIFICATIONS

Chromosome 13 Abnormalities

About 50% of MM tumors (17,22,26,61,62) and 40% to 50% of MGUS (20,26,63) tumors have deletion of chromosome 13 (Δ13) in most tumor cells, suggesting that this is often an early event in pathogenesis. In most cases, Δ13 represents whole chromosome monosomy (19,64), but in a subset of tumors the common deleted region seems to be located at 13q14 (2,8,19,29,64,65). The retinoblastoma (RB) gene falls within the minimally deleted region, however, inactivating mutations of the remaining allele are not commonly seen. Haploinsufficiency for RB1 is being investigated as a possible mechanism (Chng, unpublished). Besides coding genes, the 13q14 locus also contains miRNA. Recently, studies have shown that mir-15 and mir-16a, located on 13q14, have functional relevance in myeloma (66). Therefore, the critical molecular abnormality affected has yet to be confirmed.

Chromosome 1 Abnormalities

A number of laboratories have determined by a combination of FISH, aCGH, and GEP that there is a gain of sequences—and corresponding increased gene expression—at 1q21 in 30% to 40% of tumors. These gains are concentrated substantially in those tumors that have a t(4;14) or t(14;16), or have a high proliferation expression index (67–69). In addition, chromosome 1 abnormalities are more common in tumors with more complex karyotype and higher number of aberrations detected by aCGH. It has been proposed that the increased proliferation in tumors with gain of 1q21 sequences is due to the increased expression of *CKS1B* as a result of an increased copy number (70). However, CKS1B expression correlates closely with the expression of a number of proliferation genes in a wide variety of tumors where it appears to be a consequence rather than a cause of the proliferation. Therefore, it seems prudent to remain skeptical that *CKS1B* is the gene targeted by gain of 1q21 sequences.

Another common genetic abnormality in myeloma is 1p loss (9,71) and has been associated with poorer prognosis (9,71–74). A recently defined high-risk gene expression-based signature is composed mainly of genes located on 1q that are overexpressed and those located on 1p that are underexpressed, further highlighting the prognostic relevance of 1q gain and 1p loss (44). Whether these regions contain critical genes important for myeloma progression or these genetic abnormalities are markers of increasing genomic instability associated with more aggressive disease will need to be clarified.

Chromosome 17p13 Deletion

The 17p13 deletion, containing the p53 locus, is most likely a progression event as it is seen in only 10% of MM cases at the time of diagnosis, is significantly more common in plasma cell leukemia and myeloma cell lines, and is rarely seen in MGUS (75–80). Cases with 17p13 deletions are more frequently associated with the presence of extramedullary disease, plasmacytomas, refractory disease, hypercalcemia, plasma cell leukemia, and central nervous system involvement (75,81–83).

■ TRANSLOCATIONS

In a recent census, chromosome translocations that create a chimeric gene or appose a gene to the regulatory element of another gene are identified as the predominant mechanism of cancer gene deregulation (84) and, certainly, this mechanism is important in the pathogenesis of B-cell lymphomas (85). It is, therefore, not surprising that the translocation of oncogenes to promoters in the IgH locus on chromosome 14q32 resulting in their upregulation has received the most research efforts in MM over the years. As opposed to lymphomas, these translocations predominantly involve the switch region of the IgH locus suggesting that they occur due to errors during switch recombination in MM (86).

Several recurrent translocations and the oncogenes involved have been identified (Table 1) (87). Four partners are involved recurrently in 3% or more of MM: 11q13 (*CCND1*), about 15%; 4p16.3 (*FGFR3* and *MMSET*), about 15%; 16q23 (*MAF*), about 6%; and 6p21 (*CCND3*), about 4%. Although the actual prevalence may differ slightly between studies, these translocations affect about 40% of MM. These translocations are considered "primary" translocations because they are present in MGUS and are therefore implicated in disease initiation. They are usually balanced translocations involving B-cell–specific DNA rearrangement mechanisms and are homogenously present in the tumor population, although 20% to 30% of them will be unbalanced, always retaining one preferred derivative chromosome.

t(11;14)(q13;q32)

This translocation results in the ectopic expression of *CCND1* (encoding Cyclin D1) (88,89), although the biological consequences of this deregulation is still not well defined. In MM, high levels of *CCND1* expression are tightly linked to the presence of t(11;14)(q13;q32) (43) but positive assays by immunohistochemistry may be absent in 30% of patients with the t(11;14), possibly due to the loss of der(11) (90). There is an association between MM

TABLE 1

Prevalence of recurrent IgH translocation in multiple myeloma

IgH Translocation Gene Partner	Protein Deregulated	% of All MM	Translocation Group
11q13 (*CCND1*)	Cyclin D1	15	Cyclin D
12p13 (*CCND2*)	Cyclin D2	<1	Cyclin D
6p21 (*CCND3*)	Cyclin D3	2	Cyclin D
16q23 (*MAF*)	c-MAF	5	MAF
21q12 (*MAFB*)	MAF B	2	MAF
8q24.3 (*MAFA*)	MAF A	<1	MAF
4p16 (*WHSC1/FGFR3*)	MMSET and FGFR3	15	MMSET/FGFR3

with t(11;14)(q13;q32) with oligosecretory variant MM, CD20 expression, more bone disease, and lymphoplasmacytic morphology (16,90–94). In contrast to other genetic subtypes, clonal cells with t(11;14)(q13;q32) tend to be diploid.

t(4;14)(p16.3;q32)

This translocation was first detected by Chesi et al. who performed cloning experiments in human MM cell lines. The breakpoints at 4p16.3 are usually within the 5′ introns of *MMSET* and centromeric to *FGFR3*. This translocation uniquely deregulates two genes with *MMSET* juxtaposed to the Eμ intronic enhancer on der(4) and *FGFR3* juxtaposed to the 3′ Eα enhancer on der(14) (11,95). In 25% of MM with t(4;14)(p16.3;q32), *FGFR3* is not expressed either through loss of der(14) or expression (96,97). In a minority of human myeloma cell lines (HMCLs) and patients with t(4;14)(p16.3;q32), oncogenic activating mutation of *FGFR3* are detected (98–100). The universal overexpression of transcript originating from the *MMSET* suggests that this may be the important oncogene deregulated by the t(4;14)(p16.3;q32), even though the role of *MMSET* deregulation remains largely unknown (101). However, recent studies had pointed to possible pathogenic roles of *MMSET* in myeloma pathogenesis. In vivo animal studies showed that knockdown of MMSET

leads to xenograft regression and also changes in malignant phenotype of myeloma cell lines with *MMSET* overexpression (102,103). The functional properties of *MMSET* as a histone methyltransferase and its function in conjunction with other histone deacetylases in the regulation of gene expression mainly through gene repression have also been elucidated (104). Clinically, there is an association between t(4;14)(p16.3;q32) and IgA subtype, λ-light chain usage, and immature plasma cell morphology (22,91,94).

t(14;16)(q32;q23)

This translocation results in the upregulation of *MAF* (encoding c-MAF), which is the cellular homolog of *v-maf*, the transforming gene of the avian retrovirus AS42 (10). A recent study has elucidated the possible contribution of c-MAF overexpression to myelomagenesis. c-MAF stimulates cell cycle progression through upregulation of *CCND2* and promotes interaction with the BM microenvironment via the upregulation of integrin β7, an adhesion molecule that heterodimerizes with integrin αE to bind to E-cadherin on the surface of BM stromal cells (105). This interaction significantly increases the secretion of vascular endothelial growth factor, which is one of the key factors in the growth and survival of myeloma cells (106).

Secondary Ig Translocations

In contrast to IgH translocations involving recurrent partners, these IgH translocations, as well as most translocations involving the IgL loci, have the following features: breakpoints not in or near IgH switch or V(D)J regions; unbalanced or complex structures; and similar frequency in HRD and NHRD tumors (whereas the recurrent or primary translocations occur predominantly in NHRD tumors, see later). *MYC* rearrangements are such prototypic translocations. These translocations, often heterogeneous in primary tumors, are usually complex rearrangements or insertions, sometimes involving three different chromosomes (39,107–110). Approximately 10% to 20% of IgH translocations in MM do not involve *MYC* or one of the seven recurrent partners described earlier, but partner loci have rarely been identified (12,14,20,22,29,111).

■ OTHER ABNORMALITIES

RAS Mutations

Activating *RAS* mutations, mostly involving K- and N-*RAS* at codons 12, 13, and 61, have been found in 30% to 50% of MM patients (112–114), with increased prevalence in more advanced tumors (113). With rare exceptions, only one N- or K-*RAS* allele is mutated in a single tumor cell, although there is some evidence that subpopulations of MM tumor cells within an individual can have different *RAS* mutations (112,113). *RAS* mutations appear to be rare in MGUS, suggesting that this is a molecular marker and may be causative in the progression from MGUS to MM (112,114). Recently, it was shown that the frequency of *RAS* mutation differs between genetic subtypes. They are frequently found in patients with t(11;14)(q13;q32) but rarely in those with t(4;14)(p16.3;q32) (114). There is some conflicting data regarding the prevalence of N-*RAS* and K-*RAS* mutations. Fonseca et al. (115) found N-*RAS* and K-*RAS* mutations,

respectively, in 17% and 6% of tumors, whereas Kuehl and Shaughnessy (unpublished) found them, respectively, in 14% and 17% of tumors. The source and reasons for this discrepancy are currently unknown.

TP53 Mutations

Mutations of *TP53* (encoding p53 tumor suppressor) are relatively rare in newly diagnosed MM, occurring in approximately 5% of tumors. However, the frequency of mutations appears to increase with disease stage and is about 30% in relapse MM and 65% in HMCLs (77–79,116). Although the *TP53* locus is within the commonly deleted 17p13 region, there is no definitive evidence that the critical gene loss is *TP53*. Recently, it was shown that low expression of *TP53* correlated with 17p13 deletion and poor prognosis, suggesting that *TP53* may indeed be the important gene on 17p13 (117). Although almost all 17p13 deletions detected are monoallelic, there has been no definitive analysis of *TP53* mutation of the remaining allele in these patients to conclusively implicate *TP53* as the critical gene. In a large study comprising 268 MM patients entered into Eastern Cooperative Oncology Group combination chemotherapy studies only 5 of 31 (16%) patients with 17p13 deletion have mutation of the remaining *TP53* allele (116). However, the use of whole bone marrow DNA may have resulted in a marked reduction in sensitivity of the study. In a smaller study (24 newly diagnosed MM patients) using purified CD138+ plasma cells, no *TP53* mutations were detected, but it is unclear whether these samples also have 17p13 deletion (118). Therefore, current evidence does not exclude *TP53* as the critical gene deleted on 17p13. Furthermore, the actual impact of 17p13 monoallelic deletion on the p53 pathway and whether cooperating deregulation of various components of the pathway, for example, epigenetic silencing of p53 or increased expression of MDM2, are involved needs to be further clarified.

MYC Abnormalities

Translocations that involve the *MYC* gene are rare or absent in MGUS, but occur in 15% of MM tumors, 44% of advanced tumors, and nearly 90% of HMCL. Mostly, these rearrangements involve C-*MYC*, but about 2% of primary tumors ectopically express N-*MYC* (and presumably have N-*MYC* translocations, as confirmed in some cases), and an L-*MYC* rearrangement has been identified only in one HMCL. An Ig locus is involved in 25% (107) to 60% (119,120) of these translocations. The IgH locus is involved somewhat more than the Igλ locus, but the Igκ locus is only rarely involved.

Although abnormalities affecting MYC have conventionally been recognized as a late event in myeloma, recent studies have suggested a possible role for MYC activation in early myeloma pathogenesis. A faithful mouse model of myeloma was created by an increase in MYC translation by random reversion of an engineered stop codon in a somatic hypermutation hotspot in a mouse with background of asymptomatic monoclonal gammopathy. This raised the possibility that MYC activation may be an important event mediating transformation from MGUS to MM. A transcriptional signature for MYC activity based on published MYC network was used to interrogate published MM GEP datasets and found that the signature was present in about 60% of MM while absent from MGUS, providing intriguing evidence that MYC activation may indeed be a common mechanism mediating MGUS to MM transformation (121). Furthermore, there is a correlation between *RAS* mutation and the presence of the MYC activation signature suggesting that the secondary outcome of *RAS* mutation is MYC activation. MYC activation may therefore be a common downstream pathway of many early insults that may mediate transformation from MGUS to MM (manuscript in preparation).

Nuclear Factor-κB Abnormalities

It is widely accepted that the NFκB pathway is important in the pathogenesis of MM, but little is known about the prevalence of NFκB activation or mechanisms that cause NFκB activation. Recently, a promiscuous array of mutations that result in constitutive activation of the NFκB pathway have been identified in about 20% of patient samples, and 20 of 44 HMCL. The most common event is inactivating mutations of *TRAF3* in 13% of patients. In addition, inactivating mutations of *TRAF2*, *cIAP1/2*, and *CYLD* were identified. Chromosome translocations and amplifications resulting in activation of NFκB-inducing kinase (NIK) (122), CD40, LTBR, TACI, NFκB1, and NFκB2 were also reported (123). Although activation of both the canonical and noncanonical pathways is seen, the preponderance of mutations resulted most directly in increased processing of NFκB2 p100 to p52 (i.e., activation of the noncanonical pathway). Depletion of NIK with short hairpin RNAs resulted in the inhibition of both the classical and alternative NFκB pathways, and also growth inhibition. Half of primary MM tumors have an expression signature of NFκB target genes, with activating mutations identified in less than half of these patients. Presumably, either other mutations or ligand-dependent interactions in the BM microenvironment are responsible for the NFκB activation in the remaining patients. Clearly, we need to know more about intrinsic and extrinsic mechanisms that activate the NFκB pathway in MM, as this seems a potentially important pathway for therapeutic intervention.

RB Pathway (p16INK4A and p18INK4C)

A recent study found that universal aberrant expression of Cyclin D is already present at MGUS suggesting that it is an early pathogenic event. The mechanism of Cyclin D overexpression is not completely clear but is in some cases driven directly by IgH translocations [Cyclin D1 in t(11;14) and Cyclin D3 in t(6;14)] or indirectly as downstream target of genes involved in IgH translocations (Cyclin D2 in IgH translocations involving MAF family members) (43). Besides Cyclin D, other components of the RB pathway are also commonly dysregulated in MM. The p16INK4A and p15INK4B genes (*CDKN2A* and *CDKN2B*, respectively) are methylated in about 20% to 30% of MGUS and MM tumors, and in most HMCL (110). Two recent studies showed that most MM tumors express little or no p16INK4A regardless of whether or not the gene is methylated (124,125). This suggests that methylation of *CDKN2A* may be an epiphenomenon. Despite one example of an individual with a germline mutation and loss of the normal p16INK4A allele in MM tumor cells (126), it remains unclear if inactivation of p16INK4A is a critical and presumably early event in the pathogenesis of MM.

By contrast, it seems apparent that inactivation of *CDKN2C* (gene encoding p18INK4C), a critical gene for normal plasma cell development, is likely to contribute to increased proliferation. There is bi-allelic deletion of *CDKN2C* in 30% of HMCL, and nearly 10% of tumors in the highest quintile of proliferation, as determined by an expression-based proliferation index (127). In another study, homozygous deletion of the *CDKN2C* locus was detected in 4% of myeloma samples by high-resolution SNP array. Further screening using FISH probes specific to the *CDKN2C* locus found that hemizygous deletion is found in 4.5% of MGUS, 10.3% of SMM, and 15% of MM. Furthermore, deletion of *CDKN2C* is associated with shorter survival (55). Forced expression of p18INK4C by retroviral infection of HMCL that express little or no endogenous p18 substantially inhibits proliferation. Paradoxically, about 60% of HMCL and 60% of the more proliferative MM tumors have increased expression

of p18 compared with normal plasma cells (127). There is evidence that the E2F transcription factor, which is upregulated in association with increased proliferation, increases the expression of p18, presumably as a feedback mechanism. Apart from the lack of a functional RB protein in approximately 10% of HMCL, the mechanism(s) by which most HMCL and proliferative tumors become insensitive to increased p18INK4C levels is not yet understood.

■ MOLECULAR CLASSIFICATION: DISSECTING MYELOMA HETEROGENEITY

With the advent of GEP techniques, many investigators have studied the global transcriptional changes in myeloma and used this information to further dissect the marked heterogeneity in myeloma. It is interesting that using both unsupervised and supervised methods, different investigators seem to arrive at molecular classes that correspond to the main primary genetic abnormalities (39,43). This suggests that these genetic abnormalities are the main drivers of the predominant gene expression changes across these tumors, further highlighting the importance of these abnormalities in myeloma biology.

Translocation and Cyclin D (TC) Classification (43)

This classification is based on spiked expression of genes deregulated by primary IgH translocations and the universal overexpression of CyclinD genes either by these translocations or other mechanism. The resultant classification identifies eight groups of tumors: those with primary translocations (designated 4p16, 11q13, 6p21, and MAF), those that overexpressed *CCND1* and *CCND2* either alone or in combination (D1, D1&D2, and D2), and the rare cases that do not overexpress any cyclin D genes ("none"). Most of the patients with HRD MM fall within the D1 and D1&D2 groups.

The advantage of this classification system is that it focuses on different kinds of mechanisms that dysregulate a Cyclin D gene as an early and unifying event in pathogenesis. The underlying Cyclin D deregulation potentially has an important therapeutic implication as differential targeting of Cyclin D may be very useful and add specificity to treatment. Indeed, some potential agents targeting Cyclin D2 have been identified in a drug library screen (128).

This classification has great potential for translation into the clinic as it involves the measurement of relatively few markers, and most of the translocations can be detected by FISH.

On the downside, the TC classification does not identify patients with HRD myeloma clearly, with the majority of these patients falling into the D1 and D1&D2 group. D1&D2 HRD MM appears to have more proliferative disease, but the survival of these patients is not different from those that are D1. In addition, the clinical and biological significance of the D2 group is unclear.

UAMS Molecular Classification of Myeloma

Recently, the group from UAMS derived another MM classification using an unsupervised approach and identified seven tumor groups characterized by the coexpression of unique gene clusters (39). Interestingly, these clusters also identify tumors with t(4;14), maf translocations, t(11;14) and t(6;14), corresponding to the MS, MF, and CD1 and/or CD2 groups, respectively. In this analysis, t(11;14) and t(6;14) can belong to either the CD1 or CD2 group depending on expression of CD20 and other B-cell–related genes. This is consistent with the finding that t(11;14) and t(6;14) have very similar expression profiles, clinical profiles, and outcome. In contrast to the TC classification, the UAMS classification identifies HRD

MM as a distinct HY group. However, this may be somewhat misleading since the HY group, which is about 28% of MM tumors, includes only about 60% of HRD tumors. The distribution of the remaining HRD tumors among the other six groups has not been clarified, although most are probably in the LB and PR groups. Besides these groups that correspond to the major genetic subtypes of MM, there are two further groups: PR, defined by increased expression of proliferation-related genes; and LB, defined by low bone disease and lower expression of genes associated with bone disease in MM such as FRZB and DKK1 (129). The PR, MS, and MF groups identify patients with poor prognosis. The PR group, containing patients with t(4;14), t(11;14), and HRD patients, identifies the patients within these categories with more proliferative disease associated with poorer outcome.

The advantage of the UAMS molecular classification is that it is clinically relevant. It identifies the main genetic subtypes and other clinically relevant subtypes such as the high-risk PR subgroup and the CD20-expressing CD2 group. It is also interesting that an unsupervised analysis of GEP data essentially identifies the main genetic subtypes of MM, suggesting that the predominant transcriptional heterogeneity seen within MM is driven by these pivotal primary genetic events and/or by progression events such as proliferation in the PR group. One of the deficiencies of this classification is that samples with white cell and normal plasma cell contamination were excluded from the classification as the expression signatures from these contaminating cells may affect assignment to the different groups. Furthermore, classification is based on composite expression of large sets of genes. It is therefore uncertain how this can be applied clinically.

Classification Based on Oncogenic Pathways

Recently, it was shown that tumor heterogeneity could be dissected based on the composite of oncogenic pathways activated (130). Using such as strategy has the additional advantage of potentially providing information regarding the different pathways that can be targeted therapeutically in each tumor. These strategies were recently applied to MM and distinct subgroups that are prognostically relevant can be identified (131). The relation among this signature-based classification, the TC classification, and the UAMS classification is unclear.

Genetic Subtype-Specific Heterogeneity: HRD MM as a Model

In a recent analysis of GEP data of HRD MM, four reproducible molecular signatures could be identified: one overexpressing cancer testis antigen and proliferation genes; one overexpressing *HGF, IL-6, SOCS3,* and *PTP4A3*; another overexpressing NF-κB genes; and the last signature includes underexpressing genes associated with the first three signatures. Importantly, patients expressing different signatures have different survival. For example, after a median follow-up of 3 years, the group expressing the cancer testis antigen signature have a median survival of 27 months, whereas the median survival is not yet reached for the group expressing the NFκB signature (41). A separate study, using aCGH, identifies a group of HRD MM patients with chromosome 1q amplification, 13 deletion, and 11 trisomies that have significantly shorter progression-free survival than other HRD MM patients (132). Interestingly, 1q amplification is a common feature of both the high-risk HRD MM group identified by both the GEP and aCGH studies. These studies highlight the presence of molecular and genetic heterogeneity within HRD MM and the importance of defining genetic subtype-specific prognostic factors. Similar heterogeneity probably exists in other genetic subgroups. For example, in the UAMS classification, the t(11;14) can belong to the CD1, CD2, or PR group.

■ PATHOGENIC IMPLICATIONS

Ploidy Defines Major Subtypes With Unique Genetic Associations

Detailed analysis of numerical abnormalities reveals two broad categories of MM: HRD and NHRD MM, which have unique pattern of associations with other recurrent genetic abnormalities in MM (3,4,9). Near-tetraploid MM has been classified together with hypodiploid and pseudodiploid MM as NHRD MM as the abnormalities seen in these tumors appear to represent 4N duplications of those present in cells with pseudodiploid or hypodiploid karyotypes. The NHRD MM is characterized by a very high prevalence of IgH translocations (>85%), in particular, the three main recurrent IgH translocations involving 4p16.3, 11q13, and 16q23 as partners, whereas IgH translocations are less common in the HRD MM (<30%). Likewise, Δ13 is more common in patients with NHRD karyotype (9,23,133). On the other hand, the HRD tumors are associated with trisomies of chromosomes 3, 5, 7, 9, 11, 15, 19, and 21. Although they harbor less IgH translocations, the proportion of IgH translocations involving unknown partners is higher (4,9,23). Recently, we have shown that this HRD and NHRD dichotomy already exist in MGUS, suggesting that the mechanisms leading to the characteristic genetic abnormalities of these two subtypes (IgH translocations and trisomies) occur early (59). We also have some evidence that this early dichotomy persists throughout disease progression as the ploidy status of patients rarely changes even at progression (134). The two broad categories of MM are hence distinct and most likely to have different oncogenic mechanisms and biology.

Genomic Instability and Genetic Complexity

Most myeloma has complex genetic abnormalities at presentation. Some of these abnormalities such as 1p and 1q abnormalities are usually not detected in MGUS and gained upon progression to MM. However, whether the genetic evolution represent ongoing genomic instability of the same clone or emergence of more aggressive clone from a pool where multiple clones exist is not clear. It is likely that both scenarios coexist. As the primary genetic abnormalities such as t(4;14), t(11;14), t(14;16), and trisomies of hyperdiploidy are present in almost 100% of malignant cell and already present at MGUS, and the HRD-NHRD dichotomy rarely intersect, there is probably initially only one clone triggered by these initiating genetic events. However, it is also likely that there is ongoing genomic instability and continued selection of the fittest clone such that at diagnosis, multiple clones probably exist with some more dominant than others. With treatment, sensitive clones will be suppressed or eradicated whereas resistant clones may persist. When these clones acquire additional proliferative advantage or fitness to expand, they may then trigger relapse (Figure 1).

Current Model of the Multistep Genetic Progression of MM (Figure 1)

There are two pathways of pathogenesis: an NHRD pathway and a HRD pathway. The primary events appear in IgH translocations mediated mainly by errors in switch recombination or somatic hypermutation in germinal-center B cells for the NHRD pathway and acquisition of trisomies for the HRD pathway. Both these primary events lead to the dysregulation of a Cyclin D gene. Although the increased expression of a Cyclin D gene may

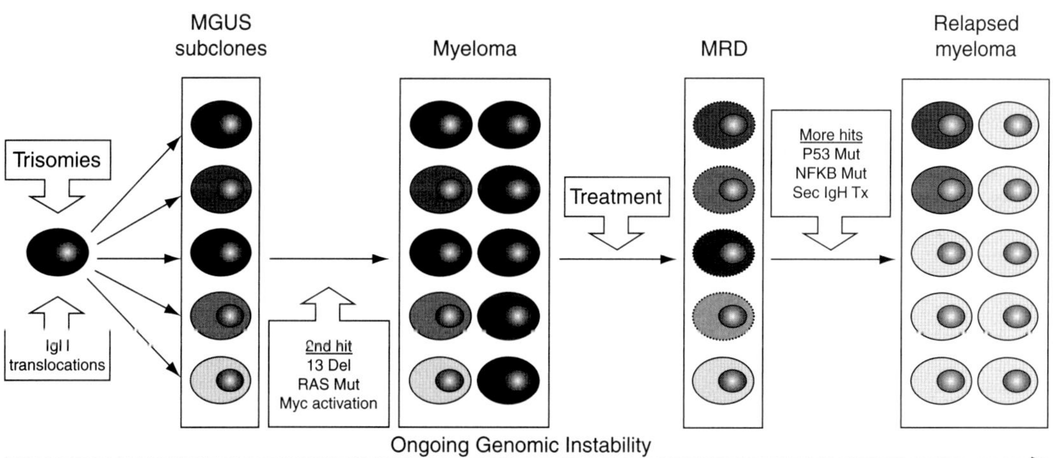

FIGURE 1

Clonal evolution of multiple myeloma (MM). The earliest clonal events are IgH translocations and trisomies, which established the NHRD and HRD pathogenic pathways, respectively. In this early phase, there is limited clonal evolution with development of subclones. One of these subclones (dark gray) may acquire a second genetic hit resulting in the expansion and dominance of the clone leading to the transformation from monoclonal gammopathy of undetermined significance to MM. As patients respond to treatment, the dominant clone (dark gray) is eradicated or suppressed to minimal residual level (clones with dotted outer lines). Similarly, some of the subclones may also be eradicated but some may be resistant and persist (light gray). This resistant clone (light gray) or the initial clone (dark gray), if not completely eradicated, may acquire further critical hits that lead to disease relapse.

not cause increased proliferation, it may make these cells more susceptible to proliferative stimuli, resulting in selective expansion of cells as a result of interaction with BM stromal cells that express IL-6, IGF-1, or other cytokines.

Early transformation events are likely to be subtype specific as they cooperate with the primary genetic events. In this regard, Δ13 is much more common in tumors that dysregulate Cyclin D2 (t(4;14) and translocations involving MAF family genes) whereas mutations of RAS are more common in D1 tumors (t(11;14) and hyperdiploidy). Expanding on this, we have recently identified that MYC activation represents a common secondary pathway for transformation from MGUS to MM. Furthermore, multiple mechanisms including RAS mutation and IgH-MYC translocations may lead to MYC activation, and there is enrichment of MYC activation among tumors that are aberrantly expressing Cyclin D1 (manuscript in preparation). This further suggests that different secondary genetic events may converge on unifying pathways. All the mechanisms activating MYC still need to be elucidated, and the other pathways activated by those tumors that do not activate MYC still need to be ascertained.

In contrast, progression events such as secondary and complex MYC rearrangements, inactivation of p53, additional inactivation of the RB pathway (inactivation of p16INK4A, p18INK4C, or RB), mutations leading to constitutive activation of the NF-κB pathway, and secondary IgH translocations have similar prevalence across the genetic subtypes. These genetic alterations predominantly result in three phenotypes, increased proliferation, independence from the BM microenvironment, and possibly genomic instability (loss of DNA damage checkpoint).

■ CLINICAL IMPLICATIONS

Genetic factors have emerged as significant prognostic factors in MM. With the further dissection of the genetic heterogeneity of MM, a hierarchical model of prognostic genetic factors is emerging. Patients with abnormal cytogenetics have poorer prognosis than those without, possibly reflecting a more proliferative clone (5). HRD MM have better survival than NHRD MM (3). Among the NHRD MM, t(11;14)(q13;q32) have better prognosis than t(4;14)(p16.3;q32) and t(14;16)(q32;q23) (22). Δ13 deletion is found in both HRD and NHRD MM (twice as many in the latter) (23). In particular, the presence of Δ13 is tightly associated with t(4;14)(p16.3;q32) and t(14;16)(q32;q23), which are poor prognostic groups (14,18). This raises the possibility that the prior observed poor prognostic impact of Δ13 is due to the presence of t(4;14)(p16.3;q32) or t(14;16)(q32;q23). Indeed, Δ13 has no prognostic impact in HRD MM (135) and in tumors without t(4;14), Δ13 also does not have prognostic impact (136). Presence of 17p13 deletion is universally associated with poor outcome. These genetic abnormalities have been utilized to stratify patients into high and standard risk groups for therapeutic decision making (137).

The International Staging System (ISS) was developed without incorporation of genetic information (138). In a large analysis of patients enrolled into Intergroupe Francophone du Myelome trials, it was shown that t(4;14) and/or 17p13 deletion have prognostic impact independent of ISS (136). This was further verified by a recent large-scale analysis involving institutions from different geographical regions and more than a thousand patients initiated by the International Myeloma Working Group. It was shown that the incorporation of t(4;14) and/or 17p13 deletion to ISS results in a powerful prognostic system where patients with ISS I or II and normal FISH have a 4-year survival of 76%; patients with ISS I and t(4;14) and/or 17p13 deletion by FISH or ISS III with normal FISH have a 4-year survival of 52%; and patients with ISS II or III and t(4;14) and/or 17p13 deletion by FISH have a 4-year survival of 32%.

Most of the studies establishing the association of t(4;14) and 17p13 deletion with poor prognosis is performed on patients treated with chemotherapy and stem cell transplantation. It has emerged that this negative prognostic implication may be reversed by certain novel agents. In particular, bortezomib has been shown to overcome poor prognosis conferred by t(4;14) in both relapse and newly diagnosed patients (139–141). However, it is presently unclear whether this is a generalized feature of bortezomib-treated patients or that chronicity of bortezomib treatment also plays an important role. On the other hand, patients with poor risk genetic features still do badly when treated with lenalidomide in an upfront setting (142) whereas Revlimid is able to overcome the poor prognosis resulting from t(4;14) but not 17p13 deletion in relapse MM (143).

The latter studies raised an important issue regarding prognostic impact of different genetic features at diagnosis and relapse. This is an important issue that needs to be further clarified. Certainly in an analysis of a cohort of relapse patients entered into bortezomib trials, patients with t(11;14), a subgroup with good prognosis at diagnosis, had the worse prognosis (139), providing intriguing evidence that prognostic impact of genetic subtypes may differ at different phases of disease.

The newer technique of GEP has been shown by a number of groups to provide extremely powerful prognostic information. Several groups have derived GEP signatures associated with poor prognosis, and these consistently have hazard ratios greater than the traditional genetic prognostic factors (42,44). The important question in the future is how to harvest the power of GEP and apply it clinically. The successful clinical translation of GEP-based signatures in breast cancer suggests that this is a distinct possibility. Another important aspect would be to identify specific pathways and targets in these high-risk cohorts that may be amenable to novel therapeutic approaches. We have used such an approach to determine aurora kinases as potential targets in high-risk patients with a high centrosome index, which identifies patients with very poor survival (144).

■ THERAPEUTIC IMPLICATIONS

The possibility of using genetic information for therapeutic risk stratification and treatment assignment stems from the availability of a wider spectrum of therapeutic strategies and differential outcome according to novel agents used. For example, a bortezomib-containing treatment seems to particularly benefit patients with t(4;14); on the other hand, patients with HRD MM have very good survival with alkylating agent–based therapy and bortezomib may be reserved for relapse. The Mayo Stratification of Myeloma and Risk-adapted Therapy treatment algorithm proposed by the Mayo Clinic is one such risk-stratified treatment strategy (145). The rationale for using different treatment strategies for different risk groups will have to be revisited constantly in light of new data of each novel treatment in different disease setting and their efficacy in relation to each risk category.

Identification of oncogenes deregulated by the genetic events in MM has started to facilitate the design of targeted therapies. A prime example is the t(4;14)(p16.3;q32) where the deregulation and overexpression of *FGFR3* represent an obvious therapeutic target. As *FGFR3* is a receptor tyrosine kinase, inhibition with small molecules akin to imatinib in chronic myeloid leukemia is an attractive possibility. Furthermore, the poor prognosis of these patients and rapid relapse after current available therapies identify them as those with unmet medical needs. Indeed, progress from proof-of-concept preclinical studies identifying *FGFR3* as a worthwhile target (146) to screening and characterization of potential compounds (147–149) has been rapid, making potential effective treatment for these patients a distinct possibility in the future.

The advent of GEP has also impacted our understanding of the therapeutic action of various drugs (150–153) and mechanism of their resistance (154,155). In addition, the use of oncogene-specific signatures (130) and also combinatory drug-sensitive signatures (156) will identify the best single drug or combination treatment using both conventional as well as novel targeted agents on an individual patient basis. This may facilitate more effective drug combinations targeting multiple critical pathways in MM. Many of the recent or ongoing clinical trials have incorporated pharmacogenomic studies (157). The outcomes of these studies are eagerly awaited and will hopefully uncover predictive gene signatures for responders and/or patients who will benefit most in terms of response duration and survival to better inform future patient selection for different treatments (Figure 2).

well-established prognostic genetic factors will have to be re-evaluated. In addition, the role of genetics in relapse disease also needs to be studied as information in this regard is lacking. In the future, expansion of studies to include microRNA and epigenetics will allow more complete understanding of myeloma genetics and integration of these data with clinical and phenotype data in a system biology approach will hopefully yield further insights into disease biology and heterogeneity that can be translated into better treatment and outcome for patients.

■ FUTURE PROSPECTS AND CONCLUSIONS

Detection of genetic abnormalities in myeloma should now be routinely performed in all newly diagnosed patients using conventional cytogenetics and FISH. Information can be used for risk stratification and therapeutic decision making. With the emergence of novel therapies,

■ REFERENCES

1. Laï JL, Zandecki M, Mary JY, et al. Improved cytogenetics in multiple myeloma: a study of 151 patients including 117 patients at diagnosis. *Blood* 1995;85(9):2490–2497.
2. Dewald GW, Kyle RA, Hicks GA, Greipp PR. The clinical significance of cytogenetic studies in 100 patients with multiple myeloma, plasma cell leukemia, or amyloidosis. *Blood* 1985;66(2):380–390.

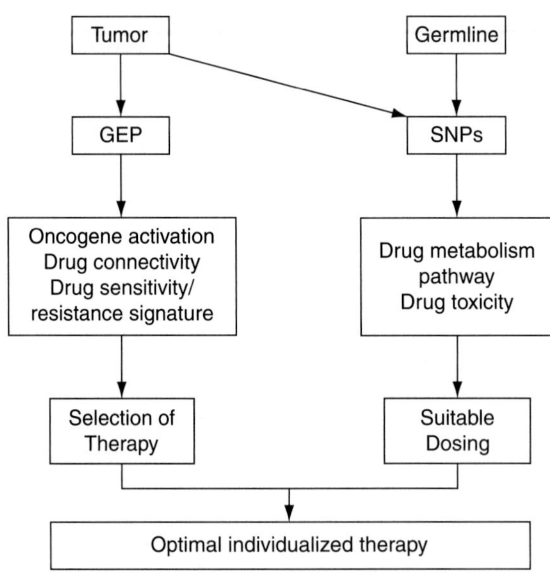

FIGURE 2
Schema toward achieving individualized therapy.

3. Smadja NV, Bastard C, Brigaudeau C, Leroux D, Fruchart C; Groupe Français de Cytogénétique Hématologique. Hypodiploidy is a major prognostic factor in multiple myeloma. *Blood* 2001; 98(7):2229–2238.

4. Smadja NV, Fruchart C, Isnard F, et al. Chromosomal analysis in multiple myeloma: cytogenetic evidence of two different diseases. *Leukemia* 1998;12(6): 960–969.

5. Rajkumar SV, Fonseca R, Dewald GW, et al. Cytogenetic abnormalities correlate with the plasma cell labeling index and extent of bone marrow involvement in myeloma. *Cancer Genet Cytogenet* 1999;113(1):73–77.

6. Gould J, Alexanian R, Goodacre A, Pathak S, Hecht B, Barlogie B. Plasma cell karyotype in multiple myeloma. *Blood* 1988;71(2):453–456.

7. Zandecki M, Laï JL, Facon T. Multiple myeloma: almost all patients are cytogenetically abnormal. *Br J Haematol* 1996;94(2):217–227.

8. Sawyer JR, Waldron JA, Jagannath S, Barlogie B. Cytogenetic findings in 200 patients with multiple myeloma. *Cancer Genet Cytogenet* 1995;82(1):41–49.

9. Debes-Marun CS, Dewald GW, Bryant S, et al. Chromosome abnormalities clustering and its implications for pathogenesis and prognosis in myeloma. *Leukemia* 2003;17(2):427–436.

10. Chesi M, Bergsagel PL, Shonukan OO, et al. Frequent dysregulation of the c-maf proto-oncogene at 16q23 by translocation to an Ig locus in multiple myeloma. *Blood* 1998;91(12):4457–4463.

11. Chesi M, Nardini E, Brents LA, et al. Frequent translocation t(4;14)(p16.3;q32.3) in multiple myeloma is associated with increased expression and activating mutations of fibroblast growth factor receptor 3. *Nat Genet* 1997;16(3):260–264.

12. Sawyer JR, Lukacs JL, Munshi N, et al. Identification of new nonrandom translocations in multiple myeloma with multicolor spectral karyotyping. *Blood* 1998;92(11):4269–4278.

13. Tabernero D, San Miguel JF, Garcia-Sanz M, et al. Incidence of chromosome numerical changes in multiple myeloma: fluorescence in situ hybridization analysis using 15 chromosome-specific probes. *Am J Pathol* 1996;149(1):153–161.

14. Avet-Loiseau H, Facon T, Grosbois B, et al.; Intergroupe Francophone du Myélome. Oncogenesis of multiple myeloma: 14q32 and 13q chromosomal abnormalities are not randomly distributed, but correlate with natural history, immunological features, and clinical presentation. *Blood* 2002;99(6):2185–2191.

15. Drach J, Schuster J, Nowotny H, et al. Multiple myeloma: high incidence of chromosomal aneuploidy as detected by interphase fluorescence in situ hybridization. *Cancer Res* 1995;55(17):3854–3859.

16. Fonseca R, Blood EA, Oken MM, et al. Myeloma and the t(11;14)(q13;q32); evidence for a biologically defined unique subset of patients. *Blood* 2002;99(10):3735–3741.

17. Fonseca R, Harrington D, Oken MM, et al. Biological and prognostic significance of interphase fluorescence in situ hybridization detection of chromosome 13 abnormalities (delta13) in multiple myeloma: an eastern cooperative oncology group study. *Cancer Res* 2002;62(3):715–720.

18. Fonseca R, Oken MM, Greipp PR; Eastern Cooperative Oncology Group Myeloma Group. The t(4;14)(p16.3;q32) is strongly associated with chromosome 13 abnormalities in both multiple myeloma and monoclonal gammopathy of undetermined significance. *Blood* 2001;98(4):1271–1272.

19. Fonseca R, Oken MM, Harrington D, et al. Deletions of chromosome 13 in multiple myeloma identified by interphase FISH usually denote large deletions of the q arm or monosomy. *Leukemia* 2001;15(6):981–986.

20. Fonseca R, Bailey RJ, Ahmann GJ, et al. Genomic abnormalities in monoclonal gammopathy of undetermined significance. *Blood* 2002;100(4):1417–1424.

21. Ahmann GJ, Jalal SM, Juneau AL, et al. A novel three-color, clone-specific fluorescence in situ hybridization procedure for monoclonal gammopathies. *Cancer Genet Cytogenet* 1998;101(1):7–11.

22. Fonseca R, Blood E, Rue M, et al. Clinical and biologic implications of recurrent genomic aberrations in myeloma. *Blood* 2003;101(11):4569–4575.

23. Fonseca R, Debes-Marun CS, Picken EB, et al. The recurrent IgH translocations are highly associated with nonhyperdiploid variant multiple myeloma. *Blood* 2003;102(7):2562–2567.

24. Avet-Loiseau H, Brigaudeau C, Morineau N, et al. High incidence of cryptic translocations involving the Ig heavy chain gene in multiple myeloma, as shown by fluorescence in situ hybridization. *Genes Chromosomes Cancer* 1999;24(1):9–15.

25. Avet-Loiseau H, Li JY, Facon T, et al. High incidence of translocations t(11;14)(q13;q32) and t(4;14) (p16;q32) in patients with plasma cell malignancies. *Cancer Res* 1998;58(24):5640–5645.

26. Avet-Loiseau H, Facon T, Daviet A, et al. 14q32 translocations and monosomy 13 observed in monoclonal gammopathy of undetermined significance delineate a multistep process for the oncogenesis of multiple

myeloma. Intergroupe Francophone du Myélome. *Cancer Res* 1999;59(18):4546–4550.

27. Fonseca R, Ahmann GJ, Jalal SM, et al. Chromosomal abnormalities in systemic amyloidosis. *Br J Haematol* 1998;103(3):704–710.

28. Hayman SR, Bailey RJ, Jalal SM, et al. Translocations involving the immunoglobulin heavy-chain locus are possible early genetic events in patients with primary systemic amyloidosis. *Blood* 2001;98(7): 2266–2268.

29. Sawyer JR, Lukacs JL, Thomas EL, et al. Multicolour spectral karyotyping identifies new translocations and a recurring pathway for chromosome loss in multiple myeloma. *Br J Haematol* 2001;112(1):167–174.

30. Rao PH, Cigudosa JC, Ning Y, et al. Multicolor spectral karyotyping identifies new recurring breakpoints and translocations in multiple myeloma. *Blood* 1998;92(5):1743–1748.

31. Avet-Loiseau H, Andree-Ashley LE, Moore D 2nd, et al. Molecular cytogenetic abnormalities in multiple myeloma and plasma cell leukemia measured using comparative genomic hybridization. *Genes Chromosomes Cancer* 1997;19(2):124–133.

32. Avet-Loiseau H, Bataille R. Detection of nonrandom chromosomal changes in multiple myeloma by comparative genomic hybridization. *Blood* 1998;92(8): 2997–2998.

33. Cigudosa JC, Rao PH, Calasanz MJ, et al. Characterization of nonrandom chromosomal gains and losses in multiple myeloma by comparative genomic hybridization. *Blood* 1998;91(8):3007–3010.

34. Gutiérrez NC, Hernández JM, García JL, et al. Differences in genetic changes between multiple myeloma and plasma cell leukemia demonstrated by comparative genomic hybridization. *Leukemia* 2001;15(5):840–845.

35. Liebisch P, Viardot A, Bassermann N, et al. Value of comparative genomic hybridization and fluorescence in situ hybridization for molecular diagnostics in multiple myeloma. *Br J Haematol* 2003;122(2):193–201.

36. Zhan F, Barlogie B, Arzoumanian V, et al. Gene-expression signature of benign monoclonal gammopathy evident in multiple myeloma is linked to good prognosis. *Blood* 2007;109(4):1692–1700.

37. Zhan F, Barlogie B, Mulligan G, Shaughnessy JD Jr, Bryant B. High-risk myeloma: a gene expression based risk-stratification model for newly diagnosed multiple myeloma treated with high-dose therapy is predictive of outcome in relapsed disease treated with single-agent bortezomib or high-dose dexamethasone. *Blood* 2008;111(2):968–969.

38. Zhan F, Hardin J, Kordsmeier B, et al. Global gene expression profiling of multiple myeloma, monoclonal gammopathy of undetermined significance, and normal bone marrow plasma cells. *Blood* 2002;99(5):1745–1757.

39. Zhan F, Huang Y, Colla S, et al. The molecular classification of multiple myeloma. *Blood* 2006; 108(6):2020–2028.

40. Zhan F, Tian E, Bumm K, Smith R, Barlogie B, Shaughnessy J Jr. Gene expression profiling of human plasma cell differentiation and classification of multiple myeloma based on similarities to distinct stages of late-stage B-cell development. *Blood* 2003;101(3):1128–1140.

41. Chng WJ, Kumar S, Vanwier S, et al. Molecular dissection of hyperdiploid multiple myeloma by gene expression profiling. *Cancer Res* 2007;67(7):2982–2989.

42. Decaux O, Lodé L, Magrangeas F, et al.; Intergroupe Francophone du Myélome. Prediction of survival in multiple myeloma based on gene expression profiles reveals cell cycle and chromosomal instability signatures in high-risk patients and hyperdiploid signatures in low-risk patients: a study of the Intergroupe Francophone du Myélome. *J Clin Oncol* 2008;26(29):4798–4805.

43. Bergsagel PL, Kuehl WM, Zhan F, Sawyer J, Barlogie B, Shaughnessy J Jr. Cyclin D dysregulation: an early and unifying pathogenic event in multiple myeloma. *Blood* 2005;106(1):296–303.

44. Shaughnessy JD Jr, Zhan F, Burington BE, et al. A validated gene expression model of high-risk multiple myeloma is defined by deregulated expression of genes mapping to chromosome 1. *Blood* 2007;109(6):2276–2284.

45. De Vos J, Thykjaer T, Tarte K, et al. Comparison of gene expression profiling between malignant and normal plasma cells with oligonucleotide arrays. *Oncogene* 2002;21(44):6848–6857.

46. Tarte K, De Vos J, Thykjaer T, et al. Generation of polyclonal plasmablasts from peripheral blood B cells: a normal counterpart of malignant plasmablasts. *Blood* 2002;100(4):1113–1122.

47. Claudio JO, Masih-Khan E, Tang H, et al. A molecular compendium of genes expressed in multiple myeloma. *Blood* 2002;100(6):2175–2186.

48. Magrangeas F, Nasser V, Avet-Loiseau H, et al. Gene expression profiling of multiple myeloma reveals molecular portraits in relation to the pathogenesis of the disease. *Blood* 2003;101(12):4998–5006.

49. Davies FE, Dring AM, Li C, et al. Insights into the multistep transformation of MGUS to myeloma using

microarray expression analysis. *Blood* 2003;102(13): 4504–4511.

50. Dring AM, Davies FE, Fenton JA, et al. A global expression-based analysis of the consequences of the t(4;14) translocation in myeloma. *Clin Cancer Res* 2004;10(17):5692–5701.

51. Agnelli L, Bicciato S, Mattioli M, et al. Molecular classification of multiple myeloma: a distinct transcriptional profile characterizes patients expressing CCND1 and negative for 14q32 translocations. *J Clin Oncol* 2005;23(29):7296–7306.

52. Mattioli M, Agnelli L, Fabris S, et al. Gene expression profiling of plasma cell dyscrasias reveals molecular patterns associated with distinct IGH translocations in multiple myeloma. *Oncogene* 2005;24(15):2461–2473.

53. Keats JJ, Fonseca R, Chesi M, et al. Promiscuous mutations activate the noncanonical NF-kappaB pathway in multiple myeloma. *Cancer Cell* 2007;12(2):131–144.

54. Annunziata CM, Davis RE, Demchenko Y, et al. Frequent engagement of the classical and alternative NF-kappaB pathways by diverse genetic abnormalities in multiple myeloma. *Cancer Cell* 2007;12(2):115–130.

55. Leone PE, Walker BA, Jenner MW, et al. Deletions of CDKN2C in multiple myeloma: biological and clinical implications. *Clin Cancer Res* 2008;14(19):6033–6041.

56. Walker BA, Leone PE, Jenner MW, et al. Integration of global SNP-based mapping and expression arrays reveals key regions, mechanisms, and genes important in the pathogenesis of multiple myeloma. *Blood* 2006;108(5):1733–1743.

57. Greipp PR, Trendle MC, Leong T, et al. Is flow cytometric DNA content hypodiploidy prognostic in multiple myeloma? *Leuk Lymphoma* 1999;35(1–2):83–89.

58. Orfão A, García-Sanz R, López-Berges MC, et al. A new method for the analysis of plasma cell DNA content in multiple myeloma samples using a CD38/propidium iodide double staining technique. *Cytometry* 1994;17(4):332–339.

59. Chng WJ, Van Wier SA, Ahmann GJ, et al. A validated FISH trisomy index demonstrates the hyperdiploid and non-hyperdiploid dichotomy in MGUS. *Blood* 2005;106:2156–2161

60. Wuilleme S, Robillard N, Lodé L, et al.; Intergroupe Francophone de Myélome. Ploidy, as detected by fluorescence in situ hybridization, defines different subgroups in multiple myeloma. *Leukemia* 2005;19(2):275–278.

61. Facon T, Avet-Loiseau H, Guillerm G, et al.; Intergroupe Francophone du Myélome. Chromosome 13 abnormalities identified by FISH analysis and serum beta2-microglobulin produce a powerful myeloma staging system for patients receiving high-dose therapy. *Blood* 2001;97(6):1566–1571.

62. Zojer N, Königsberg R, Ackermann J, et al. Deletion of 13q14 remains an independent adverse prognostic variable in multiple myeloma despite its frequent detection by interphase fluorescence in situ hybridization. *Blood* 2000;95(6):1925–1930.

63. Königsberg R, Ackermann J, Kaufmann H, et al. Deletions of chromosome 13q in monoclonal gammopathy of undetermined significance. *Leukemia* 2000;14(11):1975–1979.

64. Avet-Louseau H, Daviet A, Sauner S, Bataille R.; Intergroupe Francophone du Myélome. Chromosome 13 abnormalities in multiple myeloma are mostly monosomy 13. *Br J Haematol* 2000;111(4):1116–1117.

65. Shaughnessy J, Tian E, Sawyer J, et al. High incidence of chromosome 13 deletion in multiple myeloma detected by multiprobe interphase FISH. *Blood* 2000;96(4):1505–1511.

66. Roccaro AM, Sacco A, Thompson B, et al. MicroRNAs 15a and 16 regulate tumor proliferation in multiple myeloma. *Blood* 2009;113(26):6669–6680.

67. Chang H, Qi X, Trieu Y, et al. Multiple myeloma patients with CKS1B gene amplification have a shorter progression-free survival post-autologous stem cell transplantation. *Br J Haematol* 2006;135(4): 486–491.

68. Fonseca R, Van Wier SA, Chng WJ, et al. Prognostic value of chromosome 1q21 gain by fluorescent in situ hybridization and increase CKS1B expression in myeloma. *Leukemia* 2006;20(11):2034–2040.

69. Hanamura I, Stewart JP, Huang Y, et al. Frequent gain of chromosome band 1q21 in plasma-cell dyscrasias detected by fluorescence in situ hybridization: incidence increases from MGUS to relapsed myeloma and is related to prognosis and disease progression following tandem stem-cell transplantation. *Blood* 2006;108(5):1724–1732.

70. Zhan F, Colla S, Wu X, et al. CKS1B, overexpressed in aggressive disease, regulates multiple myeloma growth and survival through SKP2- and p27Kip1-dependent and -independent mechanisms. *Blood* 2007;109(11):4995–5001.

71. Avet-Loiseau H, Li C, Magrangeas F, et al. Prognostic significance of copy-number alterations in multiple myeloma. *J Clin Oncol* 2009;27(27): 4585–4590.

72. Chang H, Qi X, Jiang A, Xu W, Young T, Reece D. 1p21 deletions are strongly associated with 1q21 gains and are an independent adverse prognostic factor for the outcome of high-dose chemotherapy in patients with multiple myeloma. *Bone Marrow Transplant* 2010;45(1):117–121.

73. Wu KL, Beverloo B, Lokhorst HM, et al.; Dutch-Belgian Haemato-Oncology Cooperative Study Group (HOVON); Dutch Working Party on Cancer Genetics and Cytogenetics (NWCGC). Abnormalities of chromosome 1p/q are highly associated with chromosome 13/13q deletions and are an adverse prognostic factor for the outcome of high-dose chemotherapy in patients with multiple myeloma. *Br J Haematol* 2007;136(4):615–623.

74. Qazilbash MH, Saliba RM, Ahmed B, et al. Deletion of the short arm of chromosome 1 (del 1p) is a strong predictor of poor outcome in myeloma patients undergoing an autotransplant. *Biol Blood Marrow Transplant* 2007;13(9):1066–1072.

75. Drach J, Ackermann J, Fritz E, et al. Presence of a p53 gene deletion in patients with multiple myeloma predicts for short survival after conventional-dose chemotherapy. *Blood* 1998;92(3):802–809.

76. Mazars GR, Portier M, Zhang XG, et al. Mutations of the p53 gene in human myeloma cell lines. *Oncogene* 1992;7(5):1015–1018.

77. Corradini P, Inghirami G, Astolfi M, et al. Inactivation of tumor suppressor genes, p53 and Rb1, in plasma cell dyscrasias. *Leukemia* 1994;8(5):758–767.

78. Neri A, Baldini L, Trecca D, Cro L, Polli E, Maiolo AT. p53 gene mutations in multiple myeloma are associated with advanced forms of malignancy. *Blood* 1993;81(1):128–135.

79. Preudhomme C, Facon T, Zandecki M, et al. Rare occurrence of P53 gene mutations in multiple myeloma. *Br J Haematol* 1992;81(3):440–443.

80. Ackermann J, Meidlinger P, Zojer N, et al. Absence of p53 deletions in bone marrow plasma cells of patients with monoclonal gammopathy of undetermined significance. *Br J Haematol* 1998;103(4):1161–1163.

81. Avet-Loiseau H, Daviet A, Brigaudeau C, et al. Cytogenetic, interphase, and multicolor fluorescence in situ hybridization analyses in primary plasma cell leukemia: a study of 40 patients at diagnosis, on behalf of the Intergroupe Francophone du Myélome and the Groupe Français de Cytogénétique Hématologique. *Blood* 2001;97(3):822–825.

82. Chang H, Sloan S, Li D, Keith Stewart A. Multiple myeloma involving central nervous system: high frequency of chromosome 17p13.1 (p53) deletions. *Br J Haematol* 2004;127(3):280–284.

83. Tiedemann RE, Gonzalez-Paz N, Kyle RA, et al. Genetic aberrations and survival in plasma cell leukemia. *Leukemia* 2008;22(5):1044–1052.

84. Futreal PA, Coin L, Marshall M, et al. A census of human cancer genes. *Nat Rev Cancer* 2004;4(3):177–183.

85. Küppers R. Mechanisms of B-cell lymphoma pathogenesis. *Nat Rev Cancer* 2005;5(4):251–262.

86. Bergsagel PL, Chesi M, Nardini E, Brents LA, Kirby SL, Kuehl WM. Promiscuous translocations into immunoglobulin heavy chain switch regions in multiple myeloma. *Proc Natl Acad Sci USA* 1996;93(24):13931–13936.

87. Bergsagel PL, Kuehl WM. Chromosome translocations in multiple myeloma. *Oncogene* 2001;20(40):5611–5622.

88. Chesi M, Bergsagel PL, Brents LA, Smith CM, Gerhard DS, Kuehl WM. Dysregulation of cyclin D1 by translocation into an IgH gamma switch region in two multiple myeloma cell lines. *Blood* 1996;88(2):674–681.

89. Ronchetti D, Finelli P, Richelda R, et al. Molecular analysis of 11q13 breakpoints in multiple myeloma. *Blood* 1999;93(4):1330–1337.

90. Hoyer JD, Hanson CA, Fonseca R, Greipp PR, Dewald GW, Kurtin PJ. The (11;14)(q13;q32) translocation in multiple myeloma. A morphologic and immunohistochemical study. *Am J Clin Pathol* 2000;113(6):831–837.

91. Moreau P, Facon T, Leleu X, et al.; Intergroupe Francophone du Myélome. Recurrent 14q32 translocations determine the prognosis of multiple myeloma, especially in patients receiving intensive chemotherapy. *Blood* 2002;100(5):1579–1583.

92. Mateo G, Castellanos M, Rasillo A, et al. Genetic abnormalities and patterns of antigenic expression in multiple myeloma. *Clin Cancer Res* 2005;11(10):3661–3667.

93. Robbiani DF, Chesi M, Bergsagel PL. Bone lesions in molecular subtypes of multiple myeloma. *N Engl J Med* 2004;351(2):197–198.

94. Garand R, Avet-Loiseau H, Accard F, Moreau P, Harousseau JL, Bataille R. t(11;14) and t(4;14) translocations correlated with mature lymphoplasmacytoid and immature morphology, respectively, in multiple myeloma. *Leukemia* 2003;17(10):2032–2035.

95. Chesi M, Nardini E, Lim RS, Smith KD, Kuehl WM, Bergsagel PL. The t(4;14) translocation in myeloma dysregulates both FGFR3 and a novel gene,

MMSET, resulting in IgH/MMSET hybrid transcripts. *Blood* 1998;92(9):3025–3034.

96. Keats JJ, Reiman T, Maxwell CA, et al. In multiple myeloma, t(4;14)(p16;q32) is an adverse prognostic factor irrespective of FGFR3 expression. *Blood* 2003;101(4):1520–1529.

97. Santra M, Zhan F, Tian E, Barlogie B, Shaughnessy J Jr. A subset of multiple myeloma harboring the t(4;14)(p16;q32) translocation lacks FGFR3 expression but maintains an IGH/MMSET fusion transcript. *Blood* 2003;101(6):2374–2376.

98. Chesi M, Brents LA, Ely SA, et al. Activated fibroblast growth factor receptor 3 is an oncogene that contributes to tumor progression in multiple myeloma. *Blood* 2001;97(3):729–736.

99. Intini D, Baldini L, Fabris S, et al. Analysis of FGFR3 gene mutations in multiple myeloma patients with t(4;14). *Br J Haematol* 2001;114(2):362–364.

100. Onwuazor ON, Wen XY, Wang DY, et al. Mutation, SNP, and isoform analysis of fibroblast growth factor receptor 3 (FGFR3) in 150 newly diagnosed multiple myeloma patients. *Blood* 2003;102(2):772–773.

101. Keats JJ, Maxwell CA, Taylor BJ, et al. Overexpression of transcripts originating from the MMSET locus characterizes all t(4;14)(p16;q32)-positive multiple myeloma patients. *Blood* 2005;105(10): 4060–4069.

102. Lauring J, Abukhdeir AM, Konishi H, et al. The multiple myeloma associated MMSET gene contributes to cellular adhesion, clonogenic growth, and tumorigenicity. *Blood* 2008;111(2):856–864.

103. Brito JL, Walker B, Jenner M, et al. MMSET deregulation affects cell cycle progression and adhesion regulons in t(4;14) myeloma plasma cells. *Haematologica* 2009;94(1):78–86.

104. Marango J, Shimoyama M, Nishio H, et al. The MMSET protein is a histone methyltransferase with characteristics of a transcriptional corepressor. *Blood* 2008;111(6):3145–3154.

105. Hurt EM, Wiestner A, Rosenwald A, et al. Overexpression of c-maf is a frequent oncogenic event in multiple myeloma that promotes proliferation and pathological interactions with bone marrow stroma. *Cancer Cell* 2004;5(2):191–199.

106. Podar K, Anderson KC. The pathophysiologic role of VEGF in hematologic malignancies: therapeutic implications. *Blood* 2005;105(4):1383–1395.

107. Avet-Loiseau H, Gerson F, Magrangeas F, Minvielle S, Harousseau JL, Bataille R; Intergroupe Francophone du Myélome. Rearrangements of the c-myc oncogene are present in 15% of primary human multiple myeloma tumors. *Blood* 2001; 98(10):3082–3086.

108. Kuehl WM, Bergsagel PL. Multiple myeloma: evolving genetic events and host interactions. *Nat Rev Cancer* 2002;2(3):175–187.

109. Shou Y, Martelli ML, Gabrea A, et al. Diverse karyotypic abnormalities of the c-myc locus associated with c-myc dysregulation and tumor progression in multiple myeloma. *Proc Natl Acad Sci USA* 2000;97(1):228–233.

110. Gabrea A, Leif Bergsagel P, Michael Kuehl W. Distinguishing primary and secondary translocations in multiple myeloma. *DNA Repair (Amst)* 2006;5(9–10):1225–1233.

111. Fonseca R, Barlogie B, Bataille R, et al. Genetics and cytogenetics of multiple myeloma: a workshop report. *Cancer Res* 2004;64(4):1546–1558.

112. Bezieau S, Devilder MC, Avet-Loiseau H, et al. High incidence of N and K-Ras activating mutations in multiple myeloma and primary plasma cell leukemia at diagnosis. *Hum Mutat* 2001;18(3):212–224.

113. Liu P, Leong T, Quam L, et al. Activating mutations of N- and K-ras in multiple myeloma show different clinical associations: analysis of the Eastern Cooperative Oncology Group Phase III Trial. *Blood* 1996;88(7):2699–2706.

114. Rasmussen T, Kuehl M, Lodahl M, Johnsen HE, Dahl IM. Possible roles for activating RAS mutations in the MGUS to MM transition and in the intramedullary to extramedullary transition in some plasma cell tumors. *Blood* 2005;105(1):317–323.

115. Fonseca R, Price-Troska T, Blood E, et al. Implications of N-ras and K-ras mutations in clinical outcome and the biology of multiple myeloma. *Blood* 2003;102:113.

116. Chng WJ, Price-Troska T, Gonzalez-Paz N, et al. Clinical significance of TP53 mutation in myeloma. *Leukemia* 2007;21(3):582–584.

117. Xiong W, Wu X, Starnes S, et al. An analysis of the clinical and biologic significance of TP53 loss and the identification of potential novel transcriptional targets of TP53 in multiple myeloma. *Blood* 2008;112(10):4235–4246.

118. Xiong W, Zhan F, Huang Y, Barlogie B, Shaughnessy JD Jr. TP53 gene expression, correlated with 17p13 deletion, is a significant and independent adverse prognostic factor in multiple myeloma treated with high-dose therapy and auto-transplants [ASH Annual Meeting Abstracts]. *Blood* 2006;108:3394.

119. Dib A, Gabrea A, Glebov OK, Bergsagel PL, Kuehl WM. Characterization of MYC translocations

in multiple myeloma cell lines. *J Natl Cancer Inst Monographs* 2008;2008(39):25–31.

120. Gabrea A, Martelli ML, Qi Y, et al. Secondary genomic rearrangements involving immunoglobulin or MYC loci show similar prevalences in hyperdiploid and nonhyperdiploid myeloma tumors. *Genes Chromosomes Cancer* 2008;47(7):573–590.

121. Chesi M, Robbiani DF, Sebag M, et al. AID-dependent activation of a MYC transgene induces multiple myeloma in a conditional mouse model of post-germinal center malignancies. *Cancer Cell* 2008;13(2):167–180.

122. Annunziata CM, Davis RE, Gabrea A, Lenzi G, Kuehl M, Staudt LM. NF-kappaB-inducing kinase activates NF-KB signaling in multiple myeloma. *Proc Amer Assoc Cancer Res* 2006;47:426.

123. Bergsagel PL, Carpten JD, Chesi M, et al. Promiscuous mutations frequently activate the non-canonical NF-KB pathway in multiple myeloma [Abstract 109]. *Blood* 2006;108:36a.

124. Dib A, Barlogie B, Shaughnessy JD Jr, Kuehl WM. Methylation and expression of the p16INK4A tumor suppressor gene in multiple myeloma. *Blood* 2007;109(3):1337–1338.

125. Gonzalez-Paz N, Chng WJ, McClure RF, et al. Tumor suppressor p16 methylation in multiple myeloma: biological and clinical implications. *Blood* 2007;109(3):1228–1232.

126. Dilworth D, Liu L, Stewart AK, Berenson JR, Lassam N, Hogg D. Germline CDKN2A mutation implicated in predisposition to multiple myeloma. *Blood* 2000;95(5):1869–1871.

127. Dib A, Peterson TR, Raducha-Grace L, et al. Paradoxical expression of INK4c in proliferative multiple myeloma tumors: bi-allelic deletion vs increased expression. *Cell Div* 2006;1:23.

128. Tiedemann RE, Mao X, Shi CX, et al. Identification of kinetin riboside as a repressor of CCND1 and CCND2 with preclinical antimyeloma activity. *J Clin Invest* 2008;118(5):1750–1764.

129. Tian E, Zhan F, Walker R, et al. The role of the Wnt-signaling antagonist DKK1 in the development of osteolytic lesions in multiple myeloma. *N Engl J Med* 2003;349(26):2483–2494.

130. Bild AH, Yao G, Chang JT, et al. Oncogenic pathway signatures in human cancers as a guide to targeted therapies. *Nature* 2006;439(7074):353–357.

131. Anguiano A, Acharya C, Salter K, et al. Gene expression profiles for prognosis in mgus, coupled with signatures of oncogenic pathway deregulation provide a novel approach for selection of molecular targets in multiple myeloma [ASH Annual Meeting Abstracts]. *Blood* 2007;110:655.

132. Carrasco DR, Tonon G, Huang Y, et al. High-resolution genomic profiles define distinct clinico-pathogenetic subgroups of multiple myeloma patients. *Cancer Cell* 2006;9(4):313–325.

133. Smadja NV, Leroux D, Soulier J, et al. Further cytogenetic characterization of multiple myeloma confirms that 14q32 translocations are a very rare event in hyperdiploid cases. *Genes Chromosomes Cancer* 2003;38(3):234–239.

134. Chng WJ, Winkler JM, Greipp PR, et al. Ploidy status rarely changes in myeloma patients at disease progression. *Leuk Res* 2006;30(3):266–271.

135. Chng WJ, Santana-Dávila R, Van Wier SA, et al. Prognostic factors for hyperdiploid-myeloma: effects of chromosome 13 deletions and IgH translocations. *Leukemia* 2006;20(5):807–813.

136. Avet-Loiseau H, Attal M, Moreau P, et al. Genetic abnormalities and survival in multiple myeloma: the experience of the Intergroupe Francophone du Myélome. *Blood* 2007;109(8):3489–3495.

137. Stewart AK, Bergsagel PL, Greipp PR, et al. A practical guide to defining high-risk myeloma for clinical trials, patient counseling and choice of therapy. *Leukemia* 2007;21(3):529–534.

138. Greipp PR, San Miguel J, Durie BG, et al. International staging system for multiple myeloma. *J Clin Oncol* 2005;23(15):3412–3420.

139. Chng WJ, Mulligan G, Bryant B, Bergsagel L. Survival of genetic subtypes of relapsed myeloma may be modulated by secondary events. *Blood* 2007;109(8):3610–3611.

140. Chang H, Trieu Y, Qi X, Xu W, Stewart KA, Reece D. Bortezomib therapy response is independent of cytogenetic abnormalities in relapsed/refractory multiple myeloma. *Leuk Res* 2007;31(6):779–782.

141. San Miguel JF, Schlag R, Khuageva NK, et al.; VISTA Trial Investigators. Bortezomib plus melphalan and prednisone for initial treatment of multiple myeloma. *N Engl J Med* 2008;359(9):906–917.

142. Kapoor P, Kumar S, Fonseca R, et al. Impact of risk stratification on outcome among patients with multiple myeloma receiving initial therapy with lenalidomide and dexamethasone. *Blood* 2009;114(3):518–521.

143. Reece D, Song KW, Fu T, et al. Influence of cytogenetics in patients with relapsed or refractory multiple myeloma treated with lenalidomide plus dexamethasone: adverse effect of deletion 17p13. *Blood* 2009;114(3):522–525.

144. Chng WJ, Braggio E, Mulligan G, et al. The centrosome index is a powerful prognostic marker in myeloma and identifies a cohort of patients that might benefit from aurora kinase inhibition. *Blood* 2008;111(3):1603–1609.

145. Dispenzieri A, Rajkumar SV, Gertz MA, et al. Treatment of newly diagnosed multiple myeloma based on Mayo Stratification of Myeloma and Risk-adapted Therapy (mSMART): consensus statement. *Mayo Clin Proc* 2007;82(3):323–341.

146. Trudel S, Ely S, Farooqi Y, et al. Inhibition of fibroblast growth factor receptor 3 induces differentiation and apoptosis in t(4;14) myeloma. *Blood* 2004;103(9):3521–3528.

147. Paterson JL, Li Z, Wen XY, et al. Preclinical studies of fibroblast growth factor receptor 3 as a therapeutic target in multiple myeloma. *Br J Haematol* 2004;124(5):595–603.

148. Trudel S, Li ZH, Wei E, et al. CHIR-258, a novel, multitargeted tyrosine kinase inhibitor for the potential treatment of t(4;14) multiple myeloma. *Blood* 2005;105(7):2941–2948.

149. Zhu L, Somlo G, Zhou B, et al. Fibroblast growth factor receptor 3 inhibition by short hairpin RNAs leads to apoptosis in multiple myeloma. *Mol Cancer Ther* 2005;4(5):787–798.

150. Chauhan D, Auclair D, Robinson EK, et al. Identification of genes regulated by dexamethasone in multiple myeloma cells using oligonucleotide arrays. *Oncogene* 2002;21(9):1346–1358.

151. Chauhan D, Li G, Auclair D, et al. Identification of genes regulated by 2-methoxyestradiol (2ME2) in multiple myeloma cells using oligonucleotide arrays. *Blood* 2003;101(9):3606–3614.

152. Mitsiades CS, Mitsiades NS, McMullan CJ, et al. Transcriptional signature of histone deacetylase inhibition in multiple myeloma: biological and clinical implications. *Proc Natl Acad Sci USA* 2004;101(2):540–545.

153. Mitsiades N, Mitsiades CS, Poulaki V, et al. Molecular sequelae of proteasome inhibition in human multiple myeloma cells. *Proc Natl Acad Sci USA* 2002;99(22):14374–14379.

154. Hazlehurst LA, Enkemann SA, Beam CA, et al. Genotypic and phenotypic comparisons of de novo and acquired melphalan resistance in an isogenic multiple myeloma cell line model. *Cancer Res* 2003;63(22):7900–7906.

155. Zhou P, Kalakonda N, Comenzo RL. Changes in gene expression profiles of multiple myeloma cells induced by arsenic trioxide (ATO): possible mechanisms to explain ATO resistance in vivo. *Br J Haematol* 2005;128(5):636–644.

156. Potti A, Dressman HK, Bild A, et al. Genomic signatures to guide the use of chemotherapeutics. *Nat Med* 2006;12(11):1294–1300.

157. Mulligan G, Mitsiades C, Bryant B, et al. Gene expression profiling and correlation with outcome in clinical trials of the proteasome inhibitor bortezomib. *Blood* 2007;109(8):3177–3188.

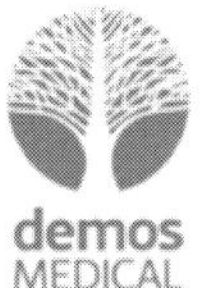

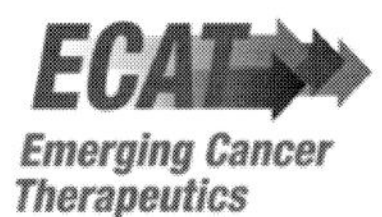

Monoclonal Gammopathy of Undetermined Significance

Sumit Madan and Vincent Rajkumar*

Mayo Clinic, Rochester, MN

■ ABSTRACT

Monoclonal gammopathy of undetermined significance (MGUS) is an asymptomatic, premalignant disease characterized by the monoclonal proliferation of bone marrow plasma cells (BMPCs) with no clinical or laboratory evidence of multiple myeloma, macroglobulinemia, light-chain amyloidosis, or related plasma-cell disorders. The identification, prevalence rates, pathogenesis, natural history, risk factors of progression, current management based on a risk-stratification model, and disease associations of MGUS are discussed.

■ INTRODUCTION

Our understanding of the pathogenesis of multiple myeloma (MM) and other plasma cell proliferative disorders underwent a paradigm shift with the recognition of the malignant potential of a presumed benign disorder (benign monoclonal gammopathy) over 30 years ago. It is now well established that a proportion of asymptomatic individuals with a small amount of serum monoclonal M-protein will progress to a symptomatic monoclonal gammopathy such as MM, light-chain (AL) amyloidosis, or Waldenström's macroglobulinemia (WM) at a fixed lifelong rate of 1% per year.

The first of the seminal series from the Mayo Clinic (Rochester, MN, US) reported progression to MM, AL, or WM in 11% of 241 patients with a serum M-protein but no initial evidence of a lymphoid or plasma cell malignancy (1). This study led to coining of the term "monoclonal gammopathy of undetermined significance" (MGUS) to highlight the long-term risk and the malignant potential of this disorder. Currently, it is widely accepted that almost all cases of MM are preceded by a premalignant disease stage termed "monoclonal gammopathy of undetermined significance" (2,3). Although MGUS is clinically under-recognized due to the asymptomatic nature of this condition, it is still the most commonly diagnosed plasma cell

*Corresponding author, Mayo Clinic, Division of Hematology, 200 First St SW, Rochester, MN 55905

E-mail address: rajkumar.vincent@mayo.edu

Emerging Cancer Therapeutics 1:2 (2010) 237–260.
© 2010 Demos Medical Publishing LLC. All rights reserved.
DOI: 10.5003/2151–4194.1.2.237

dyscrasia. It is usually diagnosed in an outpatient setting as a chance finding of an M-protein during the evaluation of an unrelated disease or in an apparently healthy individual undergoing general health examination. MGUS is defined by the presence of an M-protein less than 3 g/dL, less than 10% clonal plasma cells in the bone marrow (BM), and the absence of lytic bone lesions, anemia, hypercalcemia, or renal insufficiency that can be directly attributed to the plasma cell proliferative process (Table 1) (4).

■ EPIDEMIOLOGY

There is considerable variation in the prevalence of MGUS based on geographical region and ethnicity. In general, studies published in the latter half of the 20th century from the United States, France, Sweden, and Japan found MGUS in approximately 1% to 2% of the adult population (5–8). The prevalence of MGUS increases with age; initially estimated as approximately 3% in persons older than 70 years and more than 4%

in those older than 80 years (5–7). However, a recent study of a primarily white population of Olmsted County, MN, found an occurrence rate almost twice as high as what had been previously reported (9). Using sensitive laboratory techniques (agarose gel electrophoresis screening followed by immunofixation if abnormalities detected on screening) on the serum of 21,463 (77%) of the 28,038 enumerated residents older than 50 years of age, this population-based study found the prevalence of MGUS to be 3.2%, 5.3%, and 7.5% in individuals older than 50, 70, and 85 years, respectively. As noted in other studies (5,6,10), the age-adjusted rates were higher in men than in women (4% vs. 2.7%, respectively, $P < 0.001$), with the prevalence rate among men comparable to women a decade older. The concentration of monoclonal immunoglobulin was < 1.0 g/dL in 64% and > 2.0 g/dL in 4.5% of patients with MGUS. Uninvolved immunoglobulins were reduced in 28%, whereas 22% had a monoclonal urinary light chain. The type of immunoglobulin was IgG in 69% of the 694 MGUS patients, whereas IgM, IgA, and biclonal immunoglobulin

TABLE 1

Diagnostic criteria for MGUS, SMM, and MM

Disease Stage	Diagnostic Criteria
MGUS	Serum M-protein <3 g/dL BMPC <10% Absence of CRAB features
SMM	Serum M protein (IgG or IgA) ≥3 g/dL and/or BMPC ≥10% Absence of CRAB features
MM	Presence of a serum and/or urine M-protein BMPC ≥10% Presence of CRAB features directly attributable to the monoclonal plasma-cell disorder

BMPC, bone marrow plasma cell; CRAB, hypercalcemia, renal failure, anemia, and lytic bone lesions; MGUS, monoclonal gammopathy of undetermined significance; MM, multiple myeloma; SMM, smoldering multiple myeloma.

were present in 17%, 11%, and 3%, respectively. The serum light-chain type was κ in 62% and λ in the remaining 38% patients.

There are major differences in the prevalence of MGUS based on race and ethnicity. Blacks have a two- to threefold higher age-adjusted prevalence of MGUS compared with whites (11–14). In a study of more than 2,000 MGUS patients identified from a large group of men admitted to the Veterans Affairs' hospitals in the United States, the age-adjusted prevalence of MGUS was threefold higher in African Americans (AA) compared with whites (11). However, the increased prevalence of MGUS among the AA did not translate itself to a higher risk of MM during the first 10 years of follow-up, which was comparable among the two groups (17% in AA and 15% in whites). Similarly, Landgren et al. (13) observed an elevated risk of MGUS of twofold among the African men from Ghana aged 50 to 70 years compared with the white men of a similar age group from Olmsted County, MN. On the other hand, when Japanese survivors of the atomic bomb explosion were screened for an M-protein, the age-adjusted prevalence of MGUS was much lower (2.4% in persons older than 50 years) (10) compared with whites in the United States (9).

Etiology: Evidence Supporting the Role of Environmental and Genetic Factors

The etiologies of MGUS and MM are largely unclear. However, some recent reports offer important clues that point toward the interplay of environmental factors and host genetic architecture in the development of MGUS. The Ghanaian study showed a similar prevalence of MGUS in Ghanaian men and the AA population, thereby supporting the hypothesis of race-related genetic predisposition in the genesis of MGUS; however, certain key findings suggested the role of environmental influences as well. In contrast to the steadily increasing prevalence of MGUS in the AA and whites from the United States (1.83%

in those 50–54 years and 5.12% in those 70–74 years), no age-associated differences in the prevalence of MGUS were observed in the Ghanaian men (5.33% for those 50–54 years and 5.38% for those 70–74 years; $P = 0.94$) (13). The exact reason for the lack of age-dependent variation and the higher prevalence of MGUS at a younger age in Ghanaian men is unknown, but if genetic background is considered to be similar between the AA and Ghanaian populations, then these differences may be explained by the effect of the environmental factors. A familial occurrence and an increased risk in the first-degree relatives of patients with MGUS and MM have also been reported, providing further evidence of shared genetic and environmental factors (15–19).

Various immune-mediated conditions may also act as triggers for the evolution of MGUS. In a retrospective cohort of more than 4 million white and black male US veterans, specific prior autoimmune, infectious, and inflammatory conditions were associated with an elevated risk of MGUS and MM (20). In a recent series, the age-adjusted prevalence of MGUS was almost twofold higher among the 678 male pesticide applicators compared with the 9,469 men from Minnesota. The risk was significantly elevated with certain pesticide use such as dieldrin (insecticide), carbon tetrachloride/carbon disulfide (fumigant), and chlorthalonil (fungicide) (21).

■ IDENTIFICATION OF THE ABNORMAL M-PROTEIN

All sera with a suspected M component should be subject to an agarose gel electrophoresis, a rapid and sensitive screening method that allows quantification of the size of M-protein. At least 5×10^9 plasma cells should be present to identify an M spike on serum protein electrophoresis (22). The M-protein appears as a dense, localized band on the agarose gel electrophoresis, and as a tall, narrow spike in the γ, β, or β-γ region when converted to a densitometer tracing. This confirms the presence of a monoclonal gammopathy such as MGUS, MM, WM, AL, or another plasma cell proliferative disorder. On the other hand, a polyclonal proliferation of immunoglobulins (polyclonal gammopathy) usually manifests as a broad peak in the γ region, often seen in patients with liver disease, connective tissue disorders, and chronic infections (23). Upon the identification of a spike or a localized band on electrophoresis, an immunofixation with agarose gel should be performed to confirm the presence of M-protein, and to determine the heavy chain class (γ [IgG], α [IgA], μ [IgM], ε [IgE], or Δ [IgD]) and the light chain type (κ or λ). Immunoglobulin quantification should be performed using rate nephelometry, which yields results that are higher than those expected on the basis of the serum protein electrophoresis tracing, especially in the case of IgM M-protein.

In a recent report by Katzmann et al. (24), a combination of 3 serum tests—protein electrophoresis, immunofixation, and free light chain (FLC) assay (see below)—missed only 2 (0.5%) of the 428 monoclonal gammopathies with urinary M-protein (24). A 24-hour urine specimen to screen for the presence of an M-protein is not required, unless an M-protein is detected in the serum on one of these assays.

The introduction of the serum FLC assay in the early 2000s has enabled the quantitative estimation of κ and λ light chain that are not bound to the immunoglobulin heavy chain. The normal FLC ratio is 0.26 to 1.65 g/dL (25). An abnormal ratio identifies clonality, with values < 0.26 and > 1.65 indicating an excess production of monoclonal λ and monoclonal κ-light chains, respectively. The FLC ratio helps in monitoring disease activity in MM (secretory and nonsecretory) and monoclonal light chain disorders such as light chain MM, AL, and light chain deposition disease. Furthermore, an abnormal FLC ratio at baseline is an independent risk factor for progression in MGUS (26,27), smoldering multiple myeloma (SMM) (28), and solitary plasmacytoma of the bone.(29)

■ PATHOGENESIS

MGUS is a plasma cell tumor with a limited intramedullary tumor mass (<10%) characterized by an absence of end-organ damage. Both MGUS and MM develop through a multistep process, including genomic instability, resulting in a discreet proliferation and expansion of plasma cells. Although the events leading the transformation of MGUS to MM are not well understood, it is evident that alterations occur in both the abnormal plasma cell clone and the stromal component (nontumorous cells providing growth and survival factors) of the BM microenvironment. Cytogenetic changes, BM angiogenesis, and cytokines involved in myeloma bone disease may all play a role in the pathogenesis of MGUS and its progression to MM.

Cytogenetic Changes

A number of cytogenetic and molecular changes observed in MM such as immunoglobulin translocations, aneuploidy, chromosome 13 abnormalities, are also seen in MGUS. The event in almost all MGUS patients is thought to be the occurrence of either a primary translocation (approximately 45% of MGUS cases) or hyperdiploidy (approximately 40–50% of MGUS cases). Primary translocations refer to early pathogenetic events involving the immunoglobulin heavy chain (IgH) gene on chromosome 14q32, whereas secondary translocations refer to those associated with disease progression. Primary translocations usually occur due to errors in IgH switch recombination. They are observed in approximately 60% MM patients (30,31) and approximately 45% of MGUS patients (32,33). The three most common IgH translocations are t (11;14) (q13;q32) identified in 25%; t (4;14) (p16;q32) in 9%; and t (14;16) (q32;q23) in 5% of MGUS patients (33). These translocations dysregulate a variety of oncogenes present on the partner chromosome such as cyclin D1 (11q13) or D3 (6p21), fibroblast growth factor (FGF) receptor 3 combined with the nuclear protein MMSET

(4p16), and the transcription factor C-MAF (6p21). Approximately 40% to 50% of MGUS patients who lack evidence of IgH translocations (non-IgH translocated MGUS or hyperdiploid MGUS) have hyperdiploidy (usually of one or more of the odd-numbered chromosomes, except chromosome 13) as the hallmark of their disease (34,35). The deletion of chromosome 13, considered a poor prognostic feature in MM, has been reported in 50% MGUS patients (33,36), and occurs usually in hyperdiploid MGUS states (34). Studies indicate the possibility of a tumor suppressor gene on chromosome 13, the loss of which may be related to progression of MGUS. However, its role in initiation or progression of MGUS is ambiguous because the exact timing of 13q deletion is unknown (37). The deletion of chromosome 17p, associated with a shorter survival in MM, occurs rarely in MGUS (22,33,38).

Harada et al. (39) observed the coexistence of both CD56+, CD19– and CD56–, and CD19+ plasma cells in MGUS patients. Using flow cytometry, Ocqueteau et al. (40) studied the immunophenotypic profile of BMPCs from a group of 76 MGUS patients by comparing with the BMPCs of 65 MM patients and 10 control subjects. Phenotypically, MGUS was characterized by CD38+ plasma cells of the normal polyclonal (CD56–, CD19+) and the abnormal monoclonal (CD56+, CD19–) varieties. Only 1.5% MM patients had more than 3% normal plasma cells, whereas 98% MGUS patients had more than 3% normal plasma cells (40). In addition, the phenotypic profile of the clonal plasma cells in MGUS was similar to that observed in MM and that of the polyclonal plasma cells from MGUS was identical to those found in healthy individuals. In another study, the proportion of plasma cells expressing CD45 was higher among those with MGUS or SMM compared with patients with newly diagnosed or relapsed MM (43 vs. 22%, respectively, P = 0.005) (41). Furthermore, this study demonstrated an inverse relationship between the degree of BM angiogenesis and the percentage of CD45+ plasma cells. Bataille et al.

(42) identified CD117 (c-kit) expression in 50% of 12 MGUS patients, 33% of 83 newly diagnosed MM patients, although normal plasma cells did not express this receptor. The expression of CD117 in MM was associated with a more indolent disease associated with a better prognosis, thereby raising the question if this particular subset of MM arose from CD117+ MGUS.

The precise mechanism of progression from MGUS to MM is unknown. However, the evolution of MGUS to MM is strongly suggestive of a random 2-hit model resulting in a constant risk of malignant transformation, irrespective of the time period of the preceding MGUS phase. Changes in BM microenvironment including induction of angiogenesis and dysregulation of various cytokines are implicated in the transition of MGUS to MM. Interleukin (IL)-6 is a major growth factor in the pathogenesis of MM, which is produced by paracrine and autocrine pathways and acts by inducing proliferation, inhibiting apoptosis, and overriding the apoptotic signals mediated by cytotoxic drugs (43–45). A significantly higher level of IL-6 receptor α chain (CD126) is expressed in MGUS and MM (46). In a recent study, the frequency of amplification of chromosome band 1q21 was 0% in MGUS, 45% in SMM, 43% in newly diagnosed MM, 72% in relapsed MM, and 91% in human myeloma cell lines, suggesting its role in disease progression (47). Other abnormalities associated with transition to symptomatic disease include RAS (N and K RAS) mutations, p16 methylation, p53 mutations, myc abnormalities, secondary translocations, increased angiogenesis, and elevated bone turnover (48–51).

Angiogenesis

Angiogenesis favors the progression of MGUS or nonactive MM to active MM. In fact, active MM is considered the "vascular phase" of plasma cell tumor, whereas nonactive MM and MGUS are the "avascular phases." Angiogenesis is induced by plasma cells via angiogenic factors (vascular endothelial growth factor [VEGF], FGF, hepatocyte growth factor/scatter factor), associated with the concurrent loss of antiangiogenic factors (angiostatin, endostatin). The cause of the induction of the vascular phase and its effect on the transition from MGUS to MM is not completely understood. It is well known that premalignant cancer cells (such as in situ carcinomas) acquire the ability to induce microvessel formation at some point by altering the balance between pro- and antiangiogenic cytokines, a concept referred to as "angiogenic switch." This may be responsible, at least in part, for the progression of MGUS to MM. An increased expression of VEGF and/ or FGF-2, a shift from CD45+ to CD45– plasma cells that are VEGF producers, and an increasing tumor burden have been implicated as the possible causes responsible for the angiogenic switch observed in the transition of MGUS to MM (52,53). A study that compared the marrow microvessel density (MVD) with cytokine/receptor expression (percentage plasma cells expressing the respective marker) across the spectrum of plasma-cell disorders found a correlation between MVD and expression of VEGF (P = 0.02), basic FGF (bFGF) (P = 0.008), and VEGF receptor 1 (VEGFR1) (P = 0.02). However, the percentages of plasma cells expressing VEGF, bFGF, and their receptors were not significantly different among the three groups (53). In another study of 400 patients with plasma cell disorders, the median MVD per 400 high-power field was 1.3 in 42 normal controls, and progressively increased from MGUS (3.0) to SMM (4.0) to newly diagnosed MM (11.0), with the highest value associated with relapsing MM (20.0) (54). The MVD also correlated with the BM plasma cell labeling index (PCLI) and BMPC percentage. The median overall survival (OS) was 28 months in SMM and newly diagnosed MM with high-grade angiogenesis compared with 53 months with low- and intermediate-grade angiogenesis (P = 0.02). The results of this study confirmed the findings of a previous smaller study where patients with > 50 microvessels and < 50 microvessels per 400

BM field had a median survival of 2.6 years and 5.1 years, respectively (55). Other studies utilizing in vitro assays have also suggested a role of angiogenesis in the progression of MGUS to MM. Kumar et al. (53) observed a loss of angiogenesis inhibitory activity in 63% MGUS samples compared with 43% SMM and only 4% in newly diagnosed MM.

Pathophysiology of Bone Disease

Bone disease characterized by hypercalcemia and lytic bone destruction leading to pathological fractures are major clinical features of MM. However, alterations in skeletal remodeling are observed even in the MGUS phase. An excessive osteoclastic-mediated bone resorption followed by impaired osteoblastic bone formation causes skeletal involvement in MGUS. An increase in the ratio of receptor activator of nuclear factor κ-B ligand (RANKL) and its decoy receptor osteoprotegerin causes osteoclast activation and excessive bone resorption. Additionally, various cytokines such as macrophage inflammatory protein-1α, tumor necrosis factor α, IL-3, IL-1β, and IL-6 are also implicated as potential osteoclast activating factors (48). On the other hand, increased activity of IL-3, IL-7, and Dickkopf-1 (DKK1) inhibit osteoblast differentiation and affect bone formation.

In a retrospective cohort study of 488 MGUS patients with a median follow-up of 7.2 years, Melton et al. found a 2.7-fold increased risk of axial skeleton fractures compared with the peripheral fractures, even before progression to MM. Overall, 200 patients experienced a total of 385 fractures yielding a significantly elevated risk of vertebral fractures (standardized incidence ratio [SIR], 6.3; 95% confidence interval (CI), 5.2–7.5) and partially elevated risk of hip fracture (SIR, 1.6; 95% CI, 1.2–2.2), but not distal forearm fractures (SIR, 0.8; 95% CI, 0.4–1.5). In univariate analysis, patients with non-IgG (IgA and IgM) MGUS and κ light chain had an increased risk of fractures compared with IgG MGUS and λ light chain, respectively. However, a study from Denmark reported on 1,535 MGUS patients and found a relative risk of fracture of 1.4 times that seen in control population. Interestingly, both studies identified patients with a κ light chain type of M-protein at an increased risk for fracture. A similar elevated risk of axial fractures in MGUS patients has been identified in other studies (56–58), especially in patients with a reduced lumbar BM density (57).

In a study of 134 patients with back pain and magnetic resonance imaging evidence of acute vertebral fractures, MGUS and MM was found in 15% and 5% patients, respectively; however, both groups had a comparable number of vertebral fractures (56). An asymptomatic vertebral deformity is clinically significant due to its increased risk of subsequent fractures, and direct impact on mortality, particularly in patients who sustain a vertebral fracture (59). Few recent studies indicate the effectiveness of zoledronic acid and alendronate in improving the bone mineral density in MGUS patients who are at high risk for bone loss and fracture (60,61). Intravenous administration of zoledronic acid 4 mg given every 6 months for three doses improved bone mineral density in a study of 54 MGUS patients with osteopenia or osteoporosis. Similar favorable results with alendronate therapy have been reported with improvement in lumbar BM density compared to the

baseline values (61). More data are needed, and at present, we do not recommend bisphosphonates for patients with MGUS, except as needed for prevention and treatment of osteoporosis. In these circumstances, patients should receive bisphosphonates at the same dose and schedule as patients without MGUS would for osteoporosis.

■ RISK FACTORS FOR PROGRESSION

The major risk factors associated with an increased risk of progression of MGUS are listed in Table 2.

Size of M-Protein

In the Mayo Clinic series of 1,384 MGUS patients from Southeastern Minnesota with 15.4 years of median follow-up, the size of the serum M-protein at MGUS diagnosis was the most important risk factor for progression to a plasma cell cancer (62). At 10 years after the diagnosis of MGUS, the risk of progression for an initial M-protein value of 0.5 g/dL, 1.5 g/dL, and 2.5 g/dL was 6%, 11%, and 24%, respectively; corresponding risk at 20 years was 14%, 25%, and 49%. The risk of progression with an M-protein value of 1.5 g/dL and 2.5 g/dL was 1.9 times and 4.6 times, respectively, greater than the risk of progression with an initial

TABLE 2
Factors associated with increased risk of progression of MGUS

---

1. Elevated serum M-protein
2. Non-IgG (IgA or IgM) MGUS
3. Percentage of BMPCs
4. Abnormal free light chain ratio
5. Progressively increasing M-protein (Evolving MGUS)
6. Suppression of uninvolved immunoglobulins
7. Presence of circulating plasma cells or clonal B cells

BMPCs, bone marrow plasma cells; MGUS, monoclonal gammopathy of undetermined significance.

M-protein value of 0.5 g/dL or less. In the Italian series, MGUS patients with more than 1.9 g/dL of M-protein had twice the rate of progression compared with those with less than 0.95 g/dL (63). In a recent study by the Spanish group, not only the initial M-protein size but also the pattern of its progressive increment in the first few years of diagnosis ("evolving" MGUS) was the most important risk factor for progression to a malignant monoclonal gammopathy (64).

Bone Marrow Plasma Cells

Cesana et al. (63) reported on 1,104 MGUS patients and observed a marrow plasmacytosis of greater than 5% to be an independent risk factor for progression. The study noted a twofold risk of progression with 6% to 9% BMPC (event rate 1.35/100 person-years) than with 0% to 5% BMPC (event rate 0.64/100 person-years), with the highest risk associated with ≥ 10% BMPC (event rate 5.96/100 years) (63) Similarly, Baldini et al. (65) observed a malignant transformation in 6.8% patients with BMPC < 10%, whereas 37% patients with 10% to 30% BMPC (now termed smoldering multiple myeloma) showed evidence of progression. The study also identified a subset of IgG MGUS with a very low probability of progression to MM: serum M-protein ≤ 1.5 g/dL, BMPC <5%, no reduction in polyclonal immunoglobulin and no detectable light chain proteinuria (65). In fact, serum M-protein size and BMPC constitute the tumor burden in MGUS, and studies including patients with a high tumor burden (66–68) report a higher rate of malignant evolution than the studies that included patients with a lower tumor burden (62).

Type of M Protein

Several studies have reported a lower risk of progression of MGUS with an IgG M-protein. In contrast, non-IgG (IgA [62–64,69,70] or IgM [62,63]) MGUS patients have a greater likelihood of malignant evolution. In the Mayo Clinic study,

MGUS patients with IgM or IgA M-protein had a greater risk of progression than patients with an IgG M-protein (P = 0.001) (62). IgA MGUS was the only variable associated with a higher probability of progression in a study of 128 MGUS patients (69). Gregersen et al. (70) observed a relative risk of progression of 1.8 and 1.1 for IgA and IgM-MGUS, respectively, compared with the IgG MGUS type.

Serum FLC Ratio

In a study of 1,148 MGUS patients, an abnormal FLC ratio was observed in 379 (33%) patients. The risk of progression was significantly higher in patients with an abnormal serum FLC ratio (hazard ratio 3.5, P < 0.001), independent of the size and type of M-protein (27). The findings of this study confirmed the results of a previous smaller case control study. Forty-seven MGUS patients with progression to MM or related disorder served as cases, and 50 MGUS patients without evidence of disease progression served as controls. The study observed a 2.5-fold increased risk of progression in patients with an abnormal FLC ratio.

Other Factors

The suppression of the uninvolved or polyclonal immunoglobulins is characteristically seen in greater than 90% MM patients, but occurs in fewer (approximately 25–40%) patients with MGUS (62,70). Baldini et al. reported a 3.6- and 13.1-fold elevated risk of progression with reduction of one and two uninvolved immunoglobulin, respectively. However, other studies have been unable to confirm the increased risk with reduction in polyclonal immunoglobulin (65,66,71). Similarly, the presence of urine paraprotein has been inconsistently reported as a risk factor across the aforementioned studies (62,63,65) and cannot be used as a reliable predictor of progression. Using a slide-based immunofluorescence method, Kumar et al. (72) detected the presence of a median of 1%

circulating plasma cells in the peripheral blood in 19% MGUS patients who were twice as likely to progress to MM than those without circulating plasma cells. The median progression-free survival and the median OS were also shorter for MGUS patients with circulating plasma cells. Similarly, Isaksson et al. (73) demonstrated a prognostic significance for the presence of peripheral blood clonal B cells in MGUS patients. In a study of 57 MGUS patients, the presence of blood clonal B cells as determined by immunofluorescence microscopy was associated with a 3.5-fold higher risk of transformation.

Risk-Stratification Model

A model to risk-stratify MGUS based upon three important risk factors identified four cohorts of patients with significantly different rates of progression (Figure 1, Table 3). At 20 years of MGUS diagnosis, patients with non-IgG MGUS, abnormal serum FLC ratio, and serum M-protein value ≥ 1.5 g/dL have a 58% risk of progression (high risk), compared with 37% with any two risk factors (high-intermediate risk), 21% with one risk factor (low-intermediate), and 5% when no risk factor is present (low risk) (27).

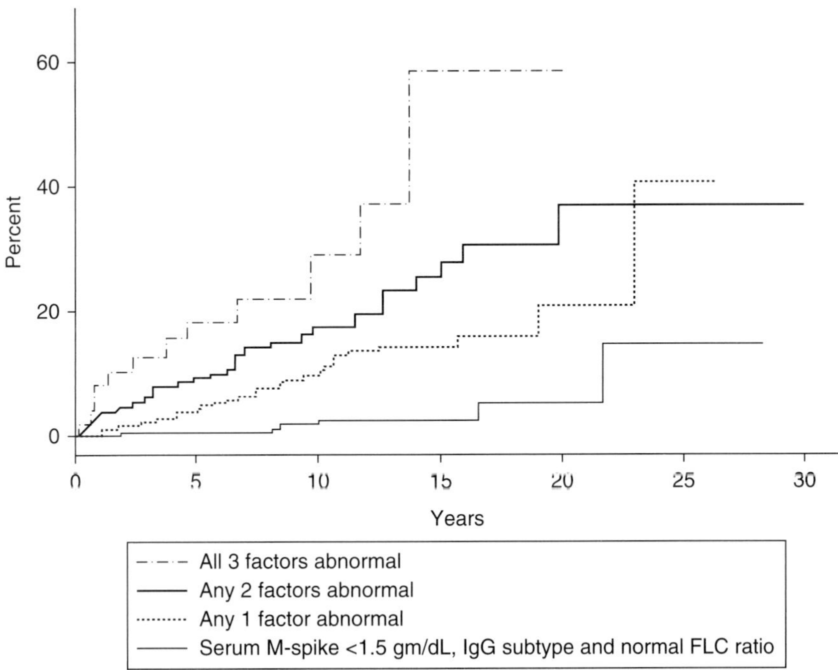

FIGURE 1

Risk of progression of monoclonal gammopathy of undetermined significance (MGUS) to myeloma or related disorder using a risk-stratification model that incorporates the free light chain (FLC) ratio and the size and type of the serum monoclonal protein. The top curve illustrates risk of progression with time in patients with all 3 risk factors, namely an abnormal serum κ-λ FLC ratio (<0.26 or >1.65), a high serum monoclonal protein level (≥1.5 g/dL), and non-IgG MGUS; the second gives the risk of progression in patients with any 2 of these risk factors; the third curve illustrates the risk of progression with one of these risk factors; the bottom curve is the risk of progression for patients with none of the risk factors. From Rajkumar et al. © The American Society of Hematology.

TABLE 3
Risk-stratification models to predict progression of MGUS to myeloma or related disorders

Risk Group	No. Patients	Relative Risk, 95% CI	Absolute Risk of Progression at 20 Years, %	Absolute Risk of Progression at 20 Years Accounting for Death as a Competing Risk, %
Addition of FLC ratio to known prognostic categories				
Low risk (serum M-protein <15 g/L and IgG subtype)				
Normal FLC ratio	449	1	5	2
Abnormal FLC ratio	142	7.4	27	12
Intermediate risk (either serum M-protein 15 g/L or non-IgG subtype)				
Normal FLC ratio	278	1	22	9
Abnormal FLC ratio	184	2.2	37	17
High risk (serum M-protein 15 g/L and non-IgG subtype)				
Normal FLC ratio	42	1	37	23
Abnormal FLC ratio	53	1.5	58	27
Risk-stratification model incorporating all 3 predictive factors				
Low risk (serum M-protein <15 g/dL, IgG subtype, normal FLC ratio [0.26-1.65])	449	1	5	2
Low-intermediate risk (any 1 factor abnormal)	420	5.4	21	10
High-intermediate risk (any 2 factors abnormal)	226	10.1	37	18
High risk (all 3 factors abnormal)	53	20.8	58	27

FLC, free light chain; MGUS, monoclonal gammopathy of undetermined significance.

■ NATURAL HISTORY

The natural history of MGUS can be best studied by following the outcomes of a group of 241 MGUS patients examined at the Mayo Clinic, Minnesota, between January 1956 and December 1970. The findings of this study were carefully updated and periodically reported; the concluding data being reported in 2004 (71). After 3,579 person-years of follow-up (median, 13.7 years; range, 0–39 years), only 14 (6%) patients with stable M-protein values were alive. Twenty five (10%) patients had an increase of M-protein of 3.0 g/dL or higher without requiring chemotherapy. However, more than half of the patients (N = 138 [57%]) died from unrelated plasma cell diseases (cardiac or cerebrovascular causes) without developing MM, AL, WM, or another lymphoid or plasma cell malignancy. MM was most commonly diagnosed in 44 of the 64 patients that developed a malignant plasma cell proliferative disorder. Another eight patients developed AL and seven patients developed WM, at a median of 9 and 10.3 years after the detection of serum M-protein, respectively. Among patients with MM, 33 patients had serum M-protein > 3 g/dL, and 30 (68%) patients developed lytic lesions or fractures. The interval from MGUS diagnosis to MM diagnosis ranged from 1 to 32 years (median, 10.6 years), including 10 patients diagnosed with MM more than 20 years after the initial MGUS diagnosis. The median survival after MM diagnosis was 33 months and all but one patient from this group had died at the time of analysis. The actuarial rate of progression to MM or a related disorder was 17% at 10 years and 34% at 20 years; a rate of approximately 1.5% per year.

To confirm the findings of this study, which may have been subjected to a referral bias, a larger series included 1,384 MGUS patients from southeastern Minnesota. The median age at MGUS diagnosis was 72 years, and only 2% patients were younger than 40 years. After a robust follow-up of 11,009 person-years (median, 15.4 years; range, 0 to 35 years), MM, lymphoma with an IgM M-protein, AL, WM, chronic lymphocytic leukemia (CLL), or plasmacytoma developed in 115 (8.3%) patients (62). Among patients who progressed to a plasma cell cancer, two thirds developed MM, including few patients (7%) who progressed after 20 years of follow-up. The cumulative probability of progression to any of these disorders was 10% at 10 years, 21% at 20 years, and 26% at 25 years. The number of patients with progression to a plasma cell neoplasm or related disorder (115 patients) was more than seven times that expected on the basis of incidence rates for these conditions in the general population. The risk of disease was increased by a factor of 25 for MM, 46 for WM, 8.4 for AL, and 2.4 for lymphoma. The overall risk of progression was about 1% per year, and patients were at risk for progression even after 25 years or more of stable MGUS (62). The rates of death due to other diseases such as cardiovascular and cerebrovascular diseases, and non–plasma cell cancers was 53% at 10 years and 76% at 25 years; corresponding rates for death due to plasma cell cancers was 6% at 10 years, and 11% at 25 years.

■ DIFFERENTIAL DIAGNOSIS

There are several diseases associated with monoclonal gammopathies. In the spectrum of plasma cell disease from MGUS to MM, is an intermediate asymptomatic stage termed "smoldering multiple myeloma" (SMM); previously referred to as "monoclonal gammopathy of borderline significance" (65). It is defined by an M-protein (IgG or IgA) of ≥ 3 g/dL and/or ≥10% clonal BMPC, without any end-organ damage (Table 1) (4). These patients often have small amounts of urine M-protein, reduction of uninvolved immunoglobulins, and a low PCLI. SMM is a clinical category that includes some patients with biological MGUS and some with early MM. SMM patients as with MGUS do not require treatment but need frequent follow-up, as their risk of progression is significantly higher than MGUS patients (10% per year for the first 5 years, approximately 3% per year for the next 5 years, and 1% per year for the next 10 years) (Figure 2) (74).

Although MGUS is the most common diagnosis in the presence of an M-protein, it is critical to rule out other incurable monoclonal plasma cell disorders. There is no one particular clinical feature that distinguishes MGUS from MM. Because MGUS is relatively common in the elderly, a number of characteristic clinical and laboratory abnormalities of MM such as anemia and renal failure may actually be due to a non–plasma cell disease with coincidental presence of an asymptomatic M-protein. In general, a serum M-protein > 3 g/dL, large amount of urine M-protein, clonal BMPC > 10%, high PCLI, and presence of end-organ damage (hypercalcemia, renal insufficiency, anemia, and bone lesions) indicates the presence of MM rather than MGUS (Table 1). However, MGUS patients can occasionally have large amounts of urine M-protein and reduction of uninvolved immunoglobulins. Normal PCLI values are also present in MGUS and a third of symptomatic MM patients.

Constitutional symptoms and lytic bone lesions in the presence of an M-protein suggests MM. However, metastatic carcinoma with coincidental MGUS should be kept high in the differential diagnosis when marrow plasmacytosis is less than 10%. Similarly, patients with a clonal plasma-cell proliferative disorder with features such as congestive heart failure, nephrotic range

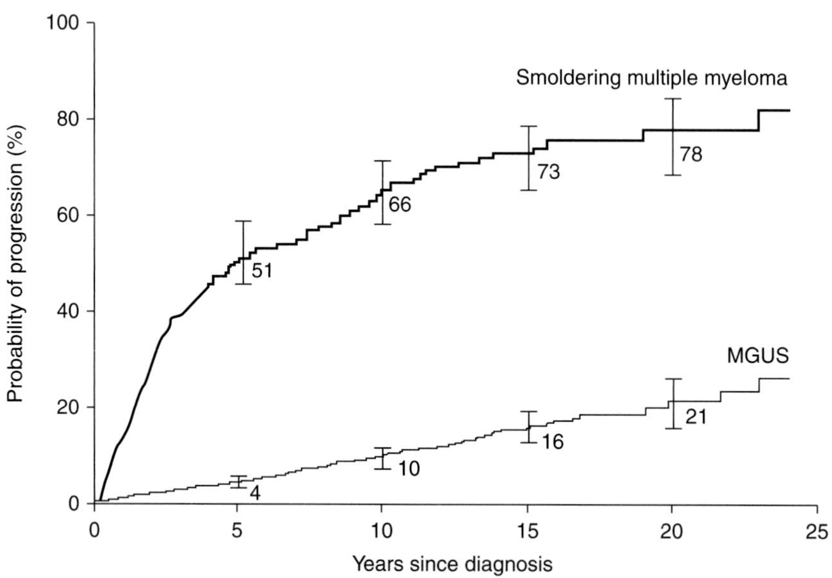

FIGURE 2

Probability of progression to active multiple myeloma or primary amyloidosis in patients with smoldering multiple myeloma or monoclonal gammopathy of undetermined significance (MGUS). I bars denote 95% confidence intervals. From Ref. 74 with permission. © Massachusetts Medical Society, 2007. All rights reserved.

albuminuria, paresthesias, hepatomegaly, macroglossia, or periorbital ecchymosis should undergo a tissue biopsy followed with Congo red staining to evaluate for the presence of AL. Patients with WM may present with weakness, fatigue, weight loss, neurologic symptoms secondary to hyperviscosity or peripheral neuropathy, and fever or night sweats. Physical examination reveals lymphadenopathy, hepatomegaly, and splenomegaly. Because IgM-MGUS can progress to WM, a BM examination and computed tomography abdomen should be obtained in these patients for evaluating the presence of retroperitoneal lymph nodes.

■ DISEASE ASSOCIATIONS

Several clinical conditions are associated with an M-protein. The presence of an M-protein should be actively sought in some diseases, which appear to be strongly linked with monoclonal gammopathies. However, a number of diseases occur more commonly in the elderly making it difficult to identify true causal associations.

M-proteins have been recognized in a variety of lymphoproliferative disorders (75–80) Azar et al. (75) recognized the presence of an abnormal serum protein of the myeloma type in a small group of patients with malignant lymphoma and lymphatic leukemia. In a study of 430 patients with an IgM M-protein, Kyle et al. (76) found MGUS in 242 (56%) patients. Another 71 (17%) patients were diagnosed with WM, 28 (7%) with lymphoma, 21 (5%) with CLL, 6 (1%) with AL, and 62 (14%) with other malignant lymphoproliferative diseases. Importantly, among those with IgM-MGUS; nearly a fifth subsequently developed a lymphoid malignant lesion highlighting the importance of lifelong surveillance among this group of patients. In another study of 1,150 consecutive patients with lymphoma or CLL, Alexanian and coworkers (77) identified an M-protein in 49 patients. Forty-four (7%) of the 640 patients with diffuse non-Hodgkin's lymphoma (NHL) or CLL had an M-protein, whereas 4 of 292 patients with nodular lymphoma and 1 of 218 patients with Hodgkin's lymphoma had a monoclonal gammopathy. Among this group, IgM and IgG M-protein were identified in 29 and 15 patients, respectively, whereas the M-protein was not typed in the remaining 5 patients.

In a study from Mayo Clinic, Noel et al. (78) reported on 100 patients with CLL and an M-protein in the serum or urine. IgG and IgM M-protein were most commonly identified in 51% and 38%, respectively, whereas others had FLCs (10%) or an IgA (1%) M-protein. However, no important differences were seen in CLL patients, whether they had an IgG or IgM M-protein, or a free monoclonal light chain. Similarly, a recent study showed no difference in survival between the 26 untreated patients with CLL and small lymphocytic lymphoma (SLL) associated with an IgM M-protein compared with 52 CLL/SLL patients without an IgM M-protein ($P = 0.60$) (80). Monoclonal gammopathy has also been reported in association with other hematological conditions such as chronic myelocytic leukemia, hairy cell leukemia (81), adult T-cell leukemia (82), and mycosis fungoides, but there is no clear evidence of an association yet.

An acquired deficiency of von Willebrand factor (vWF) (von Willebrand syndrome [vWS]) has been reported in association with monoclonal gammopathies (83–85) Lamboley et al. (83) described seven patients with a monoclonal gammopathy and vWS; an antibody that inhibited vWF was found in all. Although treatment with intravenous immunoglobulins (IVIg) had a better efficacy than vWF concentrate, the bleeding severity was similar in patients with MGUS and MM. Similarly, in a small study that compared the effectiveness of desmopressin (DDAVP), factor VIII/vWF (FVIII/vWF) concentrate, and high-dose (1 g/kg/d for 2 days) IVIg among patients with MGUS and acquired vWS, a more sustained improvement of the laboratory abnormalities was seen in IgG MGUS patients (but not with IgM-MGUS) treated with IVIg than with other therapies (86).

On the other hand, a prothrombotic state characterized by an increase in the level of FVIII and vWF has been implicated in the increased risk of venous thromboembolic disease (VTD) in MGUS (87–89). Sallah et al. (89) reported a thromboembolic event in 19 (6.1%) of 310 MGUS patients during a mean follow-up of 44 months. Srkalovic et al. (88) observed a VTD in 7.5% of MGUS patients at a median of 4 months after diagnosis. Additionally, a lower risk has been reported with IgG MGUS than with non-IgG variety of MGUS (87,88). Other hematological disorders associated with monoclonal gammopathies include pernicious anemia, polycythemia vera, idiopathic myelofibrosis, myelodysplastic syndrome, and pure red cell aplasia. The presence of a circulating lupus-like anticoagulant associated with a monoclonal gammopathy has also been described (90).

Peripheral neuropathy is commonly associated with monoclonal gammopathies (91–95) The incidence of peripheral neuropathy varies widely in different studies, likely a reflection of the patient selection, criteria (clinical vs. electrophysiological) used for diagnosis, and the meticulousness of the search for an M-protein. Approximately 10% patients diagnosed with idiopathic peripheral neuropathy have an M-protein in their serum or urine, a prevalence rate of nearly five times more common than the general population (96). Furthermore, the prevalence of MGUS is higher in patients with idiopathic neuropathy than in patients with an identifiable cause of neuropathy. The paraproteinemic neuropathy is typically a sensorimotor peripheral neuropathy, and involvement of the autonomic or cranial nerves is uncommon. It can be classified into two groups, IgM and non-IgM M-protein associated neuropathies. Patients with IgM paraproteinemic neuropathy may have a more progressive course, with significantly more weakness and sensory signs (97).

The M-protein binds to myelin associated glyco-protein (MAG) in nearly half of patients with an IgM-MGUS–associated neuropathy (98). In the Mayo Clinic series of 65 MGUS patients and sensorimotor peripheral neuropathy, 31 patients had IgM, 24 had IgG, and 10 had IgA M-proteins (91). IgM-MGUS–associated neuropathies were characterized by a higher frequency of sensory loss and ataxia, nerve conduction abnormalities, and dispersion of the compound muscle action potential. However, the size of the M-protein and the presence of anti-MAG antibodies were not associated with the severity of neuropathy. The optimum treatment is usually difficult, and the response rate varies with different therapies. In a double-blind trial of 39 MGUS patients of the IgG, IgA, or IgM types, a favorable response was observed with plasma exchange, especially among those with IgG or IgA MGUS (99). In patients with IgM paraproteinemic neuropathy, a recent double-blind, randomized, placebo-controlled study showed no benefit on the functional outcomes with oral cyclophosphamide and prednisone (100); fludarabine improved the clinical and neurophysiological parameters in one small study; α-interferon (α-IFN) therapy produced significant clinical improvement in a small cohort of patients but lacked effectiveness in a double-blind study of α-IFN versus placebo (101); and rituximab (chimeric monoclonal antibody against CD20) showed moderate benefit in one study (102), but not in others (103,104). High-dose therapy with autologous stem-cell transplantation has been used in select patients with debilitating peripheral neuropathy who are unresponsive to conventional treatment (105).

Motor neuron disease has been reported in association with MGUS. In a study of 56 patients with motor neuron disease, 6 (11%) were found to have MGUS (106). On the other hand, only 4.1% of 121 age-matched patients with other neuroimmunological disorders had an M-protein, most commonly due to MM. The presence of monoclonal gammopathy correlated with the absence of marked upper motor neuron involvement and elevated cerebrospinal fluid protein concentration.

POEMS syndrome (osteosclerotic myeloma) is a rare multisystemic disease characterized by the constellation of *p*olyneuropathy, *o*rganomegaly, *e*ndocrinopathy, *M*-proteins and *s*kin changes. The peak incidence of POEMS syndrome occurs in the 5th and 6th decades of life. The diagnosis requires the presence of a monoclonal plasma cell disorder (usually λ light-chain type), peripheral neuropathy, and at least one of the following seven features: osteosclerotic bone lesions, Castleman's disease, organomegaly, endocrinopathy (excluding diabetes mellitus or hypothyroidism), edema, typical skin changes, and papilledema (107,108). These features should have a temporal relationship to each other without other attributable cause(s). The size of the M-protein is small (median 1.1 g/dL), and the BM usually contains less than 5% plasma cells. Plasma and serum levels of VEGF are elevated and correlate with disease activity; IL-1β, TNF-α,, and IL-6 levels are also often increased. Peripheral neuropathy often dominates the clinical picture, and muscle weakness is more marked than sensory loss. Bence Jones (BJ) proteinuria, renal insufficiency, and hypercalcemia are uncommon. Skeletal fractures are rare, but sclerotic bone lesions are commonly observed on skeletal survey. Radiation therapy has been used effectively for localized lesions; alkylator-based therapy or systemic therapy with high-dose therapy and autologous stem-cell transplantation can be used for widespread bone lesions. Novel therapies such as bevacizumab (monoclonal antibody against VEGF), bortezomib, thalidomide, and lenalidomide have been used with variable efficacy. Typically, the disease runs a chronic course. Median survival was 13.8 years in a series of 99 patients with POEMS syndrome, independent of the number of syndrome features, bone lesions, or plasma cells at diagnosis (109). However, respiratory features such as pulmonary hypertension, restrictive lung disease, and respiratory muscle weakness predict a poorer prognosis. In a recent study of 137 patients with POEMS syndrome, the median survival with and without respiratory muscle weakness was 87 months and 139 months ($P < 0.05$), respectively (110).

Several skin disorders have been recognized in association with an M-protein. Daoud et al. (111) have divided skin disorders associated with monoclonal gammopathies into four distinct groups. Group 1 diseases (amyloidosis, cryoglobulinemia, plasmacytoma, POEMS syndrome, and WM cutis) are characterized by infiltration and proliferation of skin by malignant plasma cells or a product of these plasma cells; group 2 diseases have a strong association with monoclonal gammopathies (scleredema, scleromyxedema, plane xanthoma, necrobiotic xanthogranuloma, Schnitzler syndrome, Sweet's syndrome, pyoderma gangrenosum, and erythema elevatum diutinum among others); group 3 represents various dermatoses linked to a paraproteinemia without a clear association; and group 4 comprises nonspecific cutaneous conditions, symptoms, and complications related to M-protein.

Scleromyxedema (papular mucinosis, lichen myxedematosus) is a rare skin disorder characterized by macules, papules, and plaques infiltrating the skin, associated with an IgG λ paraprotein (112). Pyoderma gangrenosum is an ulcerative skin disorder that often occurs in association with other systemic diseases. In a study of 67 patients with pyoderma gangrenosum, 8 (12%) had a monoclonal gammopathy and all but one patient had an IgA M-protein (113); a finding corroborated by another study as well (114). Schnitzler syndrome is characterized by chronic urticarial rash and an IgM M-protein accompanied by intermittent fever, arthralgia or arthritis, bone pain, and lymphadenopathy. A recent review of literature observed a 15% 10-year risk of developing a lymphoproliferative disorder, most notably WM (115). Other cutaneous conditions associated with an M-protein are discoid lupus erythematosus (116), necrobiotic

xanthogranuloma (117), and erythema elevatum diutinum (118,119).

The immunosuppression at the time of transplantation causes a temporary immunodeficiency state that is, likely, responsible for the presence of a transient M-protein in patients undergoing organ transplantation (kidney [120,121], liver [122], or heart [123]), autologous stem-cell transplantation (124), or an allogeneic BM transplantation. In a small report of five MGUS patients who underwent an organ transplant, two patients developed SMM and another patient had an increase in the serum M-protein level (125). However, the M-protein in these cases usually disappears with the recovery of the immune system. In a study of 341 HIV patients, 11 (3.2%) were found to have a serum M-protein. After a mean follow-up of 50 months, the M-protein disappeared in seven patients (126).

Chronic antigenic stimulation has been implicated to play a role in the pathogenesis of MGUS. In a small series of MGUS patients, more than two thirds were found to have *Helicobacter pylori* infection. A normalization of the serum protein electrophoresis and resolution of the gammopathy with appropriate medical therapy was reported in 30% (127). However, in a large cohort of MGUS patients from the Mayo Clinic, serological testing showed identical diagnosis rates of *H pylori* in the MGUS patients and the control subjects, without any evidence of resolution of MGUS with successful treatment of *H pylori* (128).

Although, autoimmune disorders such as rheumatoid arthritis, systemic lupus erythematosus, scleroderma, polymyalgia rheumatica, and ankylosing spondylitis have been described in association with an M-protein, the supporting evidence is weak and the relationship appears to be coincidental rather than causal (129–132). Other disorders such as hepatitis C virus positive cryoglobulinemia, acquired C1 inhibitor deficiency, capillary leak syndrome, and acquired angioedema type 2 have also been described in relation with an M-protein.

■ DISEASE VARIANTS

Biclonal and Triclonal Gammopathies

Two (biclonal gammopathy) (133–135) or three (triclonal gammopathy) (133,136,137) M-proteins may be present in a single patient due to the proliferation of separate clones of plasma cells that produce M-proteins of different immunoglobulin classes, or by the production of different M-proteins by a single clone of plasma cells. Kyle et al. (133) found a biclonal gammopathy of undetermined significance in 37 of the 57 patients with a biclonal gammopathy. The remaining patients with a biclonal gammopathy had MM, WM, or another lymphoproliferative disorder. The concurrent presence of the two most common immunoglobulin classes (IgG and IgA) were observed in more than half of the patients with biclonal gammopathy, whereas another 26% had IgG and IgM M-proteins. Two localized bands were seen only in 18 patients with electrophoresis on cellulose acetate, whereas others required an immunoelectrophoresis or immunofixation for the recognition of the second M-protein. Patients with biclonal gammopathy were not clinically different from those with monoclonal gammopathy. In another series of 1,135 patients with paraproteinemias, 28 (2.5%) were found to have two M-components, of whom 6 patients had biclonal gammopathy of undetermined significance (134). A similar rate of double gammopathy has been reported in another study of 1,034 patients with gammopathy (135). Triclonal gammopathy has been described in various case reports and is rarer than biclonal gammopathy. Grosbois et al. (136) identified three distinct monoclonal gammopathies (IgM κ, IgG κ, and IgA κ) in an elderly patient with WM who later developed MM. In another report, three M-components (IgG κ, IgG λ, ang IgM λ) synthesized by three separate plasma-cell populations were identified in association with NHL (137). In a review of 26 cases of triclonal gammopathies, 16 were associated with malignant immunoproliferative diseases (NHL, WM, and MM), 5 had nonhematological diseases, and 3 cases were of undetermined significance (136).

Idiopathic Bence Jones Proteinuria

Although light-chain proteinuria occurs frequently in MM, AL, or WM, patients may occasionally present with isolated BJ proteinuria without evidence of end-organ damage (138–140). Several patients with BJ proteinuria have been recognized whose disease has remained stable over long periods of follow-up. Kyle reported seven patients with BJ proteinuria of more than 1 g/day in the absence of serum M-protein or evidence of another plasma-cell proliferative process. MM and SMM developed in three and one patient(s), respectively, whereas two patients were followed up for 12 years without any evidence of progression (139). These patients may have a stable course over a long period but carry a definite increased risk of progression requiring close follow-up. Idiopathic BJ proteinuria likely represents a more advanced stage of patients with an MGUS that involves only FLCs without expression of IgH (light-chain MGUS).

■ MANAGEMENT

MGUS patients require periodic lifelong follow-up without therapy, until evidence of progression to a plasma cell malignancy. Once the diagnosis of MGUS is established, a BM aspirate and biopsy should be performed with any one of the following high-risk features: M-protein ≥ 1.5 g/dL, IgA or IgM M-protein, abnormal FLC ratio, or a clinical suspicion of a plasma-cell malignancy (108). Additionally, a metastatic skeletal survey should also be obtained in these patients.

MGUS is a classic premalignant condition characterized by nonprogression to MM or another related disorder in the majority (approximately 75–90%) (62,71) of patients. The true lifetime probability of progression of MGUS is lower than 1% per year when competing causes of death are taken into account, approximately 11% at 25 years (27). Therefore, it is critical to identify individuals who are more likely to undergo malignant transformation. Although it is impossible to predict with certainty which patients will progress, specific risk factors have been identified that delineate the high-risk MGUS patients from the others. Patients with an M-protein > 1.5 g/dL, non-IgG M-protein, and abnormal FLC ratio have a risk of progression at 20 years of 58% (high-risk MGUS) compared with 5% when none of the risk factors are present (low-risk MGUS). Patients with high-risk MGUS should have cytogenetic studies (both conventional and fluorescence in situ hybridization), PCLI studies, and determination of circulating peripheral blood plasma cells, in addition to the tests mentioned above.

The interval of follow-up is determined by the risk factors of progression to ensure the timely institution of effective therapy before complications such as hypercalcemia, renal failure, or a pathological fracture develop. Patients with low-risk MGUS can be followed up at 6 months and every 2 years thereafter or at the time of clinical symptoms; all other subsets of MGUS patients (low-intermediate, high-intermediate, and high-risk) should be reassessed in 6 months and then yearly thereafter. A pattern of rising M-protein ("evolving" MGUS) should be monitored with more frequent follow-up testing (64). On return visits for all MGUS patients, a thorough history, physical examination, complete blood count, serum calcium and creatinine, and serum protein electrophoresis should be obtained. Further testing should be dictated by the clinical assessment and if suspicion is high, a complete workup including BM examination, skeletal survey, and urine protein electrophoresis should be obtained.

■ REFERENCES

1. Kyle RA. Monoclonal gammopathy of undetermined significance. Natural history in 241 cases. *Am J Med* 1978;64(5):814–826.

2. Landgren O, Kyle RA, Pfeiffer RM, et al. Monoclonal gammopathy of undetermined significance (MGUS) consistently precedes multiple myeloma: a prospective study. *Blood* 2009;113:5412–5417.

3. Weiss BM, Abadie J, Verma P, Howard RS, Kuehl WM. A monoclonal gammopathy precedes multiple myeloma in most patients. *Blood* 2009;113(22): 5418–5422.

4. The International Myeloma Working Group. Criteria for the classification of monoclonal gammopathies, multiple myeloma and related disorders: a report of the International Myeloma Working Group. *Br J Haematol* 2003;121(5):749–757.

5. Axelsson U, Bachmann R, Hällén J. Frequency of pathological proteins (M-components) om 6,995 sera from an adult population. *Acta Med Scand* 1966;179(2):235–247.

6. Saleun JP, Vicariot M, Deroff P, Morin JF. Monoclonal gammopathies in the adult population of Finistère, France. *J Clin Pathol* 1982;35(1):63–68.

7. Kyle RA, Finkelstein S, Elveback LR, Kurland LT. Incidence of monoclonal proteins in a Minnesota community with a cluster of multiple myeloma. *Blood* 1972;40(5):719–724.

8. Kurihara Y, Shiba K, Fukumura Y, Kobayashi I, Kamei S. Occurrence of serum M-protein species in Japanese patients older than 50 years based on relative mobility in cellulose acetate membrane electrophoresis. *J Clin Lab Anal* 2000;14(2):64–69.

9. Kyle RA, Therneau TM, Rajkumar SV, et al. Prevalence of monoclonal gammopathy of undetermined significance. *N Engl J Med* 2006;354(13): 1362–1369.

10. Iwanaga M, Tagawa M, Tsukasaki K, Kamihira S, Tomonaga M. Prevalence of monoclonal gammopathy of undetermined significance: study of 52,802 persons in Nagasaki City, Japan. *Mayo Clin Proc* 2007;82(12):1474–1479.

11. Landgren O, Gridley G, Turesson I, et al. Risk of monoclonal gammopathy of undetermined significance (MGUS) and subsequent multiple myeloma among African American and white veterans in the United States. *Blood* 2006;107(3):904–906.

12. Cohen HJ, Crawford J, Rao MK, Pieper CF, Currie MS. Racial differences in the prevalence of monoclonal gammopathy in a community-based sample of the elderly. *Am J Med* 1998;104(5):439–444.

13. Landgren O, Katzmann JA, Hsing AW, et al. Prevalence of monoclonal gammopathy of undetermined significance among men in Ghana. *Mayo Clin Proc* 2007;82(12):1468–1473.

14. Singh J, Dudley AW Jr, Kulig KA. Increased incidence of monoclonal gammopathy of undetermined significance in blacks and its age-related differences with whites on the basis of a study of 397 men and one woman in a hospital setting. *J Lab Clin Med* 1990;116(6):785–789.

15. Brown LM, Linet MS, Greenberg RS, et al. Multiple myeloma and family history of cancer among blacks and whites in the U.S. *Cancer* 1999;85(11):2385–2390.

16. Eriksson M, Hållberg B. Familial occurrence of hematologic malignancies and other diseases in multiple myeloma: a case-control study. *Cancer Causes Control* 1992;3(1):63–67.

17. Ogmundsdóttir HM, Haraldsdóttirm V, Jóhannesson GM, et al. Familiality of benign and malignant paraproteinemias. A population-based cancer-registry study of multiple myeloma families. *Haematologica* 2005;90(1):66–71.

18. Vachon CM, Kyle RA, Therneau TM, et al. Increased risk of monoclonal gammopathy in first-degree relatives of patients with multiple myeloma or monoclonal gammopathy of undetermined significance. *Blood* 2009;114(4):785–790.

19. Landgren O, Linet MS, McMaster ML, Gridley G, Hemminki K, Goldin LR. Familial characteristics of autoimmune and hematologic disorders in 8,406 multiple myeloma patients: a population-based case-control study. *Int J Cancer* 2006;118(12): 3095–3098.

20. Brown LM, Gridley G, Check D, Landgren O. Risk of multiple myeloma and monoclonal gammopathy of undetermined significance among white and black male United States veterans with prior autoimmune, infectious, inflammatory, and allergic disorders. *Blood* 2008;111(7):3388–3394.

21. Landgren O, Kyle RA, Hoppin JA, et al. Pesticide exposure and risk of monoclonal gammopathy of undetermined significance in the Agricultural Health Study. *Blood* 2009;113(25):6386–6391.

22. Fonseca R, Barlogie B, Bataille R, et al. Genetics and cytogenetics of multiple myeloma: a workshop report. *Cancer Res* 2004;64(4):1546–1558.

23. Dispenzieri A, Gertz MA, Therneau TM, Kyle RA. Retrospective cohort study of 148 patients with polyclonal gammopathy. *Mayo Clin Proc* 2001;76(5): 476–487.

24. Katzmann JA, Dispenzieri A, Kyle RA, et al. Elimination of the need for urine studies in the screening algorithm for monoclonal gammopathies by using serum immunofixation and free light chain assays. *Mayo Clin Proc* 2006;81(12):1575–1578.

25. Katzmann JA, Clark RJ, Abraham RS, et al. Serum reference intervals and diagnostic ranges for free kappa and free lambda immunoglobulin light chains: relative sensitivity for detection of monoclonal light chains. *Clin Chem* 2002;48(9): 1437–1444.

26. Rajkumar SV, Kyle RA, Therneau TM, et al. Presence of monoclonal free light chains in the serum predicts risk of progression in monoclonal gammopathy of undetermined significance. *Br J Haematol* 2004;127(3):308–310.

27. Rajkumar SV, Kyle RA, Therneau TM, et al. Serum free light chain ratio is an independent risk factor for progression in monoclonal gammopathy of undetermined significance. *Blood* 2005;106(3):812–817.

28. Dispenzieri A, Kyle RA, Katzmann JA, et al. Immunoglobulin free light chain ratio is an independent risk factor for progression of smoldering (asymptomatic) multiple myeloma. *Blood* 2008;111 (2):785–789.

29. Dingli D, Kyle RA, Rajkumar SV, et al. Immunoglobulin free light chains and solitary plasmacytoma of bone. *Blood* 2006;108(6):1979–1983.

30. Avet-Loiseau H, Li JY, Facon T, et al. High incidence of translocations t(11;14)(q13;q32) and t(4;14) (p16;q32) in patients with plasma cell malignancies. *Cancer Res* 1998;58(24):5640–5645.

31. Nishida K, Tamura A, Nakazawa N, et al. The Ig heavy chain gene is frequently involved in chromosomal translocations in multiple myeloma and plasma cell leukemia as detected by in situ hybridization. *Blood* 1997;90(2):526–534.

32. Avet-Loiseau H, Facon T, Daviet A, et al. 14q32 translocations and monosomy 13 observed in monoclonal gammopathy of undetermined significance delineate a multistep process for the oncogenesis of multiple myeloma. Intergroupe Francophone du Myélome. *Cancer Res* 1999;59(18):4546–4550.

33. Fonseca R, Bailey RJ, Ahmann GJ, et al. Genomic abnormalities in monoclonal gammopathy of undetermined significance. *Blood* 2002;100(4):1417–1424.

34. Brousseau M, Leleu X, Gerard J, et al.; Intergroupe Francophone du Myélome. Hyperdiploidy is a common finding in monoclonal gammopathy of undetermined significance and monosomy 13 is restricted to these hyperdiploid patients. *Clin Cancer Res* 2007;13(20):6026–6031.

35. Chng WJ, Van Wier SA, Ahmann GJ, et al. A validated FISH trisomy index demonstrates the hyperdiploid and nonhyperdiploid dichotomy in MGUS. *Blood* 2005;106(6):2156–2161.

36. Königsberg R, Ackermann J, Kaufmann H, et al. Deletions of chromosome 13q in monoclonal gammopathy of undetermined significance. *Leukemia* 2000;14(11):1975–1979.

37. Avet-Loiseau H, Li JY, Morineau N, et al. Monosomy 13 is associated with the transition of monoclonal gammopathy of undetermined significance to multiple myeloma. Intergroupe Francophone du Myélome. *Blood* 1999;94(8):2583–2589.

38. Ackermann J, Meidlinger P, Zojer N, et al. Absence of p53 deletions in bone marrow plasma cells of patients with monoclonal gammopathy of undetermined significance. *Br J Haematol* 1998;103(4):1161–1163.

39. Harada H, Kawano MM, Huang N, et al. Phenotypic difference of normal plasma cells from mature myeloma cells. *Blood* 1993;81(10):2658–2663.

40. Ocqueteau M, Orfao A, Almeida J, et al. Immunophenotypic characterization of plasma cells from monoclonal gammopathy of undetermined significance patients. Implications for the differential diagnosis between MGUS and multiple myeloma. *Am J Pathol* 1998;152(6):1655–1665.

41. Kumar S, Rajkumar SV, Kimlinger T, Greipp PR, Witzig TE. CD45 expression by bone marrow plasma cells in multiple myeloma: clinical and biological correlations. *Leukemia* 2005;19(8):1466–1470.

42. Bataille R, Pellat-Deceunynck C, Robillard N, Avet-Loiseau H, Harousseau JL, Moreau P. CD117 (c-kit) is aberrantly expressed in a subset of MGUS and multiple myeloma with unexpectedly good prognosis. *Leuk Res* 2008;32(3):379–382.

43. Ogata A, Anderson KC. Therapeutic strategies for inhibition of interleukin-6 mediated multiple myeloma cell growth. *Leuk Res* 1996;20(4):303–307.

44. Kawano M, Hirano T, Matsuda T, et al. Autocrine generation and requirement of BSF-2/IL-6 for human multiple myelomas. *Nature* 1988;332(6159):83–85.

45. van de Donk NW, Lokhorst HM, Bloem AC. Growth factors and antiapoptotic signaling pathways in multiple myeloma. *Leukemia* 2005;19(12):2177–2185.

46. Rawstron AC, Fenton JA, Ashcroft J, et al. The interleukin-6 receptor alpha-chain (CD126) is expressed by neoplastic but not normal plasma cells. *Blood* 2000;96(12):3880–3886.

47. Hanamura I, Stewart JP, Huang Y, et al. Frequent gain of chromosome band 1q21 in plasma-cell dyscrasias detected by fluorescence in situ hybridization: incidence increases from MGUS to relapsed myeloma and is related to prognosis and disease progression following tandem stem-cell transplantation. *Blood* 2006;108(5):1724–1732.

48. Kuehl WM, Bergsagel PL. Multiple myeloma: evolving genetic events and host interactions. *Nat Rev Cancer* 2002;2(3):175–187.

49. Bezieau S, Devilder MC, Avet-Loiseau H, et al. High incidence of N and K-Ras activating mutations in multiple myeloma and primary plasma cell leukemia at diagnosis. *Hum Mutat* 2001;18(3):212–224.

50. Liu P, Leong T, Quam L, et al. Activating mutations of N- and K-ras in multiple myeloma show different clinical associations: analysis of the Eastern Cooperative Oncology Group Phase III Trial. *Blood* 1996;88(7):2699–2706.

51. Corradini P, Ladetto M, Voena C, et al. Mutational activation of N- and K-ras oncogenes in plasma cell dyscrasias. *Blood* 1993;81(10):2708–2713.

52. Ribatti D, Vacca A. The role of microenvironment in tumor angiogenesis. *Genes Nutr* 2008;3(1):29–34.

53. Kumar S, Witzig TE, Timm M, et al. Bone marrow angiogenic ability and expression of angiogenic cytokines in myeloma: evidence favoring loss of marrow angiogenesis inhibitory activity with disease progression. *Blood* 2004;104(4):1159–1165.

54. Rajkumar SV, Mesa RA, Fonseca R, et al. Bone marrow angiogenesis in 400 patients with monoclonal gammopathy of undetermined significance, multiple myeloma, and primary amyloidosis. *Clin Cancer Res* 2002;8(7):2210–2216.

55. Rajkumar SV, Leong T, Roche PC, et al. Prognostic value of bone marrow angiogenesis in multiple myeloma. *Clin Cancer Res* 2000;6(8):3111–3116.

56. Golombick T, Diamond T. Prevalence of monoclonal gammopathy of undetermined significance/myeloma in patients with acute osteoporotic vertebral fractures. *Acta Haematol* 2008;120(2):87–90.

57. Pepe J, Petrucci MT, Nofroni I, et al. Lumbar bone mineral density as the major factor determining increased prevalence of vertebral fractures in monoclonal gammopathy of undetermined significance. *Br J Haematol* 2006;134(5):485–490.

58. Melton LJ 3rd, Rajkumar SV, Khosla S, Achenbach SJ, Oberg AL, Kyle RA. Fracture risk in monoclonal gammopathy of undetermined significance. *J Bone Miner Res* 2004;19(1):25–30.

59. Pongchaiyakul C, Nguyen ND, Jones G, Center JR, Eisman JA, Nguyen TV. Asymptomatic vertebral deformity as a major risk factor for subsequent fractures and mortality: a long-term prospective study. *J Bone Miner Res* 2005;20(8):1349–1355.

60. Berenson JR, Yellin O, Boccia RV, et al. Zoledronic acid markedly improves bone mineral density for patients with monoclonal gammopathy of undetermined

significance and bone loss. *Clin Cancer Res* 2008; 14(19):6289–6295.

61. Pepe J, Petrucci MT, Mascia ML, et al. The effects of alendronate treatment in osteoporotic patients affected by monoclonal gammopathy of undetermined significance. *Calcif Tissue Int* 2008;82(6):418–426.

62. Kyle RA, Therneau TM, Rajkumar SV, et al. A long-term study of prognosis in monoclonal gammopathy of undetermined significance. *N Engl J Med* 2002;346(8):564–569.

63. Cesana C, Klersy C, Barbarano L, et al. Prognostic factors for malignant transformation in monoclonal gammopathy of undetermined significance and smoldering multiple myeloma. *J Clin Oncol* 2002;20(6):1625–1634.

64. Rosiñol L, Cibeira MT, Montoto S, et al. Monoclonal gammopathy of undetermined significance: predictors of malignant transformation and recognition of an evolving type characterized by a progressive increase in M protein size. *Mayo Clin Proc* 2007;82(4):428–434.

65. Baldini L, Guffanti A, Cesana BM, et al. Role of different hematologic variables in defining the risk of malignant transformation in monoclonal gammopathy. *Blood* 1996;87(3):912–918.

66. Kyle RA. "Benign" monoclonal gammopathy–after 20 to 35 years of follow-up. *Mayo Clin Proc* 1993;68(1):26–36.

67. Montoto S, Bladé J, Montserrat E. Monoclonal gammopathy of undetermined significance. *N Engl J Med* 2002;346(26):2087–8; author reply 2087.

68. Bladé J. On the "significance" of monoclonal gammopathy of undetermined significance. *Mayo Clin Proc* 2004;79(7):855–856.

69. Blade J, Lopez-Guillermo A, Rozman C, et al. Malignant transformation and life expectancy in monoclonal gammopathy of undetermined significance. *Br J Haematol* 1992;81(3):391–394.

70. Gregersen H, Mellemkjaer L, Ibsen JS, Dahlerup JF, Thomassen L, Sørensen HT. The impact of M-component type and immunoglobulin concentration on the risk of malignant transformation in patients with monoclonal gammopathy of undetermined significance. *Haematologica* 2001;86(11):1172–1179.

71. Kyle RA, Therneau TM, Rajkumar SV, Larson DR, Plevak MF, Melton LJ 3rd. Long-term follow-up of 241 patients with monoclonal gammopathy of undetermined significance: the original Mayo Clinic series 25 years later. *Mayo Clin Proc* 2004;79(7):859–866.

72. Kumar S, Rajkumar SV, Kyle RA, et al. Prognostic value of circulating plasma cells in monoclonal

gammopathy of undetermined significance. *J Clin Oncol* 2005;23(24):5668–5674.

73. Isaksson E, Björkholm M, Holm G, et al. Blood clonal B-cell excess in patients with monoclonal gammopathy of undetermined significance (MGUS): association with malignant transformation. *Br J Haematol* 1996;92(1):71–76.

74. Kyle RA, Remstein ED, Therneau TM, et al. Clinical course and prognosis of smoldering (asymptomatic) multiple myeloma. *N Engl J Med* 2007; 356(25):2582–2590.

75. Azar HA, Hill WT, Osserman EF. Malignant lymphoma and lymphatic leukemia associated with myeloma-type serum proteins. *Am J Med* 1957;23(2):239–249.

76. Kyle RA, Garton JP. The spectrum of IgM monoclonal gammopathy in 430 cases. *Mayo Clin Proc* 1987;62(8):719–731.

77. Alexanian R. Monoclonal gammopathy in lymphoma. *Arch Intern Med* 1975;135(1):62–66.

78. Noel P, Kyle RA. Monoclonal proteins in chronic lymphocytic leukemia. *Am J Clin Pathol* 1987;87(3): 385–388.

79. Kim H, Heller P, Rappaport H. Monoclonal gammopathies associated with lymphoproliferative disorders: a morphologic study. *Am J Clin Pathol* 1973; 59(3):282–294.

80. Yin CC, Lin P, Carney DA, et al. Chronic lymphocytic leukemia/small lymphocytic lymphoma associated with IgM paraprotein. *Am J Clin Pathol* 2005; 123(4):594–602.

81. Jansen J, Bolhuis RL, van Nieuwkoop JA, Schuit HR, Kroese WF. Paraproteinaemia plus osteolytic lesions in typical hairy-cell leukaemia. *Br J Haematol* 1983;54(4):531–541.

82. Matsuzaki H, Yamaguchi K, Kagimoto T, Nakai R, Takatsuki K, Oyama W. Monoclonal gammopathies in adult T-cell leukemia. *Cancer* 1985;56(6): 1380–1383.

83. Lamboley V, Zabraniecki L, Sie P, Pourrat J, Fournié B. Myeloma and monoclonal gammopathy of uncertain significance associated with acquired von Willebrand's syndrome. Seven new cases with a literature review. *Joint Bone Spine* 2002;69(1):62–67.

84. Mant MJ, Hirsh J, Gauldie J, Bienenstock J, Pineo GF, Luke KH. Von Willebrand's syndrome presenting as an acquired bleeding disorder in association with a monoclonal gammopathy. *Blood* 1973;42(3):429–436.

85. Mannucci PM, Lombardi R, Bader R, et al. Studies of the pathophysiology of acquired von Willebrand's

disease in seven patients with lymphoproliferative disorders or benign monoclonal gammopathies. *Blood* 1984;64(3):614–621.

86. Federici AB, Stabile F, Castaman G, Canciani MT, Mannucci PM. Treatment of acquired von Willebrand syndrome in patients with monoclonal gammopathy of uncertain significance: comparison of three different therapeutic approaches. *Blood* 1998;92(8):2707–2711.

87. Kristinsson SY, Fears TR, Gridley G, et al. Deep vein thrombosis after monoclonal gammopathy of undetermined significance and multiple myeloma. *Blood* 2008;112(9):3582–3586.

88. Srkalovic G, Cameron MG, Rybicki L, Deitcher SR, Kattke-Marchant K, Hussein MA. Monoclonal gammopathy of undetermined significance and multiple myeloma are associated with an increased incidence of venothromboembolic disease. *Cancer* 2004;101(3):558–566.

89. Sallah S, Husain A, Wan J, Vos P, Nguyen NP. The risk of venous thromboembolic disease in patients with monoclonal gammopathy of undetermined significance. *Ann Oncol* 2004;15(10):1490–1494.

90. Bellotti V, Gamba G, Merlini G, et al. Study of three patients with monoclonal gammopathies and "lupus-like" anticoagulants. *Br J Haematol* 1989;73(2):221–227.

91. Gosselin S, Kyle RA, Dyck PJ. Neuropathy associated with monoclonal gammopathies of undetermined significance. *Ann Neurol* 1991;30(1):54–61.

92. Kyle RA. Monoclonal proteins in neuropathy. *Neurol Clin* 1992;10(3):713–734.

93. Kelly JJ. Peripheral neuropathies associated with monoclonal gammopathies of undetermined significance. *Rev Neurol Dis* 2008;5(1):14–22.

94. Kelly JJ. Neuropathies of monoclonal gammopathies of undetermined significance. *Hematol Oncol Clin North Am* 1999;13(6):1203–1210.

95. Gorson KC. Clinical features, evaluation, and treatment of patients with polyneuropathy associated with monoclonal gammopathy of undetermined significance (MGUS). *J Clin Apher* 1999;14(3):149–153.

96. Kissel JT, Mendell JR. Neuropathies associated with monoclonal gammopathies. *Neuromuscul Disord* 1996;6(1):3–18.

97. Notermans NC, Wokke JH, Lokhorst HM, Franssen H, van der Graaf Y, Jennekens FG. Polyneuropathy associated with monoclonal gammopathy of undetermined significance. A prospective study of the prognostic value of clinical and laboratory abnormalities. *Brain* 1994;117 (Pt 6):1385–1393.

98. Nobile-Orazio E, Barbieri S, Baldini L, et al. Peripheral neuropathy in monoclonal gammopathy of undetermined significance: prevalence and immunopathogenetic studies. *Acta Neurol Scand* 1992;85(6):383–390.

99. Dyck PJ, Low PA, Windebank AJ, et al. Plasma exchange in polyneuropathy associated with monoclonal gammopathy of undetermined significance. *N Engl J Med* 1991;325(21):1482–1486.

100. Niermeijer JM, Eurelings M, van der Linden MW, et al. Intermittent cyclophosphamide with prednisone versus placebo for polyneuropathy with IgM monoclonal gammopathy. *Neurology* 2007;69(1):50–59.

101. Mariette X, Brouet JC, Chevret S, et al. A randomised double blind trial versus placebo does not confirm the benefit of alpha-interferon in polyneuropathy associated with monoclonal IgM. *J Neurol Neurosurg Psychiatr* 2000;69(2):279–280.

102. Kilidireas C, Anagnostopoulos A, Karandreas N, Mouselimi L, Dimopoulos MA. Rituximab therapy in monoclonal IgM-related neuropathies. *Leuk Lymphoma* 2006;47(5):859–864.

103. Broglio L, Lauria G. Worsening after rituximab treatment in anti-mag neuropathy. *Muscle Nerve* 2005;32(3):378–379.

104. Rojas-García R, Gallardo E, de Andrés I, et al. Chronic neuropathy with IgM anti-ganglioside antibodies: lack of long term response to rituximab. *Neurology* 2003;61(12):1814–1816.

105. Lee YC, Came N, Schwarer A, Day B. Autologous peripheral blood stem cell transplantation for peripheral neuropathy secondary to monoclonal gammopathy of unknown significance. *Bone Marrow Transplant* 2002;30(1):53–56.

106. Lavrnic D, Vidakovic A, Miletic V, et al. Motor neuron disease and monoclonal gammopathy. *Eur Neurol* 1995;35(2):104–107.

107. Dispenzieri A. POEMS syndrome. *Blood Rev* 2007;21(6):285–299.

108. Madan S, Greipp PR. The incidental monoclonal protein: current approach to management of monoclonal gammopathy of undetermined significance (MGUS). *Blood Rev* 2009;23(6):257–265.

109. Dispenzieri A, Kyle RA, Lacy MQ, et al. POEMS syndrome: definitions and long-term outcome. *Blood* 2003;101(7):2496–2506.

110. Allam JS, Kennedy CC, Aksamit TR, Dispenzieri A. Pulmonary manifestations in patients with POEMS syndrome: a retrospective review of 137 patients. *Chest* 2008;133(4):969–974.

111. Daoud MS, Lust JA, Kyle RA, Pittelkow MR. Monoclonal gammopathies and associated skin disorders. *J Am Acad Dermatol* 1999;40(4):507–35; quiz 536.

112. James K, Fudenberg H, Epstein WL, Shuster J. Studies on a unique diagnostic serum globulin in papular mucinosis (lichen myxedematosus). *Clin Exp Immunol* 1967;2(2):153–166.

113. Powell FC, Schroeter AL, Su WP, Perry HO. Pyoderma gangrenosum and monoclonal gammopathy. *Arch Dermatol* 1983;119(6):468–472.

114. Holt PJ, Davies MG, Saunders KC, Nuki G. Pyoderma gangrenosum: clinical and laboratory findings in 15 patients with special reference to polyarthritis. *Medicine (Baltimore)* 1980;59(2):114–133.

115. de Koning HD, Bodar EJ, van der Meer JW, Simon A; Schnitzler Syndrome Study Group. Schnitzler syndrome: beyond the case reports: review and follow-up of 94 patients with an emphasis on prognosis and treatment. *Semin Arthritis Rheum* 2007;37(3):137–148.

116. Powell FC, Greipp PR, Su WP. Discoid lupus erythematosus and monoclonal gammopathy. *Br J Dermatol* 1983;109(3):355–360.

117. Nestle FO, Hofbauer G, Burg G. Necrobiotic xanthogranuloma with monoclonal gammopathy of the IgG lambda type. *Dermatology (Basel)* 1999;198(4):434–435.

118. Kövary PM, Dhonau H, Happle R. Paraproteinaemia in erythema elevatum diutinum. *Arch Dermatol Res* 1977;260(2):155–158.

119. Chowdhury MM, Inaloz HS, Motley RJ, Knight AG. Erythema elevatum diutinum and IgA paraproteinaemia: "a preclinical iceberg." *Int J Dermatol* 2002;41(6):368–370.

120. Renoult E, Bertrand F, Kessler M. Monoclonal gammopathies in HBsAg-positive patients with renal transplants. *N Engl J Med* 1988;318(18):1205.

121. Ducloux D, Carron P, Racadot E, et al. T-cell immune defect and B-cell activation in renal transplant recipients with monoclonal gammopathies. *Transpl Int* 1999;12(4):250–253.

122. Badley AD, Portela DF, Patel R, et al. Development of monoclonal gammopathy precedes the development of Epstein-Barr virus-induced posttransplant lymphoproliferative disorder. *Liver Transpl Surg* 1996;2(5):375–382.

123. Caforio AL, Gambino A, Belloni Fortina A, et al. Monoclonal gammopathy in heart transplantation: risk factor analysis and relevance of immunosuppressive load. *Transplant Proc* 2001;33(1–2):1583–1584.

124. Zent CS, Wilson CS, Tricot G, et al. Oligoclonal protein bands and Ig isotype switching in multiple myeloma treated with high-dose therapy and hematopoietic cell transplantation. *Blood* 1998;91(9):3518–3523.

125. Rostaing L, Modesto A, Abbal M, Durand D. Long-term follow-up of monoclonal gammopathy of undetermined significance in transplant patients. *Am J Nephrol* 1994;14(3):187–191.

126. Lefrère JJ, Debbia M, Lambin P. Prospective follow-up of monoclonal gammopathies in HIV-infected individuals. *Br J Haematol* 1993;84(1):151–155.

127. Malik AA, Ganti AK, Potti A, Levitt R, Hanley JF. Role of Helicobacter pylori infection in the incidence and clinical course of monoclonal gammopathy of undetermined significance. *Am J Gastroenterol* 2002;97(6):1371–1374.

128. Rajkumar SV, Kyle RA, Plevak MF, Murray JA, Therneau TM. Helicobacter pylori infection and monoclonal gammopathy of undetermined significance. *Br J Haematol* 2002;119(3):706–708.

129. Zawadzki ZA, Benedek TG. Rheumatoid arthritis, dysproteinemic arthropathy, and paraproteinemia. *Arthritis Rheum* 1969;12(6):555–568.

130. Renier G, Renier JC, Gardembas-Pain M, Chevailler A, Boasson M, Hurez D. Ankylosing spondylitis and monoclonal gammopathies. *Ann Rheum Dis* 1992;51(8):951–954.

131. Ilfeld D, Barzilay J, Vana D, Ben-Bassat M, Joshua H, Pick I. IgG monoclonal gammopathy in four patients with polymyalgia rheumatica. *Ann Rheum Dis* 1985;44(7):501.

132. Porcel JM, Ordi J, Tolosa C, Selva A, Castro-Salomo A, Vilardell M. Monoclonal gammopathy in systemic lupus erythematosus. *Lupus* 1992;1(4):263–264.

133. Kyle RA, Robinson RA, Katzmann JA. The clinical aspects of biclonal gammopathies. Review of 57 cases. *Am J Med* 1981;71(6):999–1008.

134. Riddell S, Traczyk Z, Paraskevas F, Israels LG. The double gammopathies. Clinical and immunological studies. *Medicine (Baltimore)* 1986;65(3):135–142.

135. Nilsson T, Norberg B, Rudolphi O, Jacobsson L. Double gammopathies: incidence and clinical course of 20 patients. *Scand J Haematol* 1986;36(1):103–106.

136. Grosbois B, Jégo P, de Rosa H, et al. [Triclonal gammopathy and malignant immunoproliferative syndrome]. *Rev Med Interne* 1997;18(6):470–473.

137. Tirelli A, Guastafierro S, Cava B, Lucivero G. Triclonal gammopathy in an extranodal non-Hodgkin lymphoma patient. *Am J Hematol* 2003;73(4):273–275.

138. Kyle RA, Maldonado JE, Bayrd ED. Idiopathic Bence Jones proteinuria–a distinct entity? *Am J Med* 1973;55(2):222–226.

139. Kyle RA, Greipp PR. "Idiopathic" Bence Jones proteinuria: long-term follow-up in seven patients. *N Engl J Med* 1982;306(10):564–567.

140. Kanoh T, Ohnaka T, Uchino H, Fujii H. The outcome of idiopathic Bence Jones proteinuria. *Tohoku J Exp Med* 1987;151(1):121–126.

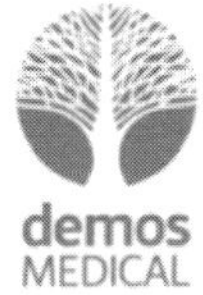

demos
MEDICAL

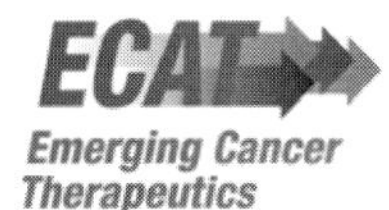

Emerging Cancer
Therapeutics

Smoldering Multiple Myeloma

John A. Lust* and Kathleen A. Donovan

Mayo Clinic, Rochester, MN

■ ABSTRACT

In this review, we will discuss the diagnosis, pathogenesis, adverse prognostic factors, and clinical trials involving smoldering multiple myeloma (SMM). Most, if not all, patients with active multiple myeloma (MM) have a pre-existing monoclonal gammopathy of undetermined significance (MGUS) and may have transitioned through an SMM phase prior to the development of active MM. It will be important for patients with SMM to be differentiated from patients with MGUS because the risk of progression from SMM to active MM is higher in this group of patients. A potential role for the acquired expression of various cytokines, chromosomal changes, and other cellular factors in the monoclonal plasma cells that modulate the interactions between the monoclonal plasma cells and the bone marrow (BM) microenvironment have been implicated in the progression of MGUS to SMM to active MM and are highlighted. Alterations in cytokine production such as (interleukin-1) IL-1, a high myeloma cell growth rate, the percentage of plasma cells in the BM and the level of the serum monoclonal protein, the serum free light chain assay, and several other markers may identify individuals with SMM at high risk for progression. Because of the wide range of time to progression (2–19 years) in this patient population, the current standard of care for patients with asymptomatic myeloma is observation. However, many patients with SMM/indolent MM are uncomfortable with this approach due to the likelihood of progression and several recent clinical trials that have included SMM patients in an attempt to delay/prevent active MM are discussed. The role of chronic inflammation driven by an IL-1/IL-6 pathway as a potential unifying mechanism for the progression of MGUS/SMM to active MM is discussed.

*Corresponding author, Mayo Clinic, Division of Hematology, 200 First St SW, Rochester, MN 55905
E-mail address: lust.john@mayo.edu

Emerging Cancer Therapeutics 1:2 (2010) 261–282.
© 2010 Demos Medical Publishing LLC. All rights reserved.
DOI: 10.5003/2151–4194.1.2.261

demosmedpub.com/ecat

SMM comprises approximately 15% of all cases of newly diagnosed MM (1). Some patients remain stable for many years during which there is little change in their M-protein; however, most SMM patients eventually progress to active (MM) (1–5). In this chapter, we will discuss the diagnosis, pathogenesis, adverse prognostic factors, and clinical trials of SMM and a potential role for chronic inflammation in the progression from SMM to active MM.

■ DIAGNOSIS

Multiple myeloma (MM) is recognized clinically by the proliferation of malignant plasma cells in the bone marrow (BM). Specific criteria exist that have been established by the International Myeloma Working Group that serve as useful guidelines to allow clinicians to differentiate among MM, monoclonal gammopathy of undetermined significance (MGUS), and other related plasma cell proliferative disorders (6). Patients with MGUS usually have less than 10% marrow plasma cells, a serum monoclonal protein < 3 g/dL, <1 g Bence Jones protein/24-hour urine, no anemia, renal failure, lytic bone lesions, or hypercalcemia. In contrast, patients with active myeloma typically present with a marrow plasmacytosis of ≥ 10%, a serum monoclonal protein of ≥ 3 g/dL, a 24-hour urine monoclonal protein of ≥ 1 g, anemia, hypercalcemia, renal insufficiency, and lytic bone lesions (7). Between these two extremes of the disease, two clinically intermediate stages have been described called smoldering MM (SMM) and indolent MM (IMM). Patients with SMM are usually asymptomatic. They have a marrow plasmacytosis of ≥ 10% and/or a serum monoclonal protein of ≥ 3 g/dL. Lytic bone lesions are absent (2,6,8). Patients with IMM are similar to those with SMM except that, with IMM, a small number of bone lesions may be present on bone survey studies. Individuals with SMM and IMM are often referred to as asymptomatic MM patients. The accurate classification of patients is crucial in balancing the risks versus

benefits of a given treatment and the appropriate targeting of novel therapies to specific patient populations.

■ PATHOGENESIS OF MYELOMA

In this section, we will review the biology of the transition from smoldering myeloma to active myeloma. At times we will refer to MGUS and MM, since in many of the studies SMM patients have been grouped into these patient populations. In addition, it appears that most, if not all, patients with active MM had a pre-existing MGUS and may have transitioned through a SMM phase prior to the development of active MM if they are followed sequentially (9,10). It is during this transition process that many of the characteristics distinguishing MGUS from MM such as an increase in paracrine (interleukin-6) IL-6 production, a key plasma cell proliferative cytokine, and certain genetic alterations are acquired. It will be important for patients with SMM to be differentiated from patients with MGUS because the risk of progression from SMM to active MM is higher.

Genetic and Phenotypic Differences in MGUS/SMM and Myeloma

With the advent of fluorescence in situ hybridization (FISH), it has been shown that virtually all patients have some myeloma cells that are cytogenetically abnormal, and aneuploidy is the most common abnormality (11–15). Plasma cells in myeloma frequently have trisomy of chromosomes 7, 9, 11, 15, and 18 (11,13,14). Additional data suggest that most MGUS plasma cells are aneuploid as well (16–18). The incidence of trisomy for at least one chromosome was 61% in one study of MGUS cells using four chromosomal probes by FISH analysis (17) and 100% in a second study that used six probes to analyze MGUS cells (15,18). Variations in the results from these types of studies are often a result of differences in the design and number of probes used. By FISH analysis, myeloma cells appear to differ from those found in patients with MGUS in that the results for myeloma may be somewhat more heterogeneous for a given patient. In any event, it does appear that karyotypic instability begins in MGUS and continues throughout the course of the disease. Chromosome 13 deletions (13q⁻) by FISH or by karyotype has been associated with an adverse prognosis in myeloma (19,20). This abnormality can be present in up to 50% of patients, and the pathogenetic mechanism remains to be determined (19–22). For MGUS, chromosome 13 abnormalities appear to be restricted primarily to a small subpopulation of clonal cells suggesting that it may be a secondary genetic event in the disease process (15,23,24).

It has been hypothesized that a translocation involving an immunoglobulin heavy or light chain gene may be the initial cause of MGUS in many patients and that other genotypic and phenotypic changes that subsequently develop in the monoclonal plasma cell are important in the clinical manifestation of the plasma cell process (15). Chromosomal translocations into the immunoglobulin heavy chain locus on chromosome 14q32 are seen in approximately 60% to 70% of cases of myeloma (12,15,25,26). Errors in VDJ recombination, somatic hypermutation, or switch recombination can mediate the immunoglobulin translocation (12,15). Translocations may occur involving the light chain loci as well, although less frequently. The incidence of IgL translocations in advanced tumors and human myeloma cell line (HMCL) is in the range of 20% while IgK rearrangements seem to be very rare (27). Most of the IgH translocations usually involve the IgH switch regions (12). These translocation move several loci including 11q13 (cyclin D1), 4p16 (FGFR3/MMSET), 16q23 (c-*maf*), 6p21 (cyclin D3), and several other chromosome partners into close proximity to the active immunoglobulin (Ig) enhancer sequences (15,28,29). By interface FISH analysis it has been reported that IgH translocations are present in approximately 47% of MGUS tumors, in 60% to 70% of patients with intramedullary MM,

and in more than 80% of patients with plasma cell leukemia (15). This increase in frequency is partially reflecting a rising number of secondary IgH translocations that is virtually absent in MGUS and SMM (30). The clinical relevance for some of these translocations remains to be elucidated. The t(11;14), which is responsible for the overexpression of cyclin D1, has been shown to be unvarying over the course of patients disease, is insufficient to promote G1 progression (unless in conjunction with cdk4 expression alone which is less common than the cyclin D2/cdk4/6 pathway in myeloma), and has been linked to a more favorable prognosis in MM (31). Unlike t(11;14), there appears to be an increase in t(4;14) positive patients as the disease progresses from MGUS to SMM with SMM cohorts having an incidence of 35.7% or 68.4% depending on the study versus a cumulative incidence of 3.3% for MGUS (32). This translocation is associated with a poor prognosis in MM and yet the underlying mechanism of how the affected genes contribute to this is unclear.

Plasma cells from patients with MGUS and MM have also been analyzed by gene expression profiling (33). In an early study using CD138+ selected MGUS or MM plasma cells, it was found that only 28 genes were differentially expressed suggesting that MGUS plasma cells are more like myeloma plasma cells than normal plasma cells (34). Using clustering analysis, normal and MM plasma cells were differentiated and four sub groups were identified. The expression pattern of MM-1 was similar to normal and MGUS plasma cells whereas MM-4 was similar to MM cell lines. Clinical parameters linked to poor prognosis such as abnormal karyotype and high serum β2 microglobulin were most prevalent in MM-4 (33). A 50-gene panel has also been reported that can distinguish "MGUS-like multiple myeloma" from "non–MGUS-like multiple myeloma" (35).

In addition to large structural abnormalities, individual genetic alterations such as point mutations or changes in methylation status play a significant role in disease progression. A higher percentage of myeloma patients appear to have activating mutations of N-*ras* or K-*ras* when compared to individuals with MGUS (36). In a study, the incidence of N- and K-*ras* mutations was found to be 39% in 160 newly diagnosed patients (37). No significant association was observed between any *ras* mutation and stage of disease, β2 microglobulin, labeling index, or survival. However, the median survival of patients with a K-*ras* mutation was significantly shorter compared to patients with no *ras* mutation (37). In another study, N-*ras* and K-*ras* mutations were found in 55% of myeloma patients at diagnosis but in only 12.5% of patients with MGUS and IMM. K-*ras* mutations were more frequent than N-*ras* mutations (38). More recently, a large study combining a 439 patient Eastern Cooperative Oncology Group (ECOG) cohort with a 96 patient Mayo cohort demonstrates a difference in incidence in mutation between MGUS (7%), newly diagnosed MM (25%) and relapsed MM (45%) patients confirming *ras* mutations as a progressive event in MM (39). In addition, the prevalence of N-*ras* over K-*ras* was shown to be 17% versus 6% in the ECOG cohort and N-*ras* mutations were more common in the Mayo cohort as well. Interestingly, in this study, there is an association with increased plasma cell percentage in the marrow, B2M more than 2.5 g/L, greater percentage of International Staging System stage II and III disease, κ light chain secretion, lower hemoglobin level and more frequent lytic bone lesions, and in the K-*ras* group a plasma cell labeling index (PCLI) > 1%. Similar to other studies *ras* mutations lead to shorter overall survival but only K-*ras* mutations were associated with a significantly shorter overall survival and progression-free survival (PFS). The association of *ras* mutation with other chromosomal abnormalities was telling about potential mechanisms of disease progression. In this study, a significant number of patients had both *ras* mutations and the t(11;14) genetic subtype but *ras* mutations were rarely found in tumors carrying the t(4;14). Patients with *ras* mutations have features associated with greater tumor burden rather than increased proliferation in MM (39).

De novo methylation of the tumor suppressor gene p16/INK4a is a frequent finding in MM patients at diagnosis (40). The inactivating mechanism of the *p16* gene in MM is associated with a high plasma cell proliferation and short survival (41). Hypermethylation of CpG islands in tumor DNA from many different neoplasias have been detected on chromosome 11p at the calcitonin locus. These sites are unmethylated in DNA from all normal tissues. There is significant evidence now that abnormal CpG island methylation at sites of tumor suppressor genes may be an important factor in altered gene expression (42). Continued DNA methylation imbalances could lead to aberrant expression of critical genes leading to overt myeloma.

Phenotypic alterations in this disease for which the underlying cellular mechanisms have not been determined are an equally important aspect of progressive disease. A striking clinical feature of myeloma cells relates to their tendency to remain in the BM environment until the very end stage of the disease (43). This clinical observation may suggest that myeloma cells exhibit increased adherence to marrow stromal elements relative to normal plasma cells (43). Marrow stromal cells from myeloma patients express intracellular adhesion molecule-1 (ICAM-1) and vascular cell adhesion molecule-1 (VCAM-1) whereas myeloma cells demonstrate lymphocyte function-associated antigen-1 (LFA-1), very late antigen-4 (VLA-4), or neural cell adhesion molecule (NCAM) (43,44). Since ICAM-1 is a ligand for the receptor LFA-1 and VCAM-1 is a ligand for the receptor VLA-4+CD29, these adhesion molecules may be important in myeloma cell-marrow stromal cell interactions in vitro and in vivo (43,44). This is supported by the observation that antibodies to adhesion molecules such as LFA-1 (CD11a), CD29, CD44, VLA-4 (CD49d), and ICAM-1 (CD54) have been shown to inhibit the adhesion of HMCLs or patient myeloma cells to marrow stromal cells (44–47). Furthermore, adhesion of HMCLs to BM stromal cells stimulates IL-6 secretion, the central growth factor for myeloma cells (47,48). This adhesion-induced IL-6 expression in marrow stromal cells involves activation of NF-κB (49).

It has been hypothesized that the acquisition of NCAM (CD56) expression in myeloma may be a malignancy-related phenomenon. CD56 is strongly expressed on most myeloma plasma cells but is not found on normal plasma cells (43,50,51) or malignant cells from other hematological disorders (43). Both CD56– and CD56+ plasma cells have been found in some patients with MGUS (52). Interestingly, NCAM is lost from the circulating plasma cells in patients with plasma cell leukemia (43). These observations on CD56 expression parallel those with IL-1β expression. Specifically, IL-1β and CD56 are absent from normal plasma cells, expressed by myeloma cells from most patients, and reduced in patients with plasma cell leukemia (or in myeloma cell lines). The aberrant IL-1 expression potentially alters multiple adhesion molecule interactions.

The PCLI, which measures synthesis of DNA, is useful for differentiating MGUS or smoldering myeloma from active myeloma (53). BM plasma cells (BMPCs) are immediately exposed to bromodeoxyuridine for 1 hour. Plasma cells are identified by intracytoplasmic immunofluorescence using anti-κ or anti-λ light chain antibodies bound to fluorescein. The percent myeloma cells in S-phase are determined using an anti-bromodeoxyuridine monoclonal antibody (BU-1) and a rhodamine labeled goat anti–mouse antibody in a double fluorescence technique. Slides are read with a fluorescence microscope containing both fluorescein and rhodamine filters. Among newly diagnosed untreated patients, a high immunofluorescence LI distinguished those with MM from those with stable monoclonal gammopathies ($P < 0.002$) (53). An increased PCLI is good evidence that myeloma either is present or will soon develop. SMM patients with an increase in their PCLI have clearly been shown to have a shorter time to progression (TTP) making this an important tool in staging SMM patients (54).

The presence of circulating plasma cells of the same isotype in the peripheral blood is also a good marker of active myeloma. In a series of 57 patients with newly diagnosed smoldering myeloma, 16 had progression within 12 months. Sixty-three percent of patients who have progressed had an increased number of peripheral blood plasma cells. In contrast, only 4 of 41 patients who remained stable for 1 year had an increase in peripheral blood plasma cells at diagnosis (55–57).

Importance of the BM Microenvironment

Early work demonstrated that paraffin oil or pristane when injected into BALB/c mice induced plasmacytomas (58,59). The generation of the plasmacytomas was dependent on factors produced by the inflammatory cells. These cells were subsequently shown to produce IL-6, a potent growth factor for plasmacytomas (59). Transgenic mice (C57BL/6) carrying the human IL-6 gene fused to a human immunoglobulin heavy chain enhancer developed a massive plasmacytosis (60). The plasma cells were not transplantable to syngeneic mice and were found not to contain *c-myc* gene rearrangements, characteristic of pristane-induced plasmacytomas (60). However, introduction of the BALB/c genetic background into IL-6 transgenic mice could generate monoclonal transplantable plasmacytomas with *c-myc* translocations (61). Finally, animal studies utilizing IL-6 knockout mice have shown that IL-6 is an essential requirement for the development of B lineage neoplasms (62). The above results provide firm evidence for the critical role of IL-6 in plasmacytoma development.

IL-6 is an autocrine growth factor for human myeloma cells (63). They have shown that myeloma cells freshly isolated from patients produce IL-6 and express its receptor. Exogenous IL-6 augments the in vitro growth of myeloma cells and anti-IL-6 antibody inhibits their growth (63). A myeloma cell line U266 expresses mRNA for both IL-6 and IL-6R. The proliferation of this cell line can be inhibited using anti-IL-6 antibody or antisense

IL-6 oligonucleotides further supporting the critical role of IL-6 in the growth of these cells (64). Significantly elevated serum IL-6 levels have been detected in 3% of MGUS/SMM patients, 35% of overt myeloma patients and in 100% of a plasma cell leukemia group (65). Reverse transcriptase/polymerase chain reaction (RT-PCR) studies on CD38+ sorted MM plasma cells confirmed the production of IL-6 in plasma cells from MM patients (66). Using an anti-bromodeoxyuridine monoclonal antibody to specifically count myeloma cells in S-phase (i.e., the labeling index), the IL-6 responsiveness of myeloma cells in vitro correlates with their labeling index in vivo, and hence to the severity of the disease emphasizing the importance of IL-6 in driving the proliferating MM plasma cell (67). An antibody to IL-6 administered in vivo has been shown to dramatically decrease the labeling index of the tumor cells in patients with aggressive MM (68). Alterations in IL-6R α-chain (CD126) expression demonstrated in MGUS stage plasma cells appears to be one of the first steps in this IL-6 driven proliferative pathway in MM (69).

The source of the IL-6 in this disease is both autocrine (especially in advanced stage MM) and paracrine in nature. The paracrine IL-6 has been demonstrated to be induced by aberrant IL-1 production driving stromal cell secretion of large amounts of IL-6 (48,70) as well as by other IL-1–induced cytokines such as tumor necrosis factor-α (TNF-α) and macrophage inflammatory protein-1α (MIP-1α) (71).

In addition to its role as the major growth factor for myeloma cells, IL-6 also protects myeloma cells from apoptosis and is essential for the terminal differentiation of normal B cells into antibody secreting plasma cells (72–74). Grigorieva et al. (72) showed that marrow stromal cell IL-6 protects myeloma cells from dexamethasone-induced apoptosis. This protective effect could be abrogated by anti-IL-6 antibody. Anti-IL-6 antibody was also effective at inhibiting pokeweed mitogen (PWM)-induced immunoglobulin production by normal mononuclear cells but not PWM-induced proliferation (74).

Studies on normal BM cells underscore the importance of IL-6 as a key growth factor for plasmablasts. Anti-IL-6 antibodies prevented Ig secretion and cell differentiation of normal plasmablasts obtained from patients with reactive plasmacytoses by inducing apoptosis of the plasmablasts (75). Perhaps the reason that IL-6 is the major growth factor for myeloma cells is because it is a bifunctional cytokine modulating both growth and differentiation of normal plasmablasts.

Role of Other Regulators/Other Cytokines in MM Growth

The IL-6 receptor consists of an 80-kD IL-6 binding molecule (gp80) and a 130-kD signal-transducing chain (gp130) (76). gp130 also serves as the signal-transducing chain for leukemia inhibitory factor, oncostain M, ciliary neurotophic factor, and IL-11 (77). Therefore, all of these factors have been shown to stimulate myeloma cell growth (78,79). However, the observed responsiveness of most myeloma cells to these growth factors is variable when compared to IL-6 because the ligand-binding receptors for these cytokines are not as consistently expressed on myeloma cells as the IL-6 binding gp80 receptor.

Other cytokines such as insulin-like growth factor I, IL-10, and hepatocyte growth factor have also been shown to stimulate myeloma cell line growth (80–82). Myeloma cells produce vascular endothelial growth factor (VEGF) that can stimulate IL-6 in a paracrine fashion leading to myeloma cell growth (83). Another study showed that proliferation of purified myeloma cells from patients was induced by IL-6 in 6 of 10 patients but not to GM-CSF, G-CSF, M-CSF, IL-1α, IL-1β, IL-2, or IL-4 (84).

Angiogenesis in Myeloma

Angiogenesis plays an important role in both hematological malignancies and solid tumors (85,86).

We investigated the production of the chemokine IL-8 by stromal cells cocultured with supernatants from BM cells of patients with MGUS, SMM, and active myeloma (87). IL-8 was detected in samples from patients with active MM or high risk SMM and was dependent upon simultaneous IL-1β production. Consistent with the proangiogenic activity of IL-8, increased BM microvessel density (MVD) correlated with stimulation of stromal cell IL-8 production (87).

In addition to stimulating IL-8, myeloma cells produce VEGF that also stimulates IL-6 in a paracrine fashion leading to myeloma cell growth (83). There is evidence that increased BM angiogenesis occurs in myeloma and is related to disease activity (86,88–91). Rajkumar et al. studied 400 patients with MGUS, SMM, MM, and primary amyloidosis. The median MVD per high power field was 1.3 in controls, 3 in MGUS, 4 in SMM, 11 in newly diagnosed MM, and 20 in relapsed MM. BM angiogenesis progressively increases from MGUS to advanced myeloma, indicating that angiogenesis may be related to disease progression (92). Angiogenesis in myeloma also appears to be correlated with the plasma cell labeling index (93), a measure of the proliferative activity of the neoplastic plasma cells, as described above, and is an independent predictor of poor survival in myeloma (94).

Studies on the IL-1/IL-6 Axis in the Pathogenesis of Myeloma

IL-6 has clearly been shown to be one of the central growth factors driving myeloma cell proliferation whose levels and activity can be monitored through the high sensitivity C-reactive protein (CRP) assay and the PCLI. We have investigated the differences in IL-6 and IL-1β expression in monoclonal plasma cells from patients with MGUS or MM (66). Expression of IL-6 and IL-1β in BM cells was determined using cell sorting to enrich for plasma cells followed by RT/PCR. IL-6 mRNA expression was detectable in the sorted CD38+/ CD45– plasma cell populations from 0/6 MGUS and 5/11 MM patients. All five MM patients with autocrine IL-6 expression demonstrated an elevated PCLI. IL-1β mRNA was detectable in the sorted CD38+/CD45– plasma cell populations from 1/6 MGUS and 10/11 MM patients. In situ hybridization (ISH) confirmed that the IL-1β producing cells were plasma cells (66). These results suggested that autocrine IL-6 production was associated with late stage MM plasma cells and was not a distinguishing characteristic between the MGUS/SMM transition to MM. Because the aberrant IL-1β expression appeared to distinguish MGUS from MM better than IL-6, we focused our investigations on this aberrant IL-1β expression.

ISH for IL-1β using BM aspirates from 51 MM, 7 smoldering MM, 21 MGUS, and 5 normal control samples (95) demonstrated the presence of IL-1β mRNA in the plasma cells from 49 of 51 patients with active myeloma and 7 of 7 patients with smoldering myeloma. In contrast, 5 of 21 patients with MGUS and 0 of 5 normal controls had detectable IL-1β message. Bone lesions were present in 40 of the 51 MM patients analyzed and all 40 patients had IL-1β mRNA by ISH. These results demonstrate that > 95% of MM patients but < 25% of MGUS patients are positive for IL-1β production (95).

Although the ISH was very useful at detecting IL-1β, it did not allow us to differentiate SMM from active MM or to determine the significance of the IL-1 positivity in MGUS patients. Therefore, we developed a functional assay that measures the IL-1–induced IL-6 production by BM stromal cells that serves as a highly sensitive surrogate marker for IL-1β functional activity in BM samples from patients with monoclonal plasma proliferative disorders. We hypothesized that patients with MM or SMM at risk for progression to active MM may have higher IL-1β bioactivity than patients with stable SMM or MGUS. IL-1β bioactivity was determined by quantitating IL-1β specific IL-6 production by cultured BM stromal cells, in the presence or absence of an IL-1 inhibitor, using an IL-6 enzyme linked immunosorbent assay (70).

Using this IL-1β bioassay, myeloma patient BM cells stimulated a higher level of IL-6 when compared with normal or MGUS patients. The degree of IL-1 specificity for each patient was determined by inhibiting the IL-6 production with IL-1Ra or IL-1 trap (Figure 1). In the three patients (SMM-3, MM-1, and MM-2) with an elevated IL-6 level, both IL-1Ra and IL-1 trap were able to inhibit the stromal cell IL-6 production by ≥ 95%. In contrast, the VEGF trap had no effect. Similar inhibitory results have been obtained using anti-IL-1β antibodies with matched isotype control antibodies causing no inhibition (data not shown). These results demonstrate that the in vitro stromal cell IL-6 production induced by BM cells from patients with active disease is IL-1 mediated. Most importantly, the SMM/IMM patients that eventually progressed to active disease induced a higher level of IL-6 compared with the SMM/IMM patients with stable disease (70). This study divides SMM patients into two groups based on paracrine IL-6 production and emphasizes the importance of inhibiting the proliferating myeloma cells at this stage of disease.

Correlation Between IL-1β Production and the Clinical Features of MM

Normal plasma cells do not produce IL-1β, however, IL-1β is detectable in the culture supernatants of BM cells from patients with MM

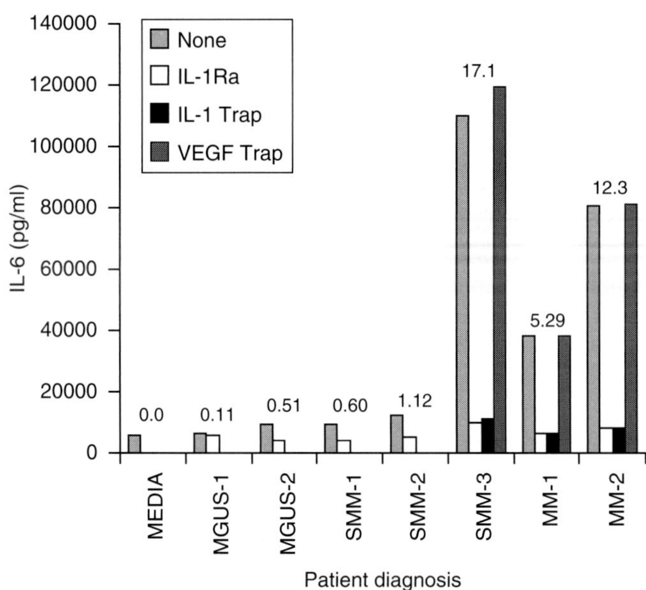

FIGURE 1

IL-6 production by supernatants from bone marrow (BM) cells of patients with monoclonal gammopathy of undetermined significance (MGUS), smoldering multiple myeloma (SMM), or multiple myeloma (MM) cocultured with marrow stromal cells. Supernatants from Ficoll purified, unsorted BM cells from seven representative patients with MGUS, SMM, or MM were cocultured with BM stromal cells. The bar graphs represent the levels of IL-6 production. Cocultures were performed in the presence and absence of IL-1Ra, IL-1 trap, or vascular endothelial growth factor (VEGF) trap. The number at the top of each bar is the IL-6 level converted to the IL-6 fold increase (IL-6 FI). The IL-6 fold increase = (patient IL-6 value—media control value)/media control value. From Ref. 70 with permission.

(48). IL-1β has potent osteoclast activating factor (OAF) activity and can induce the paracrine expression of IL-6 and several adhesion molecules such as ICAM-1, VCAM-1, and endothelial-leukocyte adhesion molecule (ELAM) in other cellular systems (48,96–100). These biological effects of IL-1β closely parallel several of the clinical features of human myeloma such as osteolytic bone lesions, IL-6–induced cell growth, and "homing" of myeloma cells to the BM (7,101). In addition, IL-1 is a known stimulator of many of the other cytokines relevant in the myeloma cytokine cascade such as IL-8, TNF-α, MIP-1α (71) having demonstrated powerful effects at extremely low concentrations.

The development of osteolytic lesions is an important clinical finding that clearly distinguishes MGUS/SMM from myeloma. Initially, two different groups had shown that the bone resorbing activity in supernatants of myeloma cell cultures was likely due to IL-1β and not to IL-1α, TNF, or lymphotoxin (100,102). Torcia et al. have clearly shown a critical role for IL-1β in the pathogenesis of bone disease (99). Using the fetal rat long-bone tissue culture assay, they demonstrated that the OAF activity of culture supernatants from unfractionated BM cells from myeloma patients correlated with the IL-1β content (r = 0.949). Furthermore, the OAF activity could be completely abolished by IL-1 receptor antagonist, sIL-1R type I or II, or neutralizing anti-IL-1β antibodies but not anti-IL-6 antibodies (99). These results suggest that the OAF activity of myeloma cells from patients is predominantly related to IL-1β.

The paracrine production of IL-6 by the IL-1β produced by myeloma cells stimulates myeloma cell proliferation (103). In addition, IL-1β can act as an autocrine growth factor for myeloma cells in rare cases (104). The ability of IL-1Ra to inhibit paracrine IL-6 production by BM cultures from myeloma patients has been reported (103). Using the bromodeoxyuridine method, they also demonstrated that IL-1Ra inhibited the percentage of myeloma cells in S-phase (103).

IL-1β has the ability to upregulate adhesion molecule expression and/or function as we have shown with CD56 expression. In the murine systems, plasmacytoma (B9) cells, that had been transfected with an IL-1α cDNA and injected intravenously into syngeneic mice, "homed" to the BM and produced metastatic bone lesions (105). (Unlike human cells, mouse cells produce and release IL-1α which is functionally homologous to human IL-1β.) By comparison, intravenous injection of autonomously growing B-cell lines generated in vitro by retroviral insertion of an IL-6 cDNA did not result in BM or bone metastases (105). Alterations in CD54 expression were identified between the parent line and the IL-1α transfected mouse plasmacytoma cells (106). In human disease, IL-1β activated BM endothelial cells (BMEC), but not unstimulated BMEC, adhered to myeloma cells. This binding was inhibited by monoclonal antibodies against E-selectin (ELAM-1), however, antibodies to IL-1β were not tested. It is of note that transcription of ELAM-1 (or CD62E), as well as VCAM-1 (or CD 106) and ICAM-1 (or CD54) can be induced by IL-1β via a nuclear factor-κB (NF-κB) intermediate. The positive regulatory domains required for maximal levels of cytokine induction have been defined in the promoters of all three genes and DNA binding studies reveal a requirement for NF-κB (96). In summary, IL-1β has potent OAF activity and can upregulate both adhesion molecules and IL-6 production contributing to the pathogenesis of MM.

The biological effects of IL-1β closely parallel several of the clinical features of human myeloma. IL-1β has potent osteoclast activating factor activity, can increase the expression of adhesion molecules, and can induce paracrine IL-6 production (70,95,101). The increased production of adhesion molecules could explain why myeloma cells are found predominantly in the BM. Subsequently, these "fixed" monoclonal plasma cells could now stimulate osteoclasts through the production of IL-1β and paracrine generation of IL-6 resulting in osteolytic disease. The paracrine generation of IL-6 by marrow stromal cells may further support the growth and survival of the myeloma cells. The importance of IL-1β in myeloma pathogenesis is a result of its ability to induce IL-6. Because femtogram amounts of IL-1β can stimulate IL-6 production (70), IL-1β may act as a "trigger" to induce IL-6 and other cytokine cascades, resulting in progression to active myeloma. This paracrine model of IL-6 production also suggests a rational therapeutic approach for myeloma prevention, that is, inhibit the IL-1β–induced IL-6 production with a potent IL-1β inhibitor.

■ ADVERSE PROGNOSTIC FACTORS IN THE PROGRESSION OF SMM/IMM

Asymptomatic MM to Active Myeloma

Several different adverse prognostic factors have been shown to assist in the identification of those individuals with SMM/IMM that may be at risk for progression. The finding of alterations in IL-1–induced paracrine IL-6 production separating SMM into high and low producers (70) has been followed up by newer efforts at stratifying SMM patients. A report on 276 patients with smoldering myeloma found that the overall risk of progression was 10% per year for the first 5 years, approximately 3% per year for the next 5 years, and 1% per year for the last 10 years (2). The proportion of plasma cells in the BM and the serum monoclonal protein were combined to create a model with three distinct prognostic groups. The median TTP was 2 years for the 106 patients in group 1 (BMPC ≥ 10%, M-spike ≥ 3 g/dL), 8 years for the 142 patients in group 2 (BMPC ≥ 10%, M-spike ≤ 3 g/dL) and 19 years for the 27 patients in group 3 (BMPC ≤ 10%, M-spike ≥ 3 g/dL) (2). This study emphasizes the importance of carefully categorizing patients into the SMM groups when evaluating future treatments as the ranges for the median TTP (2–19 years between groups) can easily cloud results and underlines the difficulty of interpreting previous SMM studies where the grouping of patients has been variable. Because it was a retrospective study, PCLI, high sensitivity CRP, and

IL-1 functional activity were unable to be quantitated precluding an evaluation of the proliferative component of the disease.

The free light chain (FLC) ratio is an independent risk factor for progression of SMM (107). The best breakpoint for predicting risk of progression was an FLC ratio of 0.125 or less or 8 or more (107). The extent of abnormality of the FLC ratio was independent of the SMM risk categories defined above by the number of BMPCs and the size of the serum M-protein. Incorporating the FLC ratio into the risk model, the 5-year progression rates in high, intermediate and low risk groups were 76%, 51%, and 25% respectively (107). Again, due to the retrospective nature of this study other relevant parameters to SMM disease were not able to be evaluated. These may be important additions to the classification of SMM patients and a prospective study including these other important features of this stage of disease is warranted.

Other efforts at distinguishing this group of patients include a study that patients with a marked predominance of aberrant plasma cells (aPCs) at diagnosis displayed a significantly higher risk of progression both in MGUS and SMM (108). Sixty-one percent of patients showed an aPC phenotype of CD19–CD56+ and 24% were CD19–CD56– (normal plasma cells were CD19+CD56–). Multivariate analysis for PFS showed the aPC/BMPC (> 95%) as the most important independent variable together with DNA aneuploidy and immunoparesis for MGUS and SMM (108).

In another report, two variants of SMM were recognized: an evolving type characterized by a progressive increase in the M-protein and a short TTP versus a nonevolving type with a stable M-protein and a long TTP (109). Comparative genomic hybridization showed 1q gains and chromosome 13 deletions in the evolving subtype consistent with active disease while the nonevolving subtype showed no gains or deletions (110).

In several studies, patients with IMM that had the presence of one or more lytic bone lesions were found to have a short median time to progression of 8 to 10 months (3–5). A study on 101 patients with stage I asymptomatic MM out of a total of 695 consecutive, previously untreated patients with MM evaluated between October 1974 and October 1995 was reported (1). Patients with MGUS were excluded. Factors associated with disease progression included a serum M-protein > 3.0 g/dL, IgA heavy chain type, and Bence Jones protein excretion > 50 mg/24-hour urine collection. Patients with at least two of these risk factors (high risk) had a median time to disease progression of 17 months. In contrast, patients with none of the risk factors (low risk) had a median time to progression of 95 months. Patients with one risk factor (intermediate risk) had a median time to progression of 39 months and could be further subclassified based on magnetic resonance imaging (MRI) of the thoracic and lumbar spine. Patients with abnormal MRI imaging had significantly earlier disease progression (median 21 months) than those with a normal pattern (median 57 months) (1).

Other adverse factors in asymptomatic myeloma include an increase in the number of circulating plasma cells, IgA subtype, and urinary M-protein > 50 mg/day (1,54,57). A 50-gene panel that can distinguish "MGUS-like multiple myeloma" from "non–MGUS-like multiple myeloma" (35) has also been reported. Gene expression data may be useful in the differentiation of smoldering and indolent myeloma from active disease (35,111). The PCLI, a marker of myeloma cell growth, has been shown to be an important prognostic factor in several myeloma studies where patients with a high labeling index have a shortened overall survival and patients with asymptomatic myeloma have a reduced TTP (53,54,94,112,113). Using an IL-1 bioassay, we have shown that two groups of SMM/IMM patients may be distinguished; those with IL-1 levels > 1 similar to patients with active myeloma and those < 1 comparable to MGUS patients (70). This altered IL-1 production could possibly explain some of the previous differences seen in the subgroups of SMM patients and it generated the hypothesis that anti-IL-1 therapies may be useful in patients with SMM at risk for progression.

■ CLINICAL TRIALS IN SMM/IMM (ASYMPTOMATIC MM)

The current standard of care for patients with asymptomatic myeloma is observation. However many patients with SMM/IMM are uncomfortable with this approach due to the likelihood of progression and several clinical trials have now included these patients in an attempt to delay/prevent active MM. In an initial study of 29 patients with SMM/IMM treated with thalidomide alone, Kaplan-Meier estimates of PFS were 63% at 2 years (114). The use of zoledronic acid alone did not influence the natural history of asymptomatic myeloma. Randomizing patients between zoledronic acid versus observation it was shown that 44% of patients in the zoledronic acid group and 45% of the control group progressed requiring chemotherapy ($P = 0.93$) after a median follow-up of 64.7 person-months (115). A 7-year median time to progression with thalidomide for SMM was reported (116). The investigators conducted a phase 2 trial in 76 eligible patients with SMM, combining thalidomide (200 mg/day) with monthly pamidronate. Within 4 years, 63% improved including 25% qualifying for partial response; 34 patients had progressed and 17 required salvage therapy. Interestingly, attaining PR status was associated with a shorter time to salvage therapy for disease progression (116). No studies on myeloma cell growth were performed and it is possible that these responding patients were individuals with an elevated myeloma cell growth rate.

An interim analysis of a multicenter, randomized, open-label phase III trial of lenalidomide-dexamethasone (len/dex) versus therapeutic abstention in SMM at high risk of progression to symptomatic MM was recently reported (117). The high risk population was defined by the presence of BMPCs ≥ 10% and M-spike ≥ 3 g/dL or if only one criterion was present patients must have a proportion of aPCs/BMPCs by immunophenotyping > 95% plus immunoparesis. One hundred and twenty patients are planned to be recruited, and between Oct 2006 and June 2008, 80 patients were randomized. In the interim analysis, the first 40 patients were presented. According to base-line characteristics both groups were balanced. In an intent to treat analysis (n = 40), based on International Myeloma Working Group criteria, the overall response rate was 90% including 53% PR, 21% very good partial remission, 11% com-plete response (CR), and 5% sCR. After a median follow-up of 16 months no disease progression was observed in the len-dex arm while eight patients progressed to active myeloma in the therapeutic abstention arm with a median TTP from inclusion in the trial of 17.5 months ($P < 0.002$). Six of the eight patients developed bone lesions as a symptom of active MM. Serious adverse events occurred in five patients (gastrointestinal bleeding, delirium, glaucoma, and two infections). Three patients developed grade 3 deep venous thrombosis. These preliminary results may ultimately show that in SMM patients at high risk for progression to active MM, delayed treatment is associated with early progression with bone disease (117).

In a phase II trial using IL-1 receptor antag-onist (IL-1Ra) and low-dose dexamethasone, the median PFS for the 47 SMM/IMM patients treated in the trial was 3.1 years (118). IL-1Ra led to a decrease in both the high sensitivity-CRP (hs-CRP), a surrogate marker for plasma cell IL-6 levels, and correspondingly, the PCLI, a measure of the myeloma cell proliferative rate in responsive patients (118). Statistical analysis using a parti-tioning algorithm showed that the median PFS for patients without (n = 12) and with (n = 35) a ≥ 15% decrease in the baseline hs-CRP (compar-ing baseline and 6 month values) was 6 months and > 3 years, respectively ($P = 0.002$) (Figure 2). Patients with IMM were more likely to progress. Twenty percent of the 35 patients with a hs-CRP decrease presented with IMM whereas 50% of the 12 patients without a hs-CRP decrease had IMM. Stability of the M-protein also separated the two groups. The median PFS for patients with (n = 19) and without (n = 28) a ≥ 5% increase in the M-protein from baseline (comparing baseline and 6 month values) was 6 months and > 3 years, respectively ($P < 0.0001$) (118).

Myeloma cell resistance to dexamethasone-in-duced apoptosis is a well recognized in vitro and in vivo phenomenon. It occurs because of increased production of IL-6 in the myeloma microenviron-ment (72,119,120). The combination of IL-1Ra

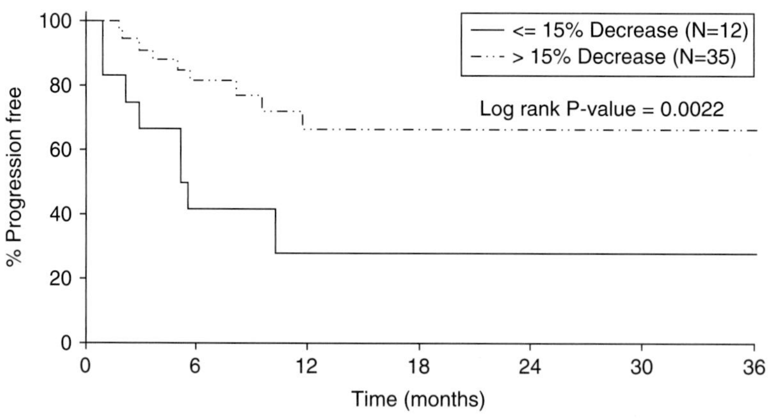

FIGURE 2

Progression-free survival (PFS). The median PFS for patients without (n = 12) and with (n = 35) a ≥ 15% de-crease in the baseline high sensitivity–C-reactive protein (hs-CRP) (comparing baseline and 6-month val-ues) was 6 months and > 3 years, respectively (P = 0.0022). Adapted from Ref. 118 with permission.

and dexamethasone minimized this problem because IL-1Ra was highly effective at inhibiting IL-6 production (Figure 3), and changed the tumor cell population back into an apoptosis-susceptible clone. The clinical trial results paralleled the in vitro findings in that there was little effect of the IL-1Ra alone on the M-protein because IL-1Ra does not induce myeloma cell apoptosis. The addition of dexamethasone synergized with the IL-1Ra by inducing myeloma cell apoptosis (Figure 3). Dexamethasone targeted the nonproliferating myeloma compartment that appeared to

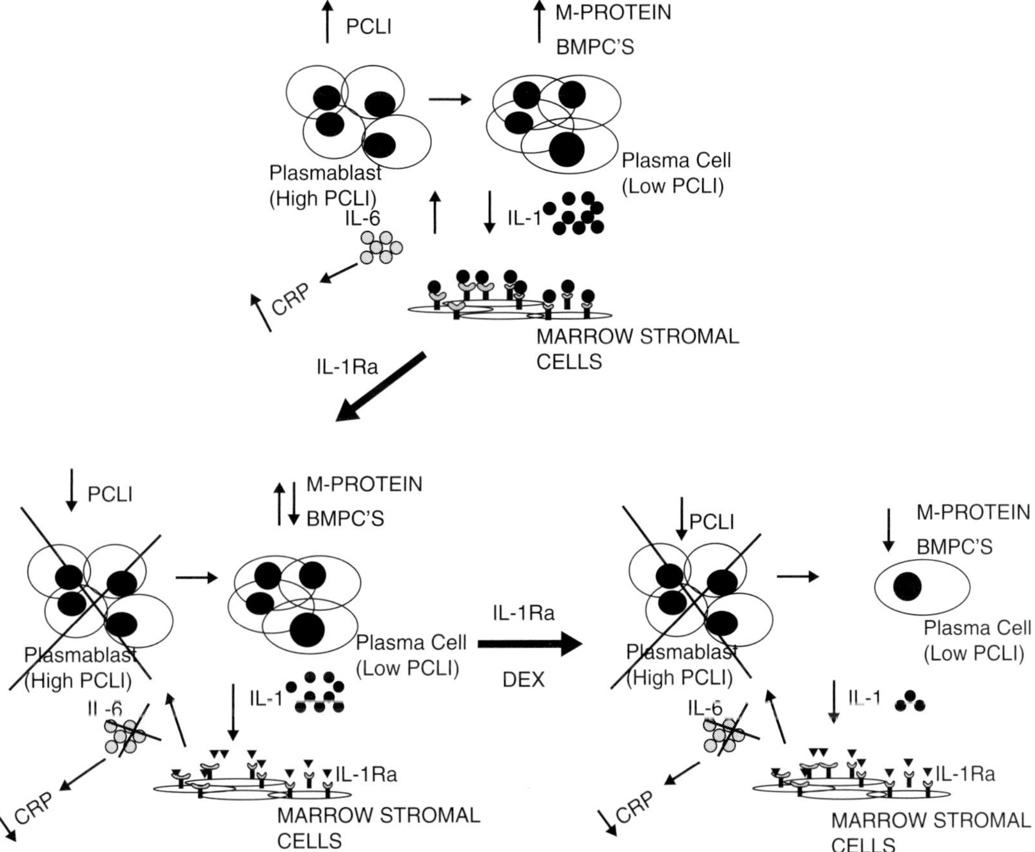

FIGURE 3

Schematic of the role of IL-1Ra and dexamethasone in the myeloma microenvironment. Bone marrow (BM) cells from patients with progressive SMM/IMM produce IL-1β that stimulates stromal cells to make IL-6 which can be monitored by the high sensitivity–C-reactive protein (hs-CRP) (upper panel). The IL-6 can then stimulate the growth of the proliferative myeloma component resulting in an elevated plasma cell labeling index (PCLI). IL-1Ra selectively targets the proliferative myeloma component resulting in a decrease in the hs-CRP and the PCLI. The proliferative component is crossed out (lower left) because it is not known whether these cells are induced into a nonproliferative state or eliminated. Dexamethasone complements IL-1Ra biologic activity by inducing myeloma cell apoptosis and decreasing the percentage of BM plasma cells (BMPCs), M-protein, and myeloma cell produced IL-1 levels (lower right). Adapted from Ref. 118 with permission.

be producing the IL-1 in addition to the secreted M-protein, while IL-1Ra reduced the elevated IL-6 levels in the microenvironment and inhibited the IL-6 responsive proliferating myeloma cell subset (Figure 3).

The IL-1Ra and dexamethasone induce a chronic disease state in responsive patients with SMM/IMM at high risk for progression. In responding patients, the PCLI and CRP have remained low, along with a stable M-protein. The goal of this study was to delay or prevent the development of active myeloma and therefore minor responses or the induction of stable disease are important in this disease group. Patients with low number of plasma cells may be controlled with IL-1Ra alone whereas patients with ≥ 20% plasma cells typically require the addition of dexamethasone. Targeting the myeloma proliferative component with IL-1Ra leads to a reduced growth rate of the proliferating plasma cells and potentially slows the acquisition of harmful genetic changes.

The in vitro biological studies and the in vivo clinical trial results demonstrate that it may be possible to delay/prevent progression to active myeloma in responsive patients by targeting the IL-1β–induced IL-6 production that stimulates the myeloma proliferative component. As previously noted, the importance of the PCLI as a prognostic factor has been reported in several myeloma studies where patients with a high labeling index have a shortened overall survival (53,54,94,112,113). The results from this trial may suggest that, in addition to the M-protein, it will be essential to monitor the proliferative myeloma population and utilize the hs-CRP to aid as predictors of progression. Currently, the M-protein is the major clinical parameter utilized as the measure of response for clinical trials and also for the selection of new therapeutic agents. Current therapies such as dexamethasone, thalidomide, Revlimid, and velcade are highly effective at targeting the monoclonal producing nonproliferative myeloma cell. However, their effect on the proliferative myeloma subset is less clear. It has been suggested that myeloma remains incurable because the stem cell/

proliferative component is not adequately targeted by current therapies (121). The IL-1Ra treatment study clearly separates the reponsiveness of the proliferative versus the nonproliferative components of this disease. It is also important to note that there is evidence to suggest that some of the newer therapies may be worsening the proliferative subset resulting in terminal disease with a high growth rate (122). Future myeloma therapies may need to employ agents that target both the IL-1β driven IL-6 responsive myeloma proliferative population as well as the IL-1β producing nonproliferative components. Targeting the proliferative myeloma component is likely to result in improved overall survival not only in patients with high risk SMM/IMM but also in patients with active disease. Of interest, the importance of the IL-1 model has been confirmed using a mathematical analysis between normal and malignant cells (123). Carefully weighing the risk versus benefits of any given treatment still needs to be evaluated within the SMM patient population given the wide range of progression (2–19 years) observed within this group.

■ CHRONIC INFLAMMATION AND CANCER: A POTENTIAL MECHANISM FOR THE PROGRESSION OF MGUS/SMM TO ACTIVE MM

There is a substantial body of literature that supports the hypothesis that chronic inflammation can predispose an individual to cancer (124–128). For example, chronic ulcerative colitis may predispose to colon cancer, hepatitis may lead to liver cancer, esophageal adenocarcinoma is associated with Barrett's esophagus, and chronic Helicobacter infection can lead to cancer of the stomach (125–128). Chronic pesticide exposure appears to result in an increased prevalence of MGUS (129). Inflammation can contribute to the development of neoplasia through the generation of reactive oxygen and nitrogen species resulting in DNA mutations and the production of inflammatory cytokines that can support and perpetuate these genetically altered cells (124,130).

Pristane can induce plasmacytomas in genetically susceptible BALB/c mice. The tumors develop in peritoneal granulomas and are characterized by *c-myc* activating t(12;15) chromosomal translocations and by secretion of IgA (59,131). Pristane induces a chronic inflammatory state leading to the production of IL-6 which has been shown to be critical for plasmacytomagenesis (59,62). Of interest, pristane can also induce rheumatoid arthritis (RA) in BALB/c mice and, in certain cases, both diseases may coexist in the same mouse (131). In humans, patients with RA often show polyclonal plasmacytosis on BM examination. RA patients have an increased risk of the development of both MGUS and MM (132–136). Agents such as prednisone, thalidomide, and anti-IL-6 monoclonal antibody therapies, which all have anti-inflammatory/anticytokine effects, have all been shown to have activity in both RA and MM (68,137–141). In the pristane mouse model, indomethacin can inhibit the development of plasmacytomas (142). The above observations suggest that chronic inflammation, typical of diseases such as RA, may play a dominant role in the pathogenesis of myeloma as well.

There are few publications in the myeloma literature that focus on the role of infectious agents in the pathogenesis of myeloma despite the fact that infection exacerbates the course of this disease (143). In one study of MGUS patients simultaneously infected with *Helicobacter pylori*, eradication of the *H pylori* with antibiotic therapy led to resolution of the monoclonal gammopathy in 28% of patients (144). The authors concluded that in a proportion of MGUS patients, *H pylori* may be implicated in the pathogenesis of the disease (144). However, these results have not been confirmed and there are no other reports on the role of specific infectious agents in myeloma.

Microorganisms share highly conserved structures called pathogen-associated molecular patterns (145). They are recognized by a family of receptors called Toll-like receptors (TLR) which are essential in host defense against infection (146,147). TLR are type I membrane proteins bearing a cytoplasmic Toll/IL-1R homology domain (147). Ten TLR and nine agonists have been characterized in humans. TLR1 and TLR2 are triggered by lipopeptides such as Pam3Cy5 (148), TLR3 by double-stranded RNA (149), TLR4 by lipopolysaccharide (150), TLR5 by flagellin (151), TLR7 and TLR8 by single-stranded RNA (152), and TLR9 by the unmethylated CpG DNA of bacteria (153). Human B cells express TLR 1,2,7,8,9, and 10 (154,155). In contrast, myeloma cells from patients with active disease express TLR 1,3,4,5,6,7,8,9 and TLR mediate proliferation of myeloma cells (156,157). However TLR expression on plasma cells from patients with MGUS and SMM has not been previously studied (158). MM is associated with immunosuppression and infection and a vicious cycle may ensue involving MM, suppression of B-cell responses, infection, and growth of MM.

Our previous studies on the role of IL-1β and IL-1 inhibitors suggest a potential mechanism for the progression of SMM/IMM to active myeloma. We have shown that two groups of SMM/IMM patients may be distinguished; those with IL-1 levels ≥ 1 similar to patients with active myeloma and those < 1 comparable to MGUS patients (70). Patients with high IL-1 levels can induce large amounts of IL-6 resulting in an elevated labeling index and CRP. These patients are at high risk for progression to active myeloma (54,70). This correlation with progression suggested that IL-1 inhibitors should be useful therapeutically. Indeed our clinical study demonstrates that IL-1Ra alone can inhibit paracrine IL-6 production as well as myeloma cell growth while dexamethasone decreases the M-protein levels and percent BMPCs. Dexamethasone lowers IL-1β production through myeloma cell apoptosis. The combination of these two agents induces a chronic disease state similar to patients with a less aggressive SMM that have a long PFS. It is notable that such patients usually do not show a decrease in their M-spike yet can have stable disease for years. One may speculate that these patients remain stable because they have low IL-1β levels or high endogenous levels of IL-1 receptor antagonist.

The etiology of the aberrant IL-1 production in the myeloma microenvironment is unclear however chronic inflammation may play an important role. After induction of a clonal initiating event (resulting in MGUS), chronic inflammation could lead to increased levels of IL-1 and IL-6 in the myeloma microenvironment resulting in myeloma cell growth and, if not adequately inhibited, eventual progression to active disease. The observation that a small group of young individuals exposed to the World Trade Center dust have developed active myeloma provides additional support for the importance of chronic inflammation in the pathogenesis of myeloma (159).

■ REFERENCES

1. Weber DM, Dimopoulos MA, Moulopoulos LA, Delasalle KB, Smith T, Alexanian R. Prognostic features of asymptomatic multiple myeloma. *Br J Haematol* 1997;97(4):810–814.
2. Kyle RA, Remstein ED, Therneau TM, et al. Clinical course and prognosis of smoldering (asymptomatic) multiple myeloma. *N Engl J Med* 2007;356(25): 2582–2590.
3. Dimopoulos MA, Moulopoulos A, Smith T, Delasalle KB, Alexanian R. Risk of disease progression in asymptomatic multiple myeloma. *Am J Med* 1993;94(1):57–61.
4. Facon T, Menard JF, Michaux JL, et al. Prognostic factors in low tumour mass asymptomatic multiple myeloma: a report on 91 patients. The Groupe d'Etudes et de Recherche sur le Myélome (GERM). *Am J Hematol* 1995;48(2):71–75.
5. Wisløff F, Andersen P, Andersson TR, et al. Incidence and follow-up of asymptomatic multiple myeloma. The myeloma project of health region I in Norway. II. *Eur J Haematol* 1991;47(5):338–341.
6. International Myeloma Working G. Criteria for the classification of monoclonal gammopathies, multiple myeloma and related disorders: a report of the International Myeloma Working Group. *Br J Haematol* 2003;121:749–757.
7. Kyle RA, Lust JA. Monoclonal gammopathies of undetermined significance. *Semin Hematol* 1989; 26(3):176–200.
8. Kyle RA, Greipp PR. Smoldering multiple myeloma. *N Engl J Med* 1980;302(24):1347–1349.
9. Landgren O, Kyle RA, Pfeiffer RM, et al. Monoclonal gammopathy of undetermined significance (MGUS) consistently precedes multiple myeloma: a prospective study. *Blood* 2009;113(22):5412–5417.
10. Weiss BM, Abadie J, Verma P, Howard RS, Kuehl WM. A monoclonal gammopathy precedes multiple myeloma in most patients. *Blood* 2009;113(22): 5418–5422.
11. Fonseca R, Coignet LJ, Dewald GW. Cytogenetic abnormalities in multiple myeloma. *Hematol Oncol Clin North Am* 1999;13(6):1169–1180, viii.
12. Hallek M, Bergsagel PL, Anderson KC. Multiple myeloma: increasing evidence for a multistep transformation process. *Blood* 1998;91(1):3–21.
13. Drach J, Schuster J, Nowotny H, et al. Multiple myeloma: high incidence of chromosomal aneuploidy as detected by interphase fluorescence in situ hybridization. *Cancer Res* 1995;55(17):3854–3859.
14. Flactif M, Zandecki M, Laï JL, et al. Interphase fluorescence in situ hybridization (FISH) as a powerful tool for the detection of aneuploidy in multiple myeloma. *Leukemia* 1995;9(12):2109–2114.
15. Dalton WS, Bergsagel PL, Kuehl WM, Anderson KC, Harousseau JL. Multiple myeloma. *Hematology Am Soc Hematol Educ Program* 2001;157–177.
16. Drach J, Angerler J, Schuster J, et al. Interphase fluorescence in situ hybridization identifies chromosomal abnormalities in plasma cells from patients with monoclonal gammopathy of undetermined significance. *Blood* 1995;86(10):3915–3921.
17. Avet-Loiseau H, Facon T, Daviet A, et al. 14q32 translocations and monosomy 13 observed in monoclonal gammopathy of undetermined significance delineate a multistep process for the oncogenesis of multiple myeloma. Intergroupe Francophone du Myélome. *Cancer Res* 1999;59(18):4546–4550.
18. Fonseca R, Ahmann GJ, Jalal SM, et al. Chromosomal abnormalities in systemic amyloidosis. *Br J Haematol* 1998;103(3):704–710.
19. Zojer N, Königsberg R, Ackermann J, et al. Deletion of 13q14 remains an independent adverse prognostic variable in multiple myeloma despite its frequent detection by interphase fluorescence in situ hybridization. *Blood* 2000;95(6):1925–1930.
20. Facon T, Avet-Loiseau H, Guillerm G, et al.; Intergroupe Francophone du Myélome. Chromosome 13 abnormalities identified by FISH analysis and serum beta2-microglobulin produce a powerful

myeloma staging system for patients receiving high-dose therapy. *Blood* 2001;97(6):1566–1571.

21. Fonseca R, Oken MM, Harrington D, et al. Deletions of chromosome 13 in multiple myeloma identified by interphase FISH usually denote large deletions of the q arm or monosomy. *Leukemia* 2001;15(6): 981–986.

22. Shaughnessy J, Barlogie B. Chromosome 13 deletion in myeloma. *Curr Top Microbiol Immunol* 1999;246:199–203.

23. Avet-Loiseau H, Li JY, Morineau N, et al. Monosomy 13 is associated with the transition of monoclonal gammopathy of undetermined significance to multiple myeloma. Intergroupe Francophone du Myélome. *Blood* 1999;94(8):2583–2589.

24. Königsberg R, Ackermann J, Kaufmann H, et al. Deletions of chromosome 13q in monoclonal gammopathy of undetermined significance. *Leukemia* 2000;14(11):1975–1979.

25. Bergsagel PL, Nardini E, Brents L, Chesi M, Kuehl WM. IgH translocations in multiple myeloma: a nearly universal event that rarely involves c-myc. *Curr Top Microbiol Immunol* 1997;224:283–287.

26. Chesi M, Kuehl WM, Bergsagel PL. Recurrent immunoglobulin gene translocations identify distinct molecular subtypes of myeloma. *Ann Oncol* 2000;11(suppl 1):131–135.

27. Kuehl WM, Bergsagel PL. Multiple myeloma: evolving genetic events and host interactions. *Nat Rev Cancer* 2002;2(3):175–187.

28. Bergsagel PL, Chesi M, Nardini E, Brents LA, Kirby SL, Kuehl WM. Promiscuous translocations into immunoglobulin heavy chain switch regions in multiple myeloma. *Proc Natl Acad Sci USA* 1996;93(24):13931–13936.

29. Chesi M, Nardini E, Brents LA, et al. Frequent translocation t(4;14)(p16.3;q32.3) in multiple myeloma is associated with increased expression and activating mutations of fibroblast growth factor receptor 3. *Nat Genet* 1997;16(3):260–264.

30. Liebisch P, Döhner H. Cytogenetics and molecular cytogenetics in multiple myeloma. *Eur J Cancer* 2006;42(11):1520–1529.

31. Ely S, Di Liberto M, Niesvizky R, et al. Mutually exclusive cyclin-dependent kinase 4/cyclin D1 and cyclin-dependent kinase 6/cyclin D2 pairing inactivates retinoblastoma protein and promotes cell cycle dysregulation in multiple myeloma. *Cancer Res* 2005;65(24):11345–11353.

32. Keats JJ, Reiman T, Belch AR, Pilarski LM. Ten years and counting: so what do we know about t(4;14)(p16;q32) multiple myeloma. *Leuk Lymphoma* 2006;47(11):2289–2300.

33. Zhan F, Hardin J, Kordsmeier B, et al. Global gene expression profiling of multiple myeloma, monoclonal gammopathy of undetermined significance, and normal bone marrow plasma cells. *Blood* 2002;99(5):1745–1757.

34. Davies FE, Dring AM, Li C, et al. The molecular basis of the transition of MGUS to multiple myeloma. *Blood* 2002;100:102a.

35. Zhan F, Barlogie B, Arzoumanian V, et al. Gene-expression signature of benign monoclonal gammopathy evident in multiple myeloma is linked to good prognosis. *Blood* 2007;109(4):1692–1700.

36. Rasmussen T, Kuehl M, Lodahl M, Johnsen HE, Dahl IM. Possible roles for activating RAS mutations in the MGUS to MM transition and in the intramedullary to extramedullary transition in some plasma cell tumors. *Blood* 2005;105(1):317–323.

37. Liu P, Leong T, Quam L, et al. Activating mutations of N- and K-ras in multiple myeloma show different clinical associations: analysis of the Eastern Cooperative Oncology Group Phase III Trial. *Blood* 1996;88(7):2699–2706.

38. Bezieau S, Devilder MC, Avet-Loiseau H, et al. High incidence of N and K-Ras activating mutations in multiple myeloma and primary plasma cell leukemia at diagnosis. *Hum Mutat* 2001;18(3):212–224.

39. Chng WJ, Gonzalez-Paz N, Price-Troska T, et al. Clinical and biological significance of RAS mutations in multiple myeloma. *Leukemia* 2008;22(12): 2280–2284.

40. González M, Mateos MV, García-Sanz R, et al. De novo methylation of tumor suppressor gene p16/INK4a is a frequent finding in multiple myeloma patients at diagnosis. *Leukemia* 2000;14(1): 183–187.

41. Mateos MV, García-Sanz R, López-Pérez R, et al. Methylation is an inactivating mechanism of the p16 gene in multiple myeloma associated with high plasma cell proliferation and short survival. *Br J Haematol* 2002;118(4):1034–1040.

42. Dhodapkar M, Grill J, Lust JA. Abnormal regional hypermethylation of the calcitonin gene in myelodysplastic syndromes. *Leuk Res* 1995;19(10):719–726.

43. Van Riet I, Van Camp B. The involvement of adhesion molecules in the biology of multiple myeloma. *Leuk Lymphoma* 1993;9(6):441–452.

44. Helfrich MH, Livingston E, Franklin IM, Soutar RL. Expression of adhesion molecules in malignant plasma cells in multiple myeloma: comparison with

normal plasma cells and functional significance. *Blood Rev* 1997;11(1):28–38.

45. Kim I, Uchiyama H, Chauhan D, Anderson KC. Cell surface expression and functional significance of adhesion molecules on human myeloma-derived cell lines. *Br J Haematol* 1994;87(3):483–493.

46. Lokhorst HM, Lamme T, de Smet M, et al. Primary tumor cells of myeloma patients induce interleukin-6 secretion in long-term bone marrow cultures. *Blood* 1994;84(7):2269–2277.

47. Uchiyama H, Barut BA, Mohrbacher AF, Chauhan D, Anderson KC. Adhesion of human myeloma-derived cell lines to bone marrow stromal cells stimulates interleukin-6 secretion. *Blood* 1993;82(12):3712–3720.

48. Carter A, Merchav S, Silvian-Draxler I, Tatarsky I. The role of interleukin-1 and tumour necrosis factor-alpha in human multiple myeloma. *Br J Haematol* 1990;74(4):424–431.

49. Chauhan D, Uchiyama H, Akbarali Y, et al. Multiple myeloma cell adhesion-induced interleukin-6 expression in bone marrow stromal cells involves activation of NF-kappa B. *Blood* 1996;87(3):1104–1112.

50. Van Camp B, Durie BG, Spier C, et al. Plasma cells in multiple myeloma express a natural killer cell-associated antigen: CD56 (NKH-1; Leu-19). *Blood* 1990;76(2):377–382.

51. Sonneveld P, Durie BG, Lokhorst HM, Frutiger Y, Schoester M, Vela EE. Analysis of multidrug-resistance (MDR-1) glycoprotein and CD56 expression to separate monoclonal gammopathy from multiple myeloma. *Br J Haematol* 1993;83(1):63–67.

52. Harada H, Kawano MM, Huang N, et al. Phenotypic difference of normal plasma cells from mature myeloma cells. *Blood* 1993;81(10):2658–2663.

53. Greipp PR, Witzig TE, Gonchoroff NJ, et al. Immunofluorescence labeling indices in myeloma and related monoclonal gammopathies. *Mayo Clin Proc* 1987;62(11):969–977.

54. Greipp PR, Kyle RA. Clinical, morphological, and cell kinetic differences among multiple myeloma, monoclonal gammopathy of undetermined significance, and smoldering multiple myeloma. *Blood* 1983;62(1):166–171.

55. Witzig TE, Gonchoroff NJ, Katzmann JA, Therneau TM, Kyle RA, Greipp PR. Peripheral blood B cell labeling indices are a measure of disease activity in patients with monoclonal gammopathies. *J Clin Oncol* 1988;6(6):1041–1046.

56. Witzig TE, Kyle RA, Greipp PR. Circulating peripheral blood plasma cells in multiple myeloma. *Curr Top Microbiol Immunol* 1992;182:195–199.

57. Witzig TE, Kyle RA, O'Fallon WM, Greipp PR. Detection of peripheral blood plasma cells as a predictor of disease course in patients with smouldering multiple myeloma. *Br J Haematol* 1994;87(2):266–272.

58. Potter M, Sklar MD, Rowe WP. Rapid viral induction of plasmacytomas in pristane-primed BALB-c mice. *Science* 1973;182(112):592–594.

59. Potter M. Perspectives on the origins of multiple myeloma and plasmacytomas in mice. *Hematol Oncol Clin North Am* 1992;6(2):211–223.

60. Suematsu S, Matsuda T, Aozasa K, et al. IgG1 plasmacytosis in interleukin 6 transgenic mice. *Proc Natl Acad Sci USA* 1989;86(19):7547–7551.

61. Suematsu S, Matsusaka T, Matsuda T, et al. Generation of plasmacytomas with the chromosomal translocation t(12;15) in interleukin 6 transgenic mice. *Proc Natl Acad Sci USA* 1992;89(1):232–235.

62. Hilbert DM, Kopf M, Mock BA, Köhler G, Rudikoff S. Interleukin 6 is essential for *in vivo* development of B lineage neoplasms. *J Exp Med* 1995;182(1):243–248.

63. Kawano M, Hirano T, Matsuda T, et al. Autocrine generation and requirement of BSF-2/IL-6 for human multiple myelomas. *Nature* 1988;332(6159):83–85.

64. Schwab G, Siegall CB, Aarden LA, Neckers LM, Nordan RP. Characterization of an interleukin-6-mediated autocrine growth loop in the human multiple myeloma cell line, U266. *Blood* 1991;77(3):587–593.

65. Bataille R, Jourdan M, Zhang XG, Klein B. Serum levels of interleukin 6, a potent myeloma cell growth factor, as a reflect of disease severity in plasma cell dyscrasias. *J Clin Invest* 1989;84(6):2008–2011.

66. Donovan KA, Lacy MQ, Kline MP, et al. Contrast in cytokine expression between patients with monoclonal gammopathy of undetermined significance or multiple myeloma. *Leukemia* 1998;12(4):593–600.

67. Zhang XG, Klein B, Bataille R. Interleukin-6 is a potent myeloma-cell growth factor in patients with aggressive multiple myeloma. *Blood* 1989;74(1):11–13.

68. Bataille R, Barlogie B, Lu ZY, et al. Biologic effects of anti-interleukin-6 murine monoclonal antibody in advanced multiple myeloma. *Blood* 1995;86(2):685–691.

69. Rawstron AC, Fenton JA, Ashcroft J, et al. The interleukin-6 receptor alpha-chain (CD126) is expressed by neoplastic but not normal plasma cells. *Blood* 2000;96(12):3880–3886.

70. Xiong Y, Donovan KA, Kline MP, et al. Identification of two groups of smoldering multiple myeloma patients who are either high or low producers of interleukin-1. *J Interferon Cytokine Res* 2006;26(2):83–95.

71. Dinarello CA. Biologic basis for interleukin-1 in disease. *Blood* 1996;87(6):2095–2147.

72. Grigorieva I, Thomas X, Epstein J. The bone marrow stromal environment is a major factor in myeloma cell resistance to dexamethasone. *Exp Hematol* 1998;26(7):597–603.

73. Lichtenstein A, Tu Y, Fady C, Vescio R, Berenson J. Interleukin-6 inhibits apoptosis of malignant plasma cells. *Cell Immunol* 1995;162(2):248–255.

74. Muraguchi A, Hirano T, Tang B, et al. The essential role of B cell stimulatory factor 2 (BSF-2/IL-6) for the terminal differentiation of B cells. *J Exp Med* 1988;167(2):332–344.

75. Jego G, Bataille R, Pellat-Deceunynck C. Interleukin-6 is a growth factor for nonmalignant human plasmablasts. *Blood* 2001;97(6):1817–1822.

76. Kishimoto T, Akira S, Taga T. Interleukin-6 and its receptor: a paradigm for cytokines. *Science* 1992;258(5082):593–597.

77. Hirano T, Matsuda T, Nakajima K. Signal transduction through gp130 that is shared among the receptors for the interleukin 6 related cytokine subfamily. *Stem Cells* 1994;12(3):262–277.

78. Westendorf JJ, Jelinek DF. Growth regulatory pathways in myeloma. Evidence for autocrine oncostatin M expression. *J Immunol* 1996;157(7):3081–3088.

79. Zhang XG, Gu JJ, Lu ZY, et al. Ciliary neurotropic factor, interleukin 11, leukemia inhibitory factor, and oncostatin M are growth factors for human myeloma cell lines using the interleukin 6 signal transducer gp130. *J Exp Med* 1994;179(4):1337–1342.

80. Lu ZY, Zhang XG, Rodriguez C, et al. Interleukin-10 is a proliferation factor but not a differentiation factor for human myeloma cells. *Blood* 1995;85(9):2521–2527.

81. Börset M, Hjorth-Hansen H, Seidel C, Sundan A, Waage A. Hepatocyte growth factor and its receptor c-met in multiple myeloma. *Blood* 1996;88(10):3998–4004.

82. Freund GG, Kulas DT, Mooney RA. Insulin and IGF-1 increase mitogenesis and glucose metabolism in the multiple myeloma cell line, RPMI 8226. *J Immunol* 1993;151(4):1811–1820.

83. Dankbar B, Padró T, Leo R, et al. Vascular endothelial growth factor and interleukin-6 in paracrine tumor-stromal cell interactions in multiple myeloma. *Blood* 2000;95(8):2630–2636.

84. Anderson KC, Jones RM, Morimoto C, Leavitt P, Barut BA. Response patterns of purified myeloma cells to hematopoietic growth factors. *Blood* 1989;73(7):1915–1924.

85. Folkman J. Angiogenesis-dependent diseases. *Semin Oncol.* 2001;28(6):536–542.

86. Rajkumar SV, Kyle RA. Angiogenesis in multiple myeloma. *Semin Oncol* 2001;28(6):560–564.

87. Kline M, Donovan K, Wellik L, et al. Cytokine and chemokine profiles in multiple myeloma; significance of stromal interaction and correlation of IL-8 production with disease progression. *Leuk Res* 2007;31(5):591–598.

88. Rajkumar SV, Witzig TE. A review of angiogenesis and antiangiogenic therapy with thalidomide in multiple myeloma. *Cancer Treat Rev* 2000;26(5):351–362.

89. Rajkumar SV, Fonseca R, Witzig TE, Gertz MA, Greipp PR. Bone marrow angiogenesis in patients achieving complete response after stem cell transplantation for multiple myeloma. *Leukemia* 1999;13(3):469–472.

90. Rajkumar SV, Leong T, Roche PC, et al. Prognostic value of bone marrow angiogenesis in multiple myeloma. *Clin Cancer Res* 2000;6(8):3111–3116.

91. Rajkumar SV, Greipp PR. Angiogenesis in multiple myeloma. *Br J Haematol* 2001;113(3):565.

92. Rajkumar SV, Mesa RA, Fonseca R, et al. Bone marrow angiogenesis in 400 patients with monoclonal gammopathy of undetermined significance, multiple myeloma, and primary amyloidosis. *Clin Cancer Res* 2002;8(7):2210–2216.

93. Vacca A, Ribatti D, Roncali L, et al. Bone marrow angiogenesis and progression in multiple myeloma. *Br J Haematol* 1994;87(3):503–508.

94. Greipp PR, Lust JA, O'Fallon WM, Katzmann JA, Witzig TE, Kyle RA. Plasma cell labeling index and beta 2-microglobulin predict survival independent of thymidine kinase and C reactive protein in multiple myeloma. *Blood* 1993;81(12):3382–3387.

95. Lacy MQ, Donovan KA, Heimbach JK, Ahmann GJ, Lust JA. Comparison of interleukin-1 beta expression by in situ hybridization in monoclonal gammopathy of undetermined significance and multiple myeloma. *Blood* 1999;93(1):300–305.

96. Collins T, Read MA, Neish AS, Whitley MZ, Thanos D, Maniatis T. Transcriptional regulation of endothelial cell adhesion molecules: NF-kappa B and cytokine-inducible enhancers. *FASEB J* 1995;9(10):899–909.

97. Dustin ML, Rothlein R, Bhan AK, Dinarello CA, Springer TA. Induction by IL 1 and interferon-gamma: tissue distribution, biochemistry, and function of a natural adherence molecule (ICAM-1). *J Immunol* 1986;137(1):245–254.

98. Terry RW, Kwee L, Levine JF, Labow MA. Cytokine induction of an alternatively spliced murine vascular cell adhesion molecule (VCAM) mRNA encoding a glycosylphosphatidylinositol-anchored VCAM protein. *Proc Natl Acad Sci USA* 1993;90(13):5919–5923.

99. Torcia M, Lucibello M, Vannier E, et al. Modulation of osteoclast-activating factor activity of multiple myeloma bone marrow cells by different interleukin-1 inhibitors. *Exp Hematol* 1996;24(8):868–874.

100. Yamamoto I, Kawano M, Sone T, et al. Production of interleukin 1 beta, a potent bone resorbing cytokine, by cultured human myeloma cells. *Cancer Res* 1989;49(15):4242–4246.

101. Lust JA, Donovan KA. The role of interleukin-1 beta in the pathogenesis of multiple myeloma. *Hematol Oncol Clin North Am* 1999;13(6):1117–1125.

102. Klein B, Lu ZY, Gaillard JP, Harousseau JL, Bataille R. Inhibiting IL-6 in human multiple myeloma. *Curr Top Microbiol Immunol* 1992;182:237–244.

103. Costes V, Portier M, Lu ZY, Rossi JF, Bataille R, Klein B. Interleukin-1 in multiple myeloma: producer cells and their role in the control of IL-6 production. *Br J Haematol* 1998;103(4):1152–1160.

104. Nagata K, Tanaka Y, Oda S, Yamashita U, Eto S. Interleukin 1 autocrine growth system in human multiple myeloma. *Jpn J Clin Oncol* 1991;21(1):22–29.

105. Hawley TS, Lach B, Burns BF, May LT, Sehgal PB, Hawley RG. Expression of retrovirally transduced IL-1 alpha in IL-6-dependent B cells: a murine model of aggressive multiple myeloma. *Growth Factors* 1991;5(4):327–338.

106. Hawley RG, Wang MH, Fong AZ, Hawley TS. Association between ICAM-1 expression and metastatic capacity of murine B-cell hybridomas. *Clin Exp Metastasis* 1993;11(2):213–226.

107. Dispenzieri A, Kyle RA, Katzmann JA, et al. Immunoglobulin free light chain ratio is an independent risk factor for progression of smoldering (asymptomatic) multiple myeloma. *Blood* 2008;111(2):785–789.

108. Pérez-Persona E, Vidriales MB, Mateo G, et al. New criteria to identify risk of progression in monoclonal gammopathy of uncertain significance and smoldering multiple myeloma based on multiparameter flow cytometry analysis of bone marrow plasma cells. *Blood* 2007;110(7):2586–2592.

109. Rosiñol L, Bladé J, Esteve J, et al. Smoldering multiple myeloma: natural history and recognition of an evolving type. *Br J Haematol* 2003;123(4):631–636.

110. Rosiñol L, Carrió A, Bladé J, et al. Comparative genomic hybridisation identifies two variants of smoldering multiple myeloma. *Br J Haematol* 2005;130(5):729–732.

111. Zhan F, Huang Y, Colla S, et al. The molecular classification of multiple myeloma. *Blood* 2006;108(6):2020–2028.

112. Greipp PR, Katzmann JA, O'Fallon WM, Kyle RA. Value of beta 2-microglobulin level and plasma cell labeling indices as prognostic factors in patients with newly diagnosed myeloma. *Blood* 1988;72(1):219–223.

113. Greipp PR, Lust JA. Pathogenetic relation between monoclonal gammopathies of undetermined significance and multiple myeloma. *Stem Cells* 1995;13 (suppl 2):10–21.

114. Rajkumar SV, Gertz MA, Lacy MQ, et al. Thalidomide as initial therapy for early-stage myeloma. *Leukemia* 2003;17(4):775–779.

115. Musto P. The role of bisphosphonates for the treatment of bone disease in multiple myeloma. *Leuk Lymphoma* 1998;31(5–6):453–462.

116. Barlogie B, van Rhee F, Shaughnessy JD Jr, et al. Seven-year median time to progression with thalidomide for smoldering myeloma: partial response identifies subset requiring earlier salvage therapy for symptomatic disease. *Blood* 2008;112(8):3122–3125.

117. Mateos M-V, Lopez-Corral L, Hernandez MT, et al. Multicenter, randomized, open-label, phase III trial of lenalidomide-dexamethasone (len/dex) vs therapeutic abstention in smoldering multiple myeloma at high risk of progression to symptomatic MM: results of the first interim analysis. ASH Annual Meeting Abstracts. *Blood* 2009;114:254.

118. Lust JA, Lacy MQ, Zeldenrust SR, et al. Induction of a chronic disease state in patients with smoldering or indolent multiple myeloma by targeting interleukin 1{beta}-induced interleukin 6 production and the myeloma proliferative component. *Mayo Clin Proc* 2009;84(2):114–122.

119. Hardin J, MacLeod S, Grigorieva I, et al. Interleukin-6 prevents dexamethasone-induced myeloma cell death. *Blood* 1994;84(9):3063–3070.

120. Rowley M, Liu P, Van Ness B. Heterogeneity in therapeutic response of genetically altered myeloma cell lines to interleukin 6, dexamethasone, doxorubicin, and melphalan. *Blood* 2000;96(9):3175–3180.

121. Huff CA, Matsui W, Smith BD, Jones RJ. The paradox of response and survival in cancer therapeutics. *Blood* 2006;107(2):431–434.

122. Balleari E, Ghio R, Falcone A, Musto P. Possible multiple myeloma dedifferentiation following thalidomide therapy: a report of four cases. *Leuk Lymphoma* 2004;45(4):735–738.

123. Dingli D, Chalub FA, Santos FC, Van Segbroeck S, Pacheco JM. Cancer phenotype as the outcome of an evolutionary game between normal and malignant cells. *Br J Cancer* 2009;101(7):1130–1136.

124. Shacter E, Weitzman SA. Chronic inflammation and cancer. *Oncology (Williston Park, NY)* 2002;16(2):217–226, 229; discussion 230.

125. Correa P. Helicobacter pylori as a pathogen and carcinogen. *J Physiol Pharmacol* 1997;48 (suppl 4)19–24.

126. Choi PM, Zelig MP. Similarity of colorectal cancer in Crohn's disease and ulcerative colitis: implications for carcinogenesis and prevention. *Gut* 1994;35(7):950–954.

127. Hayashi PH, Zeldis JB. Molecular biology of viral hepatitis and hepatocellular carcinoma. *Compr Ther* 1993;19(5):188–196.

128. Pera M, Trastek VF, Pairolero PC, Cardesa A, Allen MS, Deschamps C. Barrett's disease: pathophysiology of metaplasia and adenocarcinoma. *Ann Thorac Surg* 1993;56(5):1191–1197.

129. Landgren O, Kyle RA, Hoppin JA, et al. Pesticide exposure and risk of monoclonal gammopathy of undetermined significance in the Agricultural Health Study. *Blood* 2009;113(25):6386–6391.

130. Miwa H, Kanno H, Munakata S, Akano Y, Taniwaki M, Aozasa K. Induction of chromosomal aberrations and growth-transformation of lymphoblastoid cell lines by inhibition of reactive oxygen species-induced apoptosis with interleukin-6. *Lab Invest* 2000;80(5):725–734.

131. Potter M, Wax JS. Genetics of susceptibility to pristane-induced plasmacytomas in BALB/cAn: reduced susceptibility in BALB/cJ with a brief description of pristane-induced arthritis. *J Immunol* 1981;127(4):1591–1595.

132. Bataille R, Robinet-Levy M, Barchechath-Flaisler F, Peres S, Aznar R, Sany J. Immunofixation improves the detection of monoclonal gammopathy of undetermined significance (M.G.U.S.) in patients with rheumatoid arthritis. *Clin Exp Rheumatol* 1987;5(3):259–261.

133. Eriksson M. Rheumatoid arthritis as a risk factor for multiple myeloma: a case-control study. *Eur J Cancer* 1993;29A(2):259–263.

134. Matteson EL, Hickey AR, Maguire L, Tilson HH, Urowitz MB. Occurrence of neoplasia in patients with rheumatoid arthritis enrolled in a DMARD Registry. Rheumatoid Arthritis Azathioprine Registry Steering Committee. *J Rheumatol* 1991; 18(6):809–814.

135. Kelly C, Baird G, Foster H, Hosker H, Griffiths I. Prognostic significance of paraproteinaemia in rheumatoid arthritis. *Ann Rheum Dis* 1991;50(5): 290–294.

136. Linet MS, Mclaughlin JK, Harlow SD, Fraumeni JF. Family history of autoimmune disorders and cancer in multiple myeloma. *Int J Epidemiol* 1988;17(3):512–513.

137. Lehman TJ, Striegel KH, Onel KB. Thalidomide therapy for recalcitrant systemic onset juvenile rheumatoid arthritis. *J Pediatr* 2002;140(1):125–127.

138. Scoville CD. Pilot study using the combination of methotrexate and thalidomide in the treatment of rheumatoid arthritis. *Clin Exp Rheumatol* 2001;19(3):360–361.

139. Wendling D, Racadot E, Wijdenes J. Treatment of severe rheumatoid arthritis by anti-interleukin 6 monoclonal antibody. *J Rheumatol* 1993;20(2): 259–262.

140. Singhal S, Mehta J, Desikan R, et al. Antitumor activity of thalidomide in refractory multiple myeloma. *N Engl J Med* 1999;341(21):1565–1571.

141. Kyle RA. Diagnosis and management of multiple myeloma and related disorders. *Prog Hematol* 1986;14:257–282.

142. Potter M, Wax JS, Anderson AO, Nordan RP. Inhibition of plasmacytoma development in BALB/c mice by indomethacin. *J Exp Med* 1985;161(5). 996–1012.

143. Kyle RA, Elveback LR. Management and prognosis of multiple myeloma. *Mayo Clin Proc* 1976;51(12):751–760.

144. Malik AA, Ganti AK, Potti A, Levitt R, Hanley JF. Role of Helicobacter pylori infection in the incidence and clinical course of monoclonal gammopathy of undetermined significance. *Am J Gastroenterol* 2002;97(6):1371–1374.

145. Pétrilli V, Dostert C, Muruve DA, Tschopp J. The inflammasome: a danger sensing complex triggering innate immunity. *Curr Opin Immunol* 2007; 19(6):615–622.

146. Wolska A, Lech-Maranda E, Robak T. Toll-like receptors and their role in carcinogenesis and antitumor treatment. *Cell Mol Biol Lett* 2009;14(2): 248–272.

147. Beutler BA. TLRs and innate immunity. *Blood* 2009;113(7):1399–1407.

148. Manukyan M, Triantafilou K, Triantafilou M, et al. Binding of lipopeptide to CD14 induces physical proximity of CD14, TLR2 and TLR1. *Eur J Immunol* 2005;35(3):911–921.

149. Alexopoulou L, Holt AC, Medzhitov R, Flavell RA. Recognition of double-stranded RNA and activation of NF-kappaB by Toll-like receptor 3. *Nature* 2001;413(6857):732–738.

150. Poltorak A, He X, Smirnova I, et al. Defective LPS signaling in C3H/HeJ and C57BL/10ScCr mice: mutations in Tlr4 gene. *Science* 1998;282(5396): 2085–2088.

151. Hayashi F, Smith KD, Ozinsky A, et al. The innate immune response to bacterial flagellin is mediated by Toll-like receptor 5. *Nature* 2001;410 (6832):1099–1103.

152. Heil F, Hemmi H, Hochrein H, et al. Species-specific recognition of single-stranded RNA via toll-like receptor 7 and 8. *Science* 2004;303(5663): 1526–1529.

153. Hemmi H, Takeuchi O, Kawai T, et al. A Toll-like receptor recognizes bacterial DNA. *Nature* 2000;408(6813):740–745.

154. Bernasconi NL, Onai N, Lanzavecchia A. A role for Toll-like receptors in acquired immunity: up-regulation of TLR9 by BCR triggering in naive B cells and constitutive expression in memory B cells. *Blood* 2003;101(11):4500–4504.

155. Bourke E, Bosisio D, Golay J, Polentarutti N, Mantovani A. The toll-like receptor repertoire of human B lymphocytes: inducible and selective expression of TLR9 and TLR10 in normal and transformed cells. *Blood* 2003;102(3):956–963.

156. Jego G, Bataille R, Geffroy-Luseau A, Descamps G, Pellat-Deceunynck C. Pathogen-associated molecular patterns are growth and survival factors for human myeloma cells through Toll-like receptors. *Leukemia* 2006;20(6):1130–1137.

157. Bohnhorst J, Rasmussen T, Moen SH, et al. Toll-like receptors mediate proliferation and survival of multiple myeloma cells. *Leukemia* 2006;20(6): 1138–1144.

158. Mantovani A, Garlanda C. Inflammation and multiple myeloma: the Toll connection. *Leukemia* 2006;20(6):937–938.

159. Samet JM, Geyh AS, Utell MJ. The legacy of World Trade Center dust. *N Engl J Med* 2007;356(22):2233–2236.

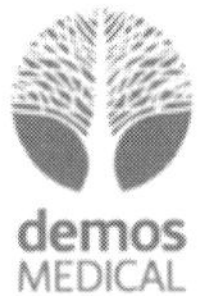 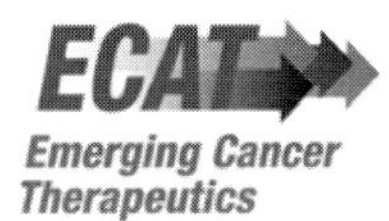

Laboratory Evaluation and Diagnosis of Monoclonal Gammopathies

Amrita Krishnan* and Myo Htut

City of Hope Medical Center, Duarte, CA

■ ABSTRACT

Multiple myeloma (MM) is characterized by a clonal proliferation of malignant plasma cells that are capable of producing immunoglobulin products of various combinations of both heavy chains and light chains. Patients with MM may produce light chains alone or rarely heavy chains alone. Demonstration of the monoclonal protein (M protein) in serum and/or urine is essential for screening and confirmation of plasma cell dyscrasia. Serum protein electrophoresis (SPEP) can detect the M protein in a majority of patients with MM. SPEP is based on the M protein's ability to migrate in an electrical field to a particular location that produces discrete band on agarose gel. Immunofixation (IFE) differentiates M protein from polyclonal protein, and it can detect smaller amount of M protein. IFE is based on reaction of different heavy and light chain antibodies to the sample that has undergone electrophoresis. The serum free light chain assay provides greater sensitivity than SPEP and IFE. It is particularly useful in light chain only plasma cell disorders such as AL amyloidosis (light chain-associated amyloid) or MM with low expression of M protein not readily detectable by SPEP and IFE. Bone marrow (BM) plasmacytosis is also a diagnostic criteria for MM. Immunostaining for light chains, heavy chains, and CD138 can document presence of clonal plasma cells in BM. Multicentric flow cytometry using CD38, 138, and 56 and other markers may also help to confirm the presence of clonal malignant plasma cells for diagnosis as well as detection of minimal residual disease in MM. Plasma cell disorders may include the following: Monoclonal gammopathy of unknown significance (MGUS) is a plasma cell disorder that can progress to MM or another malignant disease at about 1% per year at a steady rate. MGUS is associated with the absence of end-organ dysfunctions attributable to myeloma (anemia, hypercalcaemia, lytic bone lesions, and renal failure), BM plasmacytosis (<10%), and

---

*Corresponding author, City of Hope Medical Center, 1500E Duarte Road, Duarte, CA 91010
E-mail address: akrishnan@coh.org

Emerging Cancer Therapeutics 1:2 (2010) 283–298.
© 2010 Demos Medical Publishing LLC. All rights reserved.
DOI: 10.5003/2151–4194.1.2.283

demosmedpub.com/ecat

low levels of M protein (<3 g/dL). Risk of progression to MM is high if a patient with MGUS has an abnormal free light chain ratio, non-IgG subtype, and higher serum M spike (>1.5 g/dL). These risk factors will identify high-risk patients who need closer monitoring. Smoldering myeloma is also called asymptomatic MM. It is associated with an M protein 3 g/dL or higher and/or 10% or more BM clonal plasma cells without any end-organ damage related to plasma cell dyscrasia. The risk of progression to symptomatic MM from smoldering myeloma is approximately 10% per year in the first 5 years and 3% per year in the next 5 years and then down to 1% per year subsequently. So far, preemptive treatment for both MGUS and smoldering MM does not seem to improve overall survival.

The clinical presentation of myeloma may be diverse, but commonly patients have symptomatic bone or back pain and fatigue. Common laboratory findings that raise the index of suspicion of the diagnosis of myeloma include anemia, renal insufficiency, high calcium, or an elevated total protein. Any of these findings, especially in an older patient, should prompt further evaluation for the diagnosis of multiple myeloma (MM).

The presence of a monoclonal protein (M protein) in the serum or urine is one of the major criteria for diagnosis of MM. It can be detected by serum protein electrophoresis (SPEP) and/or urine protein electrophoresis (UPEP). SPEP can detect an M band or peak in 82% of patients with myeloma. Sensitivity is enhanced up to 93% if serum protein immunofixation (IFE) is added and further increased up to 97% if UPEP and IFE are done.

The malignant plasma cells can produce intact immunoglobulin (heavy chain plus light chain), light chains alone, or any with the following frequencies (1):

1. IgG—52%,
2. IgA—21%,
3. κ or λ light chain only (Bence Jones)—16%,
4. IgD—2%,
5. Biclonal—2%,
6. IgM—0.5%,
7. Negative—6.5%.

■ SERUM PROTEIN ELECTROPHORESIS

The principle of SPEP is that proteins migrate in an electrical field depending on their electrical charges. The M protein migrates to a particular location that produces a dense discrete band on the agarose gel. It also creates a narrow spike in the densitometric tracing (Figure 1).

Monoclonal immunoglobulins mainly appear in γ region but then may also be found in β globulin area. In the case of polyclonal increase of immunoglobulin, it will produce broad peaks or wide bands.

Pitfalls

A small M protein may not be visible or may be concealed by normal components. In IgD myeloma, the monoclonal peak is small and may also be overlooked. Therefore, it is prudent to do IFE whenever a plasma cell dyscrasia is suspected.

In about 20% of patients, the myeloma is characterized by only light chains in serum or urine without immunoglobulin heavy chain expression. These light chains can be detected by UPEP or urine IFE or serum free light testing, which will be discussed later.

A small percentage (approximately 3%) of patients with MM have no M protein in either serum or urine on IFE. Of these nonsecretory myelomas, a majority will have M protein in the cytoplasm of plasma cells identified by immunochemistry, but they are unable to secrete M protein (i.e., nonsecretory myeloma). A small minority do not have immunoglobulin detectable in malignant plasma cells, and they are labeled as "nonproducer myeloma." Ma et al. (2) reported a case of a nonproducer myeloma patient who presented with bone pain, anemia,

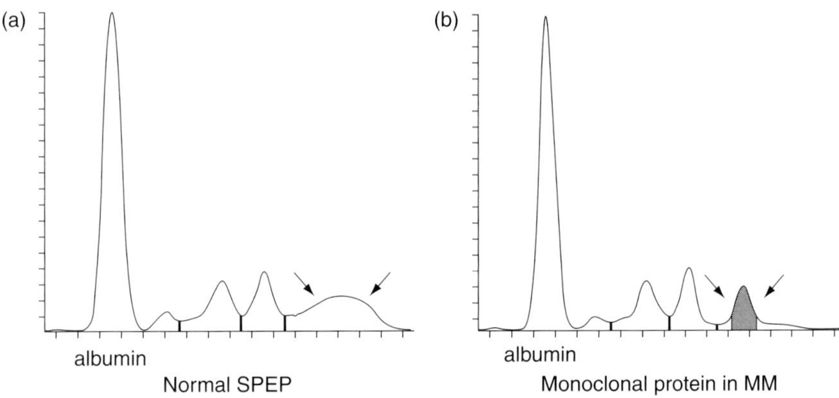

FIGURE 1

Monoclonal pattern on serum protein electrophoresis (SPEP). A dense, localized band (shaded area) representing a monoclonal protein of γ mobility is seen on SPEP. Densitometer tracing shows a narrow-based peak (shaded area) of γ mobility (B) and a reduction in the normal polyclonal γ band (solid arrows). Courtesy of Bernard R. Tegtmeier, PhD, City of Hope National Medical Center.

renal insufficiency, and high calcium (similar presentation like typical MM). Bone marrow (BM) biopsy showed sheets of CD138-positive plasma cells that were negative for κ, λ, and heavy chains. Electron microscopy of plasma cells was indistinguishable from typical secretory MM, and prominent rough endoplasmic reticulum and globules of slightly dense material morphologically consistent with immunoglobulin were identified. It was postulated that nonproducer myeloma may synthesize antigenically unrecognized immunoglobulin or its component, possibly because of somatic mutation at one of the immunoglobulin encoding genetic loci.

a localized band can be seen only in 40% of patients (3).

2. In α-HCD, which is associated with a form of small intestinal lymphoma, there is no localized band or sharp peak, probably secondary to polymerization of these chains or higher carbohydrate content (4).

3. In some IgD myelomas, the M spike may be very small.

4. In some patients with light chain disease, the light chains can be rapidly excreted in the urine, and thus a very small concentration of light chain in the serum will be visible.

5. The M protein may complex with other plasma components and form polymers or aggregates.

False-Negative Results

A small M protein may be present even when the quantitative immunoglobulin value is normal, and there are no visible abnormalities on SPEP, as in the following examples:

1. In μ-heavy chain disease (HCD), hypogammaglobulinemia is a prominent feature, but

False-Positive Results

Different serum proteins other than immunoglobulin may falsely give the impression of an M protein, as in the following examples:

1. A high concentration of transferrin in patients with iron deficiency anemia may cause a localized band in β region.

2. Hemoglobin-haptoglobin resulting from hemolysis may cause a localized band in α2 globulin section.

3. Nephrotic syndrome, which is often associated with increased α2 and β bands may be mistaken for an M protein. Serum γ globulin and albumin are usually low in nephrotic syndrome.

■ TWENTY-FOUR-HOUR UPEP

Twenty-four-hour UPEP applies the same principles as SPEP. The aim of the test is to identify presence or absence of M proteins. A 24-hour collection of urine is done to determine total protein, and then a small aliquot of the 24-hour urine is used to perform the electrophoresis. M protein measurement is done by multiplying the percentage of the monoclonal spike by total protein in the 24-hour urine specimen. Generally, the amount of urinary protein reflects the total body plasma cell burden if renal function remains relatively normal.

IFE should be done once SPEP shows a monoclonal band to identify the M protein. IgG subtype is the commonest form of M protein and IgD or E type are rare.

■ SERUM AND URINE IFE

Serum and urine IFE should be done when either the SPEP or UPEP shows monoclonal bands (dense band). IFE differentiates monoclonal from polyclonal increases in immunoglobulin by identifying monoclonal immunoglobulin. It can also detect small M proteins or multiclonal (e.g., biclonal) gammopathies.

The test is performed by placing the patient's serum sample in application slits on the electrophoretic gel and separating the proteins by electrophoresis. After electrophoresis, a specific antibody for the immunoglobulin of interest is applied to each lane. Usually, antibodies against three different heavy chain components and two for light chain components are used. For example, anti-γ, anti-μ, anti-α, anti-κ, and anti-λ, respectively, are normally used. If there is an antigen-antibody reaction, a precipitation band will be formed, and it will be stained and analyzed (Figure 2).

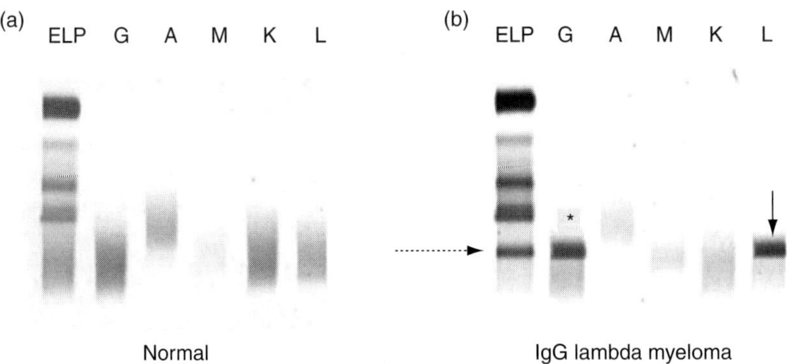

FIGURE 2

Monoclonal gammopathy on immunofixation. Each panel shows serum protein electrophoresis (SPEP) and immunofixation pattern of a normal serum sample (A) and serum from a patient with IgG λ multiple myeloma (MM) (B). Antisera to heavy chain determinants of IgG, IgA, and IgM, and to κ and λ light chains were used. It shows a discrete band on SPEP (dotted arrow) and a band (seen as a dark column) with similar mobility reacting only with the antisera to IgG (*) and the λ light chain (solid arrow), indicative of an IgG λ monoclonal protein. Courtesy of Bernard R. Tegtmeier, PhD, City of Hope National Medical Center.

An M protein is characterized by the combined presence of a sharp band in a single heavy chain class and a well-defined band with similar mobility which reacts to either κ or λ light chain antisera. IFE can detect serum M protein at a minimal concentration of 0.02 g/dL and urine M protein at a concentration of more than 0.004 g/dL (5).

Urine IFE

If UPEP shows a localized globulin band and IFE does not reveal monoclonal light chain, there is a possibility of HCD and IFE should be performed with antisera to heavy chains.

■ SERUM FREE LIGHT CHAINS

In the absence of M protein with SPEP, UPEP, and IFE of urine and serum, serum free light chains (FLCs) assays can be used to detect monoclonal FLCs. For many years, attempts to develop serum assays for FLCs failed because of their inability to produce antibodies that could differentiate between FLCs and light chain bound in intact immunoglobulin. Immunoassays using polyclonal antibodies were developed in 2001 that could detect FLCs at normal concentrations (6). The immunoassays can measure serum FLCs to a level of 2 to 4 mg/L and provide a greater sensitivity than older methods, such as IFE, that can detect FLCs at minimum concentration of 25 to 50 mg/L, depending on the position of M protein band and the content of polyclonal immunoglobulin. Nowrousian et al. (7) tested 378 paired samples of urine and serum samples from 82 patients with MM. The sensitivities of serum FLCs measurements and urine IFE in detecting FLCs were compared. Abnormal FLCs were detected in 54% of serum samples tested compared with 25% of urine tests. In abnormal serum samples for κ, urine IFE can detect Bence Jones protein in 51% of paired urine samples tested. In the case of λ serum samples, the sensitivity of urine IFE was only 35% (7). Katzman et al. (8) used an automated immunoassay for FLCs and

determined normal levels as follows (95% confidence interval [CI]):

1. free serum κ light chains—3.3 to 19.4 mg/L,
2. free serum λ light chains—5.7 to 26.3 mg/L, and
3. κ to λ ratio—0.26 to 1.65.

The same study showed that serum κ and λ FLCs increased with population age, but the κ to λ ratio did not exhibit an age-dependent trend (8).

Role of FLCs Measurement

Diagnosis and Monitoring Progression in Patients with Nonsecretory Myeloma and Oligosecretory Myeloma (<1 g/dL M Protein in the Serum and <200 mg/day M Protein in the Urine)

Nonsecretory myeloma accounts for about 3% of all myelomas and is characterized by the absence of M protein on serum and urine electrophoresis as well as IFE.

Drayson et al. reported that by using immunoassays, increased concentrations of either κ or λ FLCs (and abnormal κ/λ ratio) were detected in the serum of 19 out of 28 patients who were classified as nonsecretory myeloma. Serum FLCs can also act as a sensitive marker for monitoring disease in nonsecretory myeloma if initial levels are elevated, allowing earlier detection of responses to therapy (9).

Diagnosis and Monitoring of Patients with AL Amyloidosis and Light Chain Deposition Disease

Serum FLC assays have significantly improved the monitoring and diagnosis of patients with AL amyloidosis. As the level of intact immunoglobulin (paraprotein) is usually very low, SPEP is not helpful in monitoring AL amyloidosis. Free light levels can be used as a marker of the body amyloid load (10). In addition, it may be used to follow response to therapy. In patients with cardiac amyloid, serum FLCs and natriuretic peptide were also found to be correlated with risk of death (11). The general consensus is that the pretreatment level of serum FLCs have to be above 100 mg/L to be considered as "measurable" for monitoring patients with amyloid (12).

Predicting Risk of Progression of Monoclonal Gammopathy of Unknown Significance

Serum FLCs may also be an independent risk factor for progression to MM or related lymphoid malignancy in patients with monoclonal gammopathy of unknown significance (MGUS). Rajkumar et al. (13) showed that an abnormal FLC ratio (κ-λ ratio < 0.26 or > 1.65) was detected in 379 (33%) of 1,148 patients, and the risk of progression in patients with an abnormal FLC ratio was significantly higher and independent of the size and type of the serum M protein compared with patients with a normal ratio (hazard ratio, 3.5; 95% CI, 2.3–5.5; P < 0.001).

Risk Evaluation of Solitary Plasmacytomas of Bone

In patients with solitary bone plasmacytomas, in fact, the serum FLC is abnormal in nearly 50% of patients at diagnosis and is associated with higher risk of progression to MM (14). The same study showed that the risk of progression to MM at 5 years was 44% in patients with an abnormal serum FLC ratio at diagnosis compared with 26% in those with a normal FLC ratio. Patients with a normal FLC ratio at baseline and M protein level less than 0.5 g/dL at 1 to 2 years following diagnosis (low risk) have a progression rate at 5 years of 13%. In contrast, the high-risk group with abnormal FLC ratio at diagnosis and M protein level greater than 0.5 g/dL at 1 to 2 years following diagnosis had a progression rate of 62%.

Diagnosis, Monitoring During and After Treatment, and Perhaps Prognosis of Patients with MM with Intact Immunoglobulin

FLCs pass through the glomeruli easily, with a serum half-life of about 6 hours. In contrast, the serum half-lives of intact immunoglobulins are about 3 weeks for IgG and 6 days for IgA.

Mead et al. (15) reported that FLC concentrations fell more rapidly in response to treatment than intact IgG and showed greater concordance with serum β2 microglobulin concentrations and BM plasma cell assessments.

Van Rhee et al. (16) showed that high serum level of FLCs associated with a rapid reduction in response to therapy indicate an aggressive form of myeloma with poor prognosis in the tandem autotransplant setting.

Potentially Replacing Initial Urine Protein Studies in the Screening Algorithm for Plasma Cell Disorder When Serum FLC Analysis is Performed in Addition to SPEP and Serum Immunoelectrophoresis (17)

If an M protein is found, a urine test for electrophoresis and IFE (from an aliquot of a 24-hour urine collection) should be performed.

Notes: Renal excretion of monoclonal FLC increased with serum concentration, but excretion significantly decreased at high serum concentrations combined with renal dysfunction (7).

■ TOTAL SERUM IMMUNOGLOBULIN LEVELS

One or both of major uninvolved immunoglobulin (i.e., IgA and IgM in case of IgG myeloma) levels are reduced in 91% of patients overall. Serum immunoglobulin quantitation is done by rate nephelometry. The degree of turbidity produced by antigen-antibody reaction is measured with nephelometry. It quantitates the whole class of isotypes, so it is not limited to M protein only. Therefore, it cannot be used as a confirmatory diagnostic test for myeloma. However, depression of the levels of uninvolved immunoglobulins is a characteristic criterion of myeloma.

■ BLOOD AND BM FINDINGS

Peripheral blood smears usually show normochromic normocytic anemia in most patients at the time of diagnosis. The most frequent findings on peripheral smear are rouleaux formation (> 50%), followed by leukopenia and thrombocytopenia. Evaluation of the BM is done by aspiration and biopsy. A marrow differential is performed, and immunohistochemical staining is done (Figures 4 and 5). Marrow involvement with myeloma may be patchy and hence may not always be an accurate representation of total body myeloma burden.

BM plasmacytosis is also a diagnostic criterion for MM (Figure 3). BM plasmacytosis of more than 10% can be found in the vast majority of the patients. As an example, in the Mayo Clinic series, 96% of the patients were found to have plasma cells of more than 10%, but this value ranged from less than 5% to almost 100%, with a median value of 50% (1).

■ ROLE OF FLOW CYTOMETRY IN DIAGNOSIS OF MM

Flow cytometry has a supportive role to confirm the diagnosis of MM. Because of the patchy nature of myeloma to us involvement in BM and sample viability, flow cytometry result may not represent the actual plasma cell burden. It is mostly used as a qualitative rather than quantitative assessment of MM. Its role is mainly to establish the presence of clonal plasma cells. The plasma cells of MM typically lack surface immunoglobulin, and they have monotypic cytoplasmic immunoglobulin. They usually express CD79a and CD138 similar to normal plasma cells. In contrast, they are nearly always CD19 negative. Aberrantly, they express CD56 in 71.7% of cases (18). Myeloma cells also show moderate to bright expression of CD117, CD20, CD45, and CD52 in 17.8%, 9.3%, 8.8%, and 5.2% of the cases, respectively. Unlike most myelomas, plasma cell leukemia cells are CD56 negative (19).

Although still a research tool, the use of flow cytometry is of major interest for its ability to detect minimal residual disease (MRD). Multiparametric flow cytometry using different panels (e.g., CD38, 138, 45, 19, 56, 28, 20, 117) may be able to identify, characterize, and enumerate neoplastic cells even when few of these cells are present (20).

Immunophenotyping with multiparametric flow cytometry has been proposed as a more sensitive alternative to IFE for detecting MRD. Flow

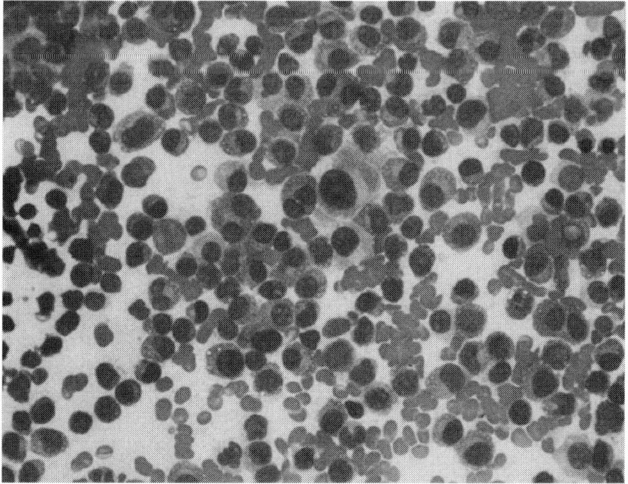

FIGURE 3
Bone marrow aspirate from a patient with multiple myeloma (MM) showing numerous plasma cells, many of which have nucleoli. Courtesy of K. Gaal, MD, City of Hope National Medical Center.

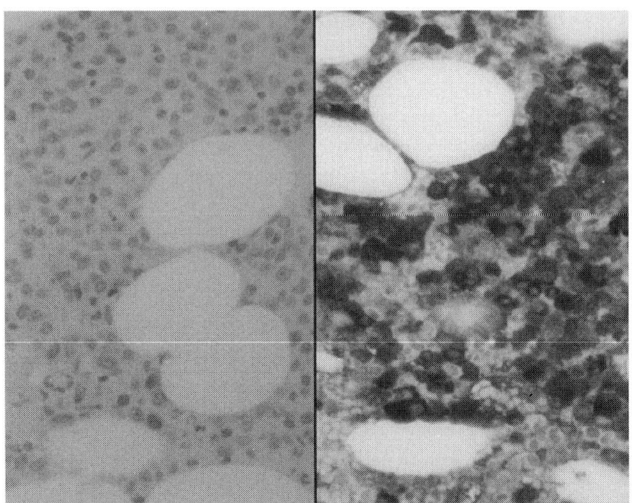

FIGURE 4

Multiple myeloma (MM) exhibiting λ light chain restriction. Bone marrow biopsy specimen from a patient with MM showing plasma cell infiltrates highlighted by immunostaining. Most of the plasma cells (left) are negative for κ and are positive for λ light chains (right) confirming monoclonality. Courtesy of K. Gaal, MD, City of Hope National Medical Center.

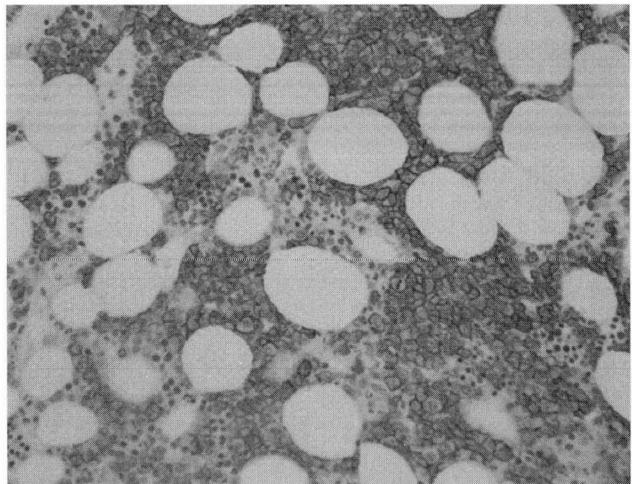

FIGURE 5

CD138+ plasma cells in bone marrow biopsy of a multiple myeloma (MM) patient highlighted by immunochemistry for CD138. Courtesy of K. Gaal, MD, City of Hope National Medical Center.

cytometry can identify a tumor surface marker profile, which in turn defines immunophenotyping of MM. In one series, patients with myeloma who have malignant plasma cells more than a specified threshold level of 0.01% (presence of $\geq$ 1 myelomatous cells per 10^4 normal hematopoietic cells) were considered to have MRD. In a small retrospective study of BM samples of 32 patients with MM who achieved complete remission after transplantation, progression-free survival was significantly longer in patients who were flow cytometry negative compared with flow cytometry-positive patients (21). The other method that can be used for MRD is quantitative polymerase chain reaction (PCR) of VDJH gene arrangement with allelic-specific oligonucleotides (ASO-PCR), which is more time consuming but has a slightly higher sensitivity compare with flow cytometry (21).

■ MONOCLONAL GAMMOPATHY

Once a plasma cell disorder has been recognized by serum electrophoresis and/or BM biopsy, it must be further characterized. Plasma cell disorders can range from monoclonal gammopathy (MGUS), which is the first pathogenetic step prior to actual active myeloma. Although patients with MGUS remain at risk of progression to myeloma or lymphoma, their median survival is long. In contrast, the median survival for patients with myeloma is only 3 to 4 years.

Initially, actual distinction between myeloma, especially smoldering myeloma, and MGUS was difficult and often fairly arbitrary. In fact, the best distinction was often retrospective, that is, observation of time to progression over the years. The International Myeloma Working Group codified a set of diagnostic criteria for MGUS in 2003, which made classification easier (22). Specifically, MGUS is defined as the presence of a low level of M protein (< 3 g/dL), BM plasmacytosis less than 10%, and the absence of end-organ dysfunction (anemia, hypercalcemia, lytic bone lesions, renal failure) attributable to the myeloma. Although

MGUS by itself is not a life-threatening condition, it is the risk of progression that remains of paramount importance. The constant rate of progression to myeloma or another malignant disease is estimated at 1% per year (23). Serum free light analysis, which will be discussed later, is also predictive of progression (Figure 6).

Approximately half of patients with both MGUS and smoldering myeloma have primary translocations in the plasma cells that involve the immunoglobulin heavy chain locus located on chromosome 14q32. The most common translocations and dysregulated genes are 11q13 (CCND1), 4p16.3 (FGFR-3 and MMSET), 6p21 (CCND3), 16q23 (c-maf), and 20q11 (mafB) (24). Microarray analysis has been performed to better characterize the genetic changes important in the multistep transformation from normal plasma cells to MGUS to frank myeloma (25). Interestingly, 380 genes were differentially expressed between normal plasma cells and myeloma. However, only 74 were differentially expressed between myeloma and MGUS. This seems to indicate that the spectrum of difference in the transformative process is much smaller between MGUS to myeloma versus that first major step from a normal plasma cell to MGUS or directly to myeloma.

The factors related to progression from MGUS to myeloma are likely related to both the plasma cell as demonstrated by the microarray analysis as well as to the marrow microenvironment (Figure 7).

The changes in the marrow microenvironment with disease progression include induction of angiogenesis and secretion of cytokines such as IL-6 and vascular endothelial growth factor (26). Studies have demonstrated an increase in BM-stimulated angiogenesis in part due to loss of angiogenesis inhibitory activity that progressively increases from MGUS to active myeloma (26).

MGUS is the most common plasma cell dyscrasia and is seen in approximately 3% of the general population. It is often diagnosed as part of routine blood work, and its prevalence increases with age, approaching 5% in individuals older than 70 years (27). Furthermore, the risk of progression

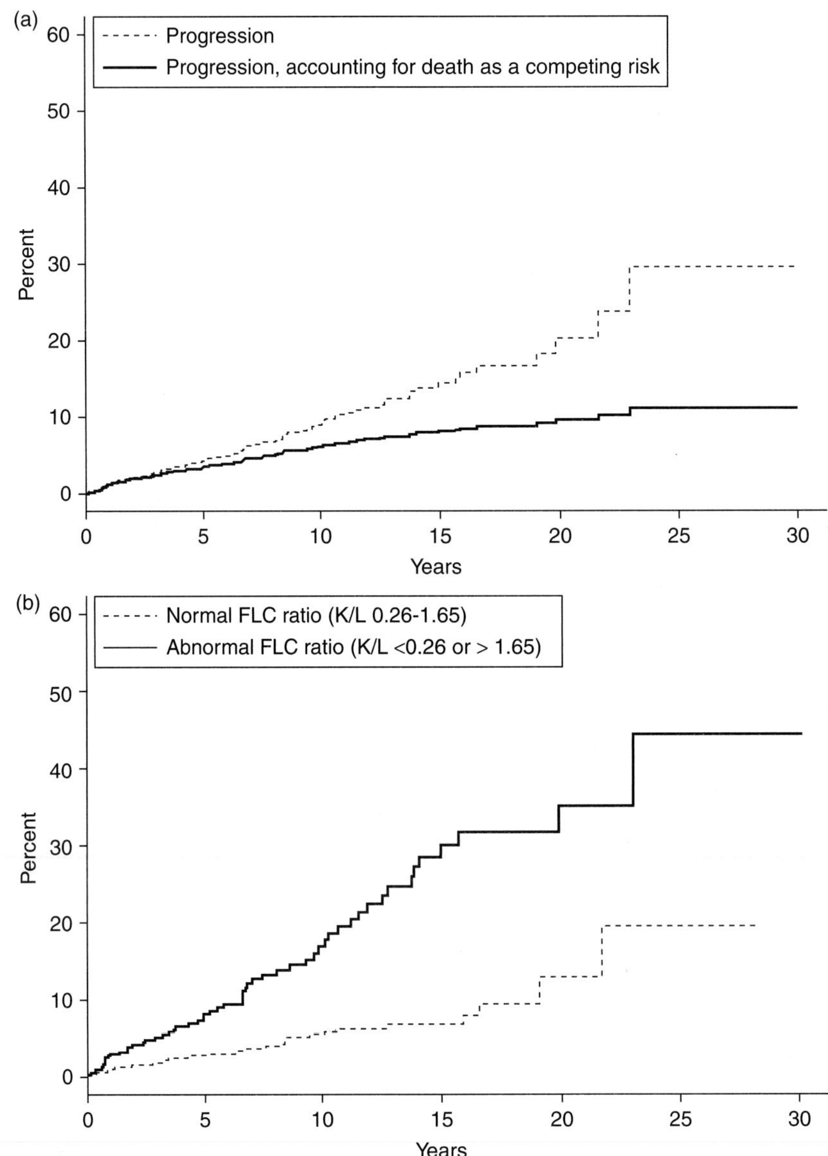

FIGURE 6

Risk of progression to myeloma or other disease in 1,148 patients with monoclonal gammopathy of unknown significance (MGUS). From Ref. 13 with permission.

to malignant disorders does not diminish with time, and thus continued follow-up of patients with MGUS is necessary. Thus, identification of factors predictive of progression is helpful in stratification of patients at higher risk of progression who might warrant closer follow-up. Identified factors include the type of M protein (IgM and IgA), level of M protein, and marrow plasmacytosis (<5% vs. 6–9%)

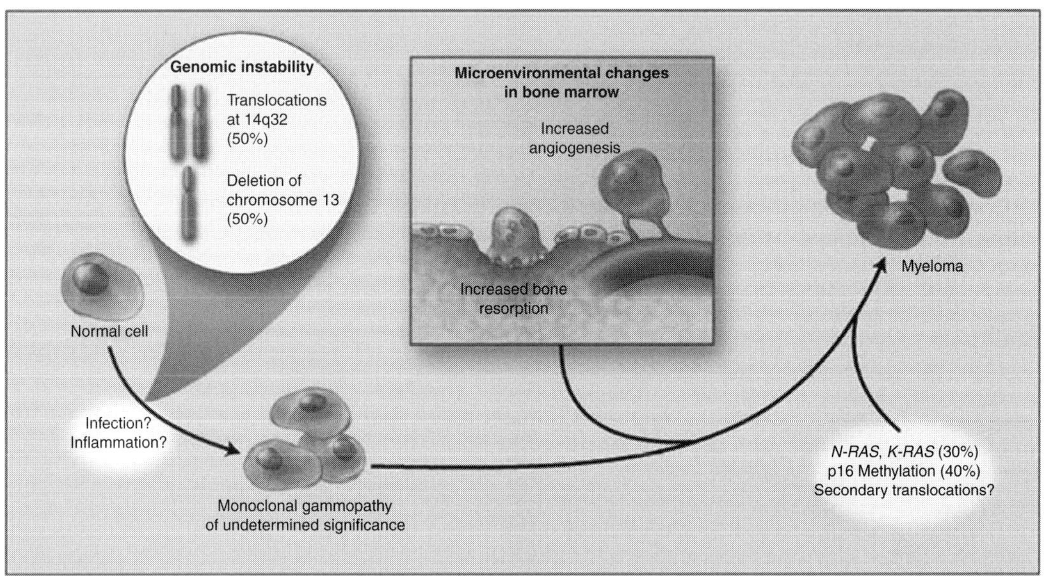

FIGURE 7

Mechanisms of disease progression in the monoclonal gammopathies. From Ref. 23 with permission.

(28,29). Recently, FLC analysis has been particularly helpful. An abnormal serum FLC ratio at baseline has been shown to correlate with an increased risk of progression (figure 6). Furthermore, the risk of progression continues to increase with increasingly abnormal free light ratio. Specifically, patients with an abnormal ratio had a risk of progression to malignancy of 17% at 10 years versus 5% for those with a normal ratio (13). All these factors except marrow plasmacytosis have been incorporated into a risk stratification model. The factors identified as low risk are serum M protein less than 1.5 g/dL, IgG subtype, and normal free light ratio. The risk of progression at 20 years ranges from 5% in patients with no risk factors to 58% in patients with all three risk factors (Figure 8).

Using this risk stratification model may be helpful for clinicians as it can serve as a guide for patient monitoring. Patients with no risk factors can be monitored yearly or even less frequently as their greatest risk of death is from other competing factors and not from MGUS progression to malignancy. In contrast, patients with three risk factors

need monitoring more akin to a patient with early stage myeloma given the high progression risk.

■ SMOLDERING MYELOMA

In contrast to MGUS, the category of smoldering myeloma represents a subset of patients with a high risk of progression to frank myeloma. In the Mayo Clinic series during the follow-up period, frank symptomatic myeloma or amyloidosis developed in 59% of the cohort diagnosed initially with smoldering myeloma. The rate of progression was approximately 10% per year in the first 5 years of follow-up (Figure 9) (30).

Similar to MGUS, older studies used various definitions of this entity that resulted in conflicting results about the clinical course. International consensus criteria were adopted in 2003, which standardized this disease category. Specifically, smoldering myeloma required the presence of a serum M protein more than 3 g/dL and more than 10% marrow plasmacytosis but no end-organ

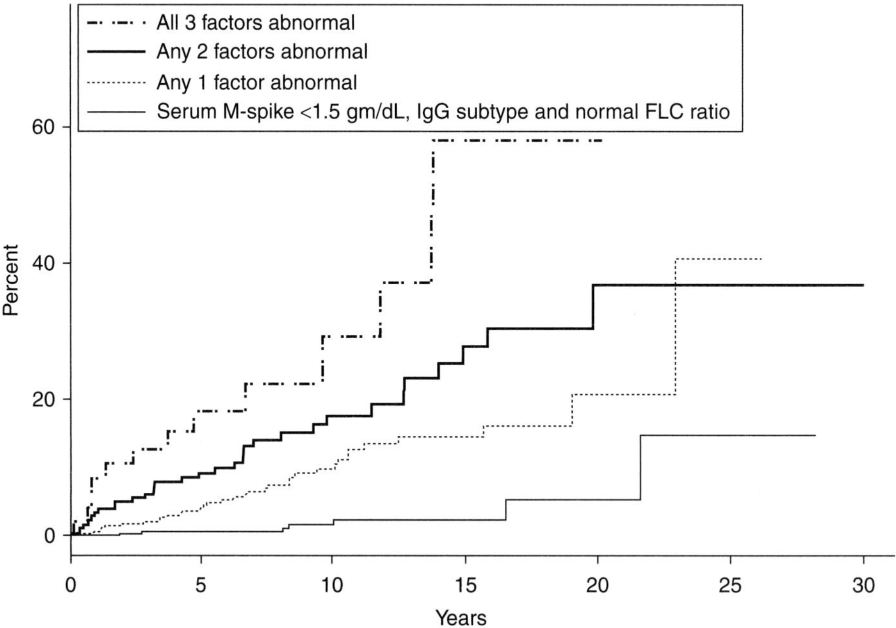

FIGURE 8

Risk of progression of monoclonal gammopathy of unknown significance (MGUS) to myeloma or other related disease using a risk-assessment model that incorporates the FLC ratio and the type and size of the serum monoclonal protein. From Ref. 13 with permission.

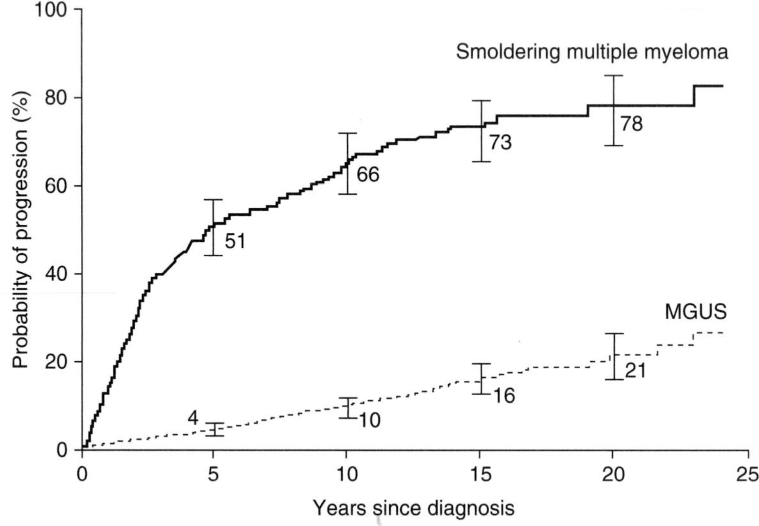

FIGURE 9

Probability of progression in cases with smoldering multiple myeloma or monoclonal gammopathy of unknown significance (MGUS) to active multiple myeloma or primary amyloidosis. From Ref. 30 with permission.

damage (defined as hypercalcemia, renal insufficiency, anemia, bone lesions, recurrent bacterial infections).

The Mayo Clinic retrospective study of 276 patients who fulfilled these criteria for smoldering myeloma identified risk factors for progression to active myeloma (30). Some factors were similar to MGUS, for example, the level and type of M protein and the extent and pattern of BM involvement. In contrast to MGUS, the presence of urinary light chains and reduction in uninvolved immunoglobulins were also prognostic. Also in contrast to MGUS, serum FLC ratios are not prognostic. A risk stratification model has been developed that divides patients into three groups. Group 1, BM plasma cells 10% or more, M protein 3g/dL or more. Group 2 plasma cells 10% or more, M protein 3 g/dL or less. Group 3 plasma cells 10% or less, M protein 3 g/dL or more (Figure 10).

A major clinical difference between smoldering myeloma and MGUS is that the risk of progression varies in smoldering myeloma, whereas it remains constant in MGUS. The risk of progression in smoldering myeloma is approximately 10% per year in the first 5 years and 3% per year in the next 5 years and then down to 1% per year subsequently.

Observation remains the standard of care for both MGUS and smoldering myeloma, although the frequency of surveillance may differ between the two entities. Use of the risk stratification models previously discussed may help guide the follow-up requirements. In general, follow-up includes complete blood counts, renal function, serum calcium, and monitoring of protein levels and watching for new symptoms. Patients with MGUS may be followed every 6 months to annually or even every 2 years for low-risk patients. Patients with smoldering myeloma need closer monitoring, up to every 2 to 3 months. There is still no conclusive proof that treatment of smoldering myeloma early will improve survival. However, one phase II trial of 31 patients treated with thalidomide did demonstrate delayed time to progression compared with historical controls (31). Progression-free survival was 63% at 2 years in the thalidomide group. More recently, a

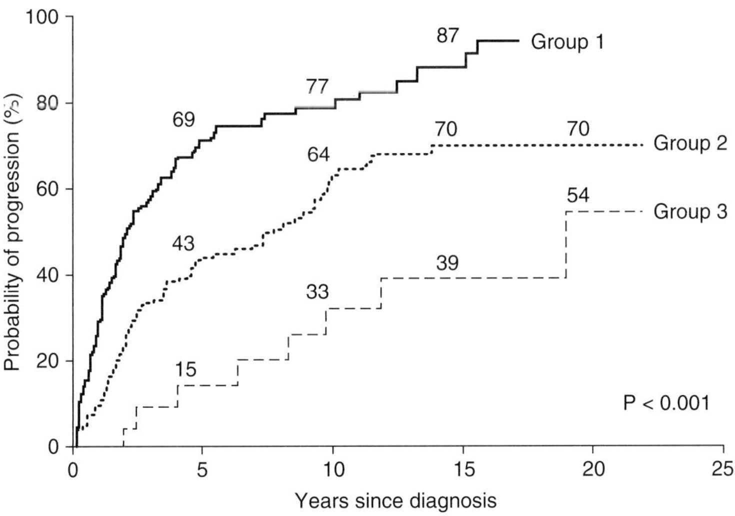

FIGURE 10

Probability of progression to active multiple myeloma or primary amyloidosis in patients with smoldering multiple myeloma among different risk groups. From Ref. 30 with permission.

phase III trial of 80 patients randomized to lenalidomide plus dexamethasone versus observation demonstrated no progression in the lenalidomide arm versus 17.5 months in the observation arm. There were no grade 4 adverse events in the lenalidomide arm. This was only an interim analysis in the first 40 patients, and thus follow-up is short. Furthermore, no survival benefit can yet be demonstrated in the lenalidomide arm; hence, this cannot be recommended as a standard approach outside of a clinical trial (32).

■ REFERENCES

1. Kyle RA, Gertz MA, Witzig TE, et al. Review of 1027 patients with newly diagnosed multiple myeloma. *Mayo Clin Proc* 2003;78(1):21–33.
2. Ma ES, Shek TW, Ma SY. Non-secretory plasma cell myeloma of the true non-producer type. *Br J Haematol* 2007;138(5):561.
3. Wahner-Roedler DL, Kyle RA. Mu-heavy chain disease: presentation as a benign monoclonal gammopathy. *Am J Hematol* 1992;40(1):56–60.
4. Al-Saleem T, Al-Mondhiry H. Immunoproliferative small intestinal disease (IPSID): a model for mature B-cell neoplasms. *Blood* 2005;105(6):2274–2280.
5. Criteria for the classification of monoclonal gammopathies, multiple myeloma and related disorders: a report of the International Myeloma Working Group. *Br J Haematol* 2003;121(5):749–757.
6. Bradwell AR, Carr-Smith HD, Mead GP, et al. Highly sensitive, automated immunoassay for immunoglobulin free light chains in serum and urine. *Clin Chem* 2001;47(4):673–680.
7. Nowrousian MR, Brandhorst D, Sammet C, et al. Serum free light chain analysis and urine immunofixation electrophoresis in patients with multiple myeloma. *Clin Cancer Res* 2005;11(24 Pt 1):8706–8714.
8. Katzmann JA, Clark RJ, Abraham RS, et al. Serum reference intervals and diagnostic ranges for free kappa and free lambda immunoglobulin light chains: relative sensitivity for detection of monoclonal light chains. *Clin Chem* 2002;48(9):1437–1444.
9. Drayson M, Tang LX, Drew R, Mead GP, Carr-Smith H, Bradwell AR. Serum free light-chain measurements for identifying and monitoring patients with nonsecretory multiple myeloma. *Blood* 2001;97(9):2900–2902.
10. Lachmann HJ, Gallimore R, Gillmore JD, et al. Outcome in systemic AL amyloidosis in relation to changes in concentration of circulating free immunoglobulin light chains following chemotherapy. *Br J Haematol* 2003;122(1):78–84.
11. Palladini G, Lavatelli F, Russo P, et al. Circulating amyloidogenic free light chains and serum N-terminal natriuretic peptide type B decrease simultaneously in association with improvement of survival in AL. *Blood* 2006;107(10):3854–3858.
12. Gertz MA, Comenzo R, Falk RH, et al. Definition of organ involvement and treatment response in immunoglobulin light chain amyloidosis (AL): a consensus opinion from the 10th International Symposium on Amyloid and Amyloidosis, Tours, France, 18–22 April 2004. *Am J Hematol* 2005;79(4):319–328.
13. Rajkumar SV, Kyle RA, Therneau TM, et al. Serum free light chain ratio is an independent risk factor for progression in monoclonal gammopathy of undetermined significance. *Blood* 2005;106:812–817.
14. Dingli D, Kyle RA, Rajkumar SV, et al. Immunoglobulin free light chains and solitary plasmacytoma of bone. *Blood* 2006;108(6):1979–1983.
15. Mead GP, Carr-Smith HD, Drayson MT, Morgan GJ, Child JA, Bradwell AR. Serum free light chains for monitoring multiple myeloma. *Br J Haematol* 2004;126(3):348–354.
16. van Rhee F, Bolejack V, Hollmig K, et al. High serum-free light chain levels and their rapid reduction in response to therapy define an aggressive multiple myeloma subtype with poor prognosis. *Blood* 2007;110(3):827–832.
17. Katzmann JA, Dispenzieri A, Kyle RA, et al. Elimination of the need for urine studies in the screening algorithm for monoclonal gammopathies by using serum immunofixation and free light chain assays. *Mayo Clin Proc* 2006;81(12):1575–1578.
18. Lin P, Owens R, Tricot G, Wilson CS. Flow cytometric immunophenotypic analysis of 306 cases of multiple myeloma. *Am J Clin Pathol* 2004;121:482–488.
19. García-Sanz R, Orfão A, González M, et al. Primary plasma cell leukemia: clinical, immunophenotypic, DNA ploidy, and cytogenetic characteristics. *Blood* 1999;93(3):1032–1037.
20. Rawstron AC, Orfao A, Beksac M, et al.; European Myeloma Network. Report of the European Myeloma Network on multiparametric flow cytometry in multiple myeloma and related disorders. *Haematologica* 2008;93(3):431–438.

21. Sarasquete ME, García-Sanz R, González D, et al. Minimal residual disease monitoring in multiple myeloma: a comparison between allelic-specific oligonucleotide real-time quantitative polymerase chain reaction and flow cytometry. *Haematologica* 2005;90(10):1365–1372.

22. The International Myeloma Working Group. Criteria for the classification of monoclonal gammopathies, multiple myeloma and related disorders: a report of the international myeloma working group. *Br J Haematol* 2003;121:749–757.

23. Kyle RA, Rajkumar SV. Multiple myeloma. *N Engl J Med* 2004;351(18):1860–1873.

24. Rajkumar SV. MGUS and smoldering myeloma update on pathogenesis, natural history and management. *Hematology Am Soc Hematol Educ Program* 2005:340–345.

25. Davies FE, Dring AM, Li C, et al. Insights into the multistep transformation of MGUS to myeloma using microarray expression analysis. *Blood* 2003;102(13): 4504–4511.

26. Kumar S, Witzig TE, Timm M, et al. Bone marrow angiogenic ability and expression of angiogenic cytokines in myeloma: evidence favoring loss of marrow angiogenesis inhibitory activity with disease progression. *Blood* 2004;104(4):1159–1165.

27. Kyle RA, Therneau TM, Rajkumar SV, et al. Prevalence of monoclonal gammopathy of undetermined significance (MGUS) among Olmstead County MN residents 50 years of age. *Blood* 2003;102:934a.

28. Kyle RA, Therneau TM, Rajkumar SV, et al. A long term study of prognosis of monoclonal gammopathy of undetermined significance. *N Engl J Med* 2002;346: 564–569.

29. Cesana C, Klersy C, Barbarano L, et al. Prognostic factors for malignant transformation in monoclonal gammopathy of undetermined significance and smoldering multiple myeloma. *J Clin Oncol* 2002;20(6):1625–1634.

30. Kyle RA, Remstein ED, Therneau TM, et al. Clinical course and prognosis of smoldering (asymptomatic) multiple myeloma. *N Engl J Med* 2007;356(25): 2582–2590.

31. Rajkumar SV, Gertz MA, Lacy MQ, et al. Thalidomide as initial therapy for early-stage myeloma. *Leukemia* 2003;17(4):775–779.

32. Mateos M, Corral LL, Hernandez M, et al. A multicenter randomized open label phase III trial of lenalidomide-dexamethasone versus therapeutic abstention in smoldering multiple myeloma at high risk of progression to symptomatic myeloma: results of the first interim analysis [Abstract 614]. *Blood* 2009.

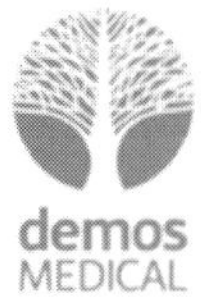

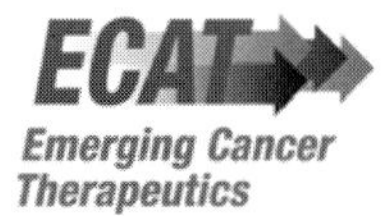

Prognostic Factors and Risk Stratification in Myeloma

Prashant Kapoor and Shaji Kumar*

Mayo Clinic, Rochester, MN

■ ABSTRACT

Increasing evidence suggests that diverse clinical outcomes in multiple myeloma (MM) are dictated by different genetic abnormalities. MM is no longer recognized as a single disease entity, and traditional parameters used to prognosticate patients with myeloma are increasingly being supplanted by models that include conventional cytogenetics and fluorescence in situ hybridization (FISH). Molecular classifications have also been described to group myeloma into subtypes with unique properties. Genetically determined risk stratification has prognostic as well as therapeutic implications. Broadly, MM can be classified into hyperdiploid and nonhyperdiploid subtypes. Chromosomal translocation involving immunoglobulin heavy chain (IgH) switch regions at chromosome 14q32 is a seminal pathogenetic event in approximately 40% to 50% of patients with MM. The cases lacking such translocations are predominantly characterized by hyperdiploidy that is predictive of superior progression-free and overall survival rates. Pathologically, both IgH translocation and hyperdiploidy are unified by the ectopic expression (upregulation) of cyclin D genes. Gene expression profiling (GEP) and array-based comparative genomic hybridization are other useful tools to identify genetic aberrations, but currently proposed molecular signatures require further validation and simplification for widespread acceptance. As such, routine use of FISH and conventional cytogenetics on bone marrow samples has become a standard of care for patients with newly diagnosed MM. This comprehensive review outlines the clinical value of conventional and novel prognostic markers in the face of emerging therapies and discusses the recently proposed framework of classification of myeloma genetic subtypes. In addition, the current clinical application of evidence-based strategies to prognosticate patients with myeloma and individualize the treatment has been outlined in this chapter.

---

*Corresponding author, Division of Hematology, Mayo Clinic, 200 First St SW, Rochester, MN 55905
E-mail address: kumar.shaji@mayo.edu

Emerging Cancer Therapeutics 1:2 (2010) 299–318.
© 2010 Demos Medical Publishing LLC. All rights reserved.
DOI: 10.5003/2151–4194.1.2.299

■ INTRODUCTION

Multiple myeloma (MM) is a hematologic malignancy characterized by the proliferation of aberrant plasma cell (PC) clone(s), leading to increased production of monoclonal protein and end-organ damage, manifesting primarily in the form of renal dysfunction, hypercalcemia, anemia, and bone lesions. The clinical course of the disease is highly heterogeneous with a wide variation in the overall survival (OS) of patients with myeloma, ranging from a few months to over a decade (1). According to the current Surveillance, Epidemiology, and End Results database, nearly 18% of patients with MM have a survival rate of more than 10 years (http://seer.cancer.gov). The reasons for such diverse outcomes are manifold and have been areas of profound interest among investigators (2). Prognosis comes from the Greek word *prognoses*, which means "foreknowledge" or "to know before," and is defined by Webster's dictionary as "the prospect of recovery as anticipated from the usual course of disease or peculiarities of the case." Identification of these disease-related "peculiarities" or prognostic factors in any patient is invaluable for both the patients who will want to know the course of the disease in future as well as the physician who will make treatment decisions based on them.

Prognostic factors should always be interpreted in the appropriate clinical context, taking into account the outcome of interest as well as the nature of therapeutic interventions. The quest for an ideal, composite prognostic marker that can universally predict outcome and assist in tailoring therapy in all cases of MM has not come to fruition, but a number of tools, including chromosomal studies, are now among the mandatory frontline investigations in the newly diagnosed patient (3–6).

The risk stratification of a patient is essential prior to initiation of therapy as it guides the clinician not only in estimating the clinical course but also in the selection of appropriate therapies (5). The clinical relevance and independence of many prognostic factors is obscured in a multivariate model. This finding has led to the development of several staging systems, utilizing only the most potent prognostic markers that can simultaneously differentiate the outcomes in large patient populations (7–13). In essence, the prognostic markers and the therapeutic agents do not act in concert as the goal of an effective drug is to overcome the adverse prognostic impact of a marker, thereby diminishing its relevance. A parameter that can distinctly segregate patient populations into the indolent (stable, standard risk) or aggressive (high risk) categories with the conventional therapy may not be applicable in the transplantation setting or the era of novel agents. It is imperative that we reassess the prognostic values of many of the current variables in the context of the paradigm shift in our approach toward patients with newly diagnosed myeloma. Therefore, a continuous evaluation of the prognostic indicators in the context of newer therapies is required.

This comprehensive review outlines the clinical value of such markers in the face of emerging therapies. In addition, we discuss the current clinical application of evidence-based strategies to prognosticate patients with myeloma and individualize the treatment (14). Besides the therapy, many factors inherent to the patient (the host factors) and the tumor (myeloma-related factors) itself independently contribute to the ultimate outcome (Figure 1) (15–17). It is also important to recognize that the utility of prognostic factors has been predominantly studied in the setting of newly diagnosed MM (NDMM), and scant evidence exists about their significance in advanced stages of the disease.

■ HOST FACTORS

Patient Demographics

The importance of host features in dictating the disease outcome cannot be overemphasized. Younger patients with MM tend to demonstrate superior OS. This observation is somewhat akin to that seen in the patients with non-Hodgkin lymphoma

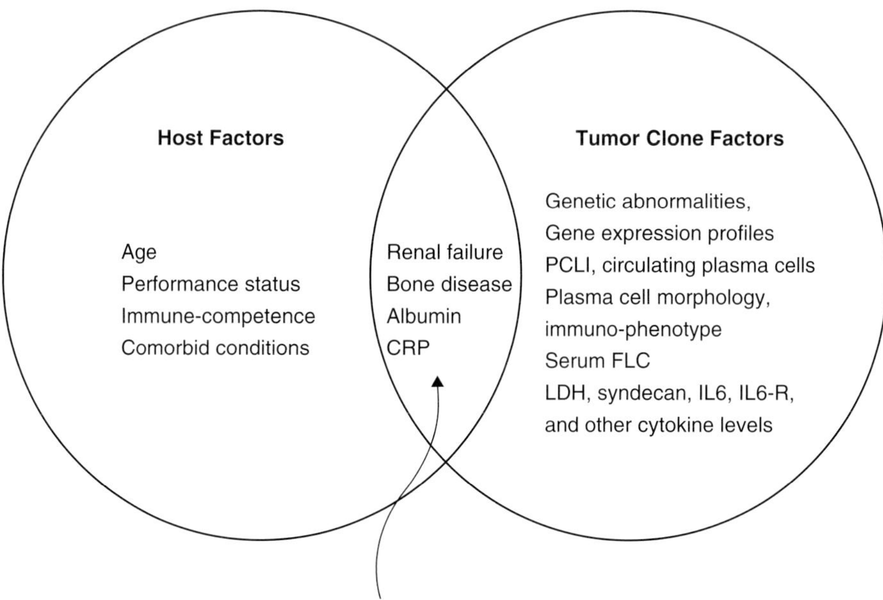

FIGURE 1
Host and tumor clone-related prognostic factors in multiple myeloma.
Abbreviations: CRP, C-reactive protein; FLC, free light chain; IL-6, interleukin-6; IL6-R, interleukin-6 receptor; LDH, lactate dehydrogenase; PCLI, plasma cell labeling index.

who have their ages factored into the calculation of the International Prognostic Index Score (18). A recent large study by the International Myeloma Working Group (IMWG) and two smaller studies have shown consistent findings with similar frequency of cytogenetic abnormalities in both younger (younger than 45–50 years) and older age groups (19–21). The results, however, differed from the findings of another study of 228 patients with MM, which concluded that the high-risk features such as nonhyperdiploidy and immunoglobulin heavy chain (IgH) translocations (discussed later) tended to cluster in the younger population (22). The IMWG study demonstrated that the patients younger than 50 years presented with more favorable prognostic features such as the low International Staging System (ISS) and the Durie-Salmon (DS) staging and better performance status, hemoglobin, and renal function. In addition, the younger patients had superior survival outcomes, even with

the adjustment for the differences in the life expectancies, both after the conventional chemotherapy (median OS, 4.5 years vs. 3.7 years; $P < 0.001$) or the high-dose therapy (HDT) with stem cell rescue (median, 7.5 years vs. 5.7 years; $P = 0.04$) (19). In a separate cohort of 415 patients older than 65 years who were treated with conventional chemotherapy, very advanced age (>80 years) appeared to be an independent prognostic factor in a multivariate model (23). The prognostic relevance of age has been questioned in a study by the Arkansas group in which the patients as old as 76 years underwent autotransplantation (ASCT) with comparable event-free survival (EFS, $P = 0.2$) and OS ($P = 0.4$) with those younger than 65 years when matched for other prognostic variables (24). Thus, in general, despite enrichment for higher risk genetic features, younger patients have a better survival rate, likely a reflection of better ability to tolerate treatments.

Although MM is more than twice as common in the African Americans (AA) as the whites (25), with a higher myeloma-related mortality in blacks, a South Western Oncology Group study of 614 patients, involving approximately 20% blacks, noted no difference in the OS by race when patients of the two races were exposed to comparable treatments (26). Another smaller study (N = 70; 38 AA vs. 32 non-AA patients) demonstrated a superior EFS for AA, without any difference in the OS between the two groups after ASCT (27). The socioeconomic factors, including access to health care rather than the racial factors per se, probably account for a higher death rate in the black population. Data comparing other population groups are currently lacking. Neither gender appears to offer a distinct survival advantage over the other in MM.

Performance Status and Comorbid Conditions

Often ignored because of the exclusion of patients with poor performance status from the clinical trials, and the subjectivity involved in its assessment, this prognostic factor, as assessed by the Eastern Cooperative Oncology Group (ECOG) score, was deemed more potent than many other predictors of OS, including the serum β_2-microglobulin (β_2M), in a univariate analysis from a series of 1,027 patients (relative risk, 1.9, confidence interval [CI], 1.6–2.4; P < 0.001) (13,28,29). Comorbid conditions, including acute renal failure, can substantially contribute to adverse outcome, irrespective of the risk stratification (5).

■ DISEASE-RELATED FACTORS

Serum β_2M

β_2M, a component of the light chain of the major histocompatibility complex I, is renally excreted and strongly correlates with the tumor load (1,8,10,12,13,28,29). A high β_2M predicts shorter survival not only in the patients receiving conventional chemotherapy but also in those undergoing ASCT. A β_2M level of 5.5 mg/L or higher stratifies a third of patients into the highest ISS 3 category with a median survival of 29 months (12). Besides the tumor growth, a deterioration of the renal function leads to an increase in the serum β_2M levels, thereby upstaging the patients. If the β_2M level is corrected for the renal function, its prognostic influence in patients of renal failure is lost. The uncorrected β_2M continues to remain one of the most powerful and reliable prognostic factors in MM, but it is not a useful parameter during clinical follow-up as patients are known to relapse in the absence of an increase in the β_2M level (12,30).

Albumin

Albumin is the other variable used in the ISS to stage patients with NDMM. Increased interleukin-6 (IL-6) level in a patient with myeloma downregulates the synthesis of albumin by the liver, and low albumin level adversely affects the survival. About 40% of patients with NDMM have low albumin (< 3.5 mg/dL), and the combination of this inexpensive laboratory test with the serum β_2M has led to widespread adoption and application of the ISS, which has now been validated in different populations (12). For staging by ISS, the serum albumin as measured by the serum protein electrophoresis is as reliable as that measured by the bromocresol green method utilized in the comprehensive metabolic panel (31).

C-Reactive Protein

The hepatic synthesis of acute phase reactants such as C-reactive protein (CRP) and α1-antitrypsin is upregulated in the presence of IL-6, a growth factor with autocrine and paracrine actions, generated in abundance in patients with myeloma (32). Increased levels of serum IL-6 have an adverse prognostic impact on patients with MM, although conflicting results have been reported (33–35).

Elevated soluble IL-6 receptors augment the proliferative activity of IL-6 (36) and are also associated with a shortened survival. The CRP serves as a surrogate for IL-6, reflecting its activity, and was first combined with β_2M by European investigators to stage patients with myeloma (8). Similarly, patients have been stratified by pairing β_2M with α1AT to generate a prognostically useful classification (32). The CRP level does not appear to correlate with disease activity and is, therefore, not useful in the clinical monitoring of patients.

The prognostic values of CRP and other laboratory parameters, such as lactate dehydrogenase enzyme, serum calcium, the level of the M protein on serum or urine electrophoresis, immunoglobulin isotype, neopterin (37), erythrocyte sedimentation rate, and thymidine kinase, do not carry as much prognostic value as the albumin combined with β_2M (12,38). In addition, the independent prognostic relevance of the measures of renal function, such as serum creatinine and blood urea nitrogen, is nullified by the use of uncorrected β_2M (12).

Serum Free Light Chain Assay

This nephelometric assay is used to primarily monitor oligosecretory MM and light chain-only MM, and the baseline free light chain (FLC) is a useful prognostic parameter in many PC disorders, including monoclonal gammopathy of undetermined significance (MGUS), smoldering myeloma (SMM), solitary plasmacytoma, and NDMM (39–42). Moreover, normal FLC ratio is required for the establishment of stringent complete remission (sCR) (43). More than 95% of patients with MM have an abnormal FLC (κ/λ) ratio, indicating clonality or a disproportionate increase in a clone of PCs (38). Snozek et al. combined the baseline FLC ratio to albumin and β_2M (the independent variables used in the ISS) and noted an improvement in the risk stratification of patients with NDMM

based on the presence of zero, one, two, and three abnormal laboratory measurements, with median survival of 51, 39, 30, and 20 months, respectively ($P < 0.001$) (39). The difference between the involved (the monoclonal light chain isotype) and the uninvolved FLC (the nondominant, polyclonal light chain isotype) is preferred over the FLC ratio for serial measurements during follow-up to predict the response to therapy (40). Although FLC assay after 2 months of alkylator-based therapy is found to be superior to early electrophoretic M protein measurement in the prediction of overall response, it does not predict OS and progression-free survival, and serial determinations do not provide additional information in evaluating patients who have a measurable M protein (40).

Complete Blood Count

Anemia (hemoglobin concentration $\leq$ 12 g/dL) is present in nearly three quarters of the patients with MM (25,28). It is usually normocytic and moderate in severity. Hemoglobin less than 10 g/dL adversely affects the outcome. However, in a multivariate analysis, its prognostic relevance is usually lost (12). Although thrombocytopenia (platelet count < 130,000) is a powerful and independent predictor of survival, its absence in nearly 88% of newly diagnosed patients severely limits its usefulness as a prognosticator (12). Absolute lymphocyte count has been found to be an independent predictor of survival, both in the post-transplant recovery period and the NDMM setting, with higher absolute lymphocyte count predicting a better outcome (41,42). With untreated advanced disease, a decrement in the memory CD4 lymphocytes is noted, a reflection of the defective immune system, and reduction in the total CD4 lymphocyte count correlates with a shorter OS (44–46). In another study of 254 patients with MM, the presence of 4% or more peripheral blood mononuclear PCs was associated with a median survival of 2.4 years compared with 4.4 years for those with less than 4% circulating PCs ($P < 0.001$) (47).

BM Biopsy Findings

The diagnosis of MM rests on the presence of bone marrow (BM) plasmacytosis of 10% or more, in addition to the presence of M protein and certain clinical features (anemia, renal failure, hypercalcemia, and lytic bone lesions) attributable to the end-organ damage due to myeloma. It is therefore mandatory to study the BM aspirate and biopsy for the diagnosis. Attempts to gather information about the prognosis and biology of the disease through the use of additional studies on the BM have been extremely successful. Indeed, the cytogenetic information and most of the information on the rate of proliferation of the PCs is obtained from the BM examination. The cytogenetic features have been discussed in a separate section.

The morphologic differences in the bone marrow plasma cells (BMPCs) of patients with MM have led to the introduction of a classification for PCs. The plasmablastic morphology, that is, PCs with a nucleolus greater than 2 μm or a nucleus greater than 10 μm with fine reticular chromatin pattern, and scant cytoplasm, one half the size of the nuclear area, with absent or minimal hof region, is of prognostic significance. Plasmablastic myeloma (PB MM), defined by the presence of 2% or higher plasmablasts, is an aggressive disease with reduced OS as shown in an ECOG trial (median OS of 1.9 for PB MM vs. 3.7 years for non-PB MM, $P <$ 0.001) and other studies (48). Furthermore, cases with plasmablastic morphology have been shown to demonstrate poorer OS after ASCT compared with non-PB MM in the relapsed or refractory setting (median survival time, 5 months vs. 24 months, respectively; $P <$ 0.001).

A massive PC load and diffuse infiltration of the BM is suggestive of a higher tumor burden, but because of the variable distribution of PCs in the BM, such histologic features and the BM characteristics proposed by Bartl et al. (7,49) have found limited practical applicability in risk stratifying the patients.

■ BM ANGIOGENESIS

Angiogenesis in myeloma refers to an abnormal multistep process that ultimately leads to increased formation of new vessels in the BM that ultimately contributes to tumor growth, invasion, and spread (50,51). The interaction between PCs and the BM microenvironment is complex (52). Compared with healthy controls, marked increase in the proliferative activity of BM endothelial cells of multiple myeloma patients is noted. This results in development of irregular blood vessels. Endothelial cells of multiple myeloma promote angiogenesis and neoplastic PC growth by virtue of enhanced expression of angiogenic receptors such as vascular endothelial growth factor receptor-2, metalloproteinases, and basic fibroblast growth factor (bFGF) and by expression of multiple other growth factors (53,54).

BM microvessel density (MVD) has been demonstrated to have prognostic value in previously untreated MM (50,51,55–57). Indeed, MM is the first hematologic malignancy to underscore the prognostic significance of increased MVD (52). The angiogenic switch that is at least in part responsible for the induction of vascular phase from MGUS to active myeloma is a consequence of imbalance between the proangiogenic and antiangiogenic factors in the tumor milieu (54,58,59).

In a cohort of 400 patients from Mayo Clinic, the MVD was shown to progressively increase from MGUS to SMM to NDMM, with the highest value associated with relapsed MM. Survival was 28 months in SMM and NDMM with high grade angiogenesis, compared with 53 months for low- and intermediate-grade angiogenesis ($P = 0.02$) (56).

MVD has been found to correlate with other prognostic markers such as plasma cell labeling index (PCLI), circulating PCs, BMPC percentage, $\beta_2 M$, lactate dehydrogenase, and del13q14 (55,60–64). Moreover, post-treatment MVD been shown to decrease considerably in patients who achieve remission after therapy (65).

In another study from Mayo Clinic, a loss of angiogenesis inhibitory activity was found along the PC disease spectrum, with samples from patients with MGUS markedly inhibiting angiogenesis compared with those of SMM and MM (59).

Although the prognostic relevance of angiogenic makers in patients with MM is still not completely understood, cytokines such as plasma vascular endothelial growth factor, serum bFGF, and hepatocyte growth factor appear to be independent prognosticators of survival (66–68).

Cytogenetics

Chromosomal analysis serves as the cornerstone of prognostic evaluation of MM which is commonly associated with aneuploidy of two major subcategories: hyperdiploidy, that is, 48 to 74 chromosomes associated with gains of many odd numbered chromosomes, or nonhyperdiploidy, comprising of hypodiploid, pseudodiploid, near-diploid or near-tetraploid PCs, and frequently associated with IgH chromosomal translocations (69). The IgH translocations, primarily involving chromosomal 14 IgH locus (q32.3), cause juxtapositioning of immunoglobulin enhancers to oncogenes on different partner chromosomes, leading to their upregulation (70). A common unifying pathway, even in the absence of translocations, is the overexpression of one of the cyclin D genes (70). Both the t(4;14)(p16.3;q32) and t(14;16)(q32;q23), present in approximately 15% and 2% to 10% of patients with MM, respectively, are associated with a dismal prognosis and highly aggressive phenotypes with shortened survival [OS, 18–36 months for t(4;14) and 16 months for t(14;16)], irrespective of the therapeutic intervention (69,71). Interestingly, a subset of patients with a low β_2M (<4 g/dL) and a relatively better hemoglobin (≥10 g/dL) has appeared to benefit from tandem transplant with EFS and OS of 26 and 54.6 months, respectively, in a French study

(72). Total Therapy 3, a double transplantation protocol incorporating bortezomib-based regimen for both induction and consolidation phase, has been shown to abrogate the poor prognostic effect of t(4;14) (*FGFR3/MMSET* on the GEP model discussed later) as opposed to Total Therapy 2. Hyperdiploid MM is slightly more common in males, older patients, and those with myeloma bone disease. Hyperdiploid MM may be a result of chromosome 5 gain. Patients with hyperdiploid MM in general have a better survival. On the other hand, a few genetic aberrations such as C-*myc* translocations, deletion of 17p13 (10% patients), and chromosome 1p deletion or 1q amplification are considered secondary genetic events that accumulate during the course of MM and are a reflection of disease progression. The tumor suppressor gene, p53, considered "the guardian of the genome," (73) resides at 17p13 locus, and its loss confers a survival disadvantage (74), irrespective of the therapy, with median OS of 14.7 months for patients on HDT (75–77). In addition to association with hypercalcemia and elevated creatinine, a predilection for the central nervous system involvement is seen in patients with deletion 17p13.1 (78).

It is believed that the increased proliferation and BM angiogenesis along with the loss of a tumor suppressor gene, *Rb-1*, play a pivotal role in adversely affecting the outcome of patients with chromosomal 13 abnormalities (Δ13) (63,69,79). Monosomy 13, partial deletion of chromosome 13, or translocations involving 13q, constitute Δ13 that are critical predictors of survival in patients with MM if detected by the conventional cytogenetics which takes into account the proliferative capacity of the clonotypic PCs during metaphase analysis. In contrast, the interphase fluorescence in situ hybridization (iFISH) studies discount the impact of proliferation, although the evidence of Δ13 by iFISH (~51%) has still been considered prognostically relevant, both in patients receiving conventional chemotherapy and HDT (67–69).

A recent multicenter study of 794 patients with myeloma addressing the discrepancies related to the detection of Δ13 found that when the cases of chromosome 13 deletion detected by both conventional cytogenetics and iFISH were separated from those detected by iFISH alone, the ability of iFISH to prognosticate the patients on the basis of this chromosomal defect was obscured (P = 0.115) (70). Furthermore, the prognostic power of deletion 13 by iFISH disappeared in a French study when patients with simultaneous t(4;14) or del(17p) were excluded, indicating that prognostic value of iFISH-detected deletion 13 was due to its frequent association with other known high-risk genetic abnormalities (74). Another study by Shaughnessy and colleagues found that the incorporation of the PCLI to iFISH could not substitute for the Δ13 detected on metaphase cytogenetics and that cytogenetic studies were imperative in the initial work-up of patients with MM (80). A total of 16% of cases with chromosomal 13 abnormalities on cytogenetics went unrecognized by iFISH in this study (80). A recent study involving the patients of APEX or SUMMIT trials elucidated the impact of bortezomib on the patients with deletion 13 detected by either method, with no survival advantage for the patients lacking Δ13, thereby suggesting that this proteosome inhibitor may effectively surmount the adverse impact of Δ13 (81). Another study with bortezomib has reported similar outcomes with no significant difference in the response rates, duration of response, and OS between the patients with and without Δ13 (82). Chromosomal translocation t(11;14)(q13,q32) is present in up to 15% to 20% of patients and confers a favorable prognosis (83), particularly in patients receiving HDT, with 88% surviving at 80 months. However, this favorable influence of t(11;14) is questioned by some investigators because a subset of long-term MM survivors (survival ≥8 years from the diagnosis) was not found to be enriched for this genetic abnormality (84) and PC leukemia has (a more aggressive form of plasma cell proliferative disorder) been associated with this abnormality. Thus, at worst it may considered a neutral prognostic factor (5,74).

Using high-density, single-nucleotide polymorphism arrays, Avet-Loiseau and colleagues identified genetic lesions associated with prognosis in 192 patients with NDMM. Their analyses revealed deletions and amplifications in 98% of patients. Amplifications in 1q and deletions in 1p, 12p, 14q, 16q, and 22q were the most common abnormalities conferring poor prognosis, whereas recurrent amplifications of chromosomes 5, 9, 11, 15, and 19 were associated with favorable prognosis. Although amp(1q23.3), amp(5q31.3), and del(12p13.31) were independent prognostic markers, the latter remained the most powerful independent adverse marker (P < 0.0001; hazard ratio [HR], 3.17), and marker amp(5q31.3) (P = 0.0005; HR, 0.37) was a favorable prognostic marker. Patients with amp (5q31.3) alone and low serum $\beta_2 M$ had an extremely favorable prognosis (5-year OS, 87%); conversely, patients with del(12p13.31) alone, or amp(5q31.3) and del(12p13.31) and high serum $\beta_2 M$ had a very poor outcome (5-year OS, 20%). This prognostic model was validated in an independent validation cohort of 273 patients (85).

The protooncogene, *ras*, was studied for activating mutations in 346 patients with previously untreated MM, enrolled in the ECOG trial E4986, and no relationship to survival was detected with the more frequent N-*ras* mutations. However, patients with K-*ras* gene mutation demonstrated a greater tumor load with a negative impact on the survival. Overall, the incidence of ras mutations was 39%.

Gene Expression Profiling

It is increasingly being recognized that the wide variation in the survival of patients with MM cannot be solely accounted for by the ISS and that the molecular signatures provide invaluable information about the disease biology, prognosis, and the best treatment options. Many hematologic malignancies have witnessed the development of prognostically relevant disease subclassification through microarray profiling. MM is no exception, and considerable progress has been made to accurately predict individual patients' clinical course and survival outcomes using a molecular classification. Zhan and colleagues have comprehensively studied the gene expression on purified (CD138 selection) PCs of 414 patients with NDMM who underwent HDT with tandem transplants (86). They introduced seven molecular subtypes of MM: PR (proliferation), LB (low bone disease), MS (*MMSET*), HY (hyperdiploid), CD-1 (*CCND1*), CD-2 (*CCND3*), and MF (MAF/MAFB). HY, CD-1, CD-2, and LB comprised the low-risk group with 3-year actuarial probabilities of 81% to 88%. The two high-risk groups, MS and PR, did not achieve a therapeutic benefit on Total Therapy 2 (87). In a cohort of 532 newly diagnosed patients who received tandem transplants, the same group of investigators identified 70

genes linked to shortened survival, with 30% of 51 overexpressing and 50% of 19 underexpressing gene mapping to chromosome 1 (a chromosome linked to many malignancies, including non-Hodgkin lymphoma, Wilms tumor, and ovarian and breast cancers). This model was supplanted by an extremely powerful and simplified 17-gene prognostic model to detect the high-risk disease. In addition, this model could successfully prognosticate the patients with relapsed disease on either single-agent bortezomib or high-dose dexamethasone (APEX phase 3 trial) (87). It has been validated using Mayo Clinic data set of 71 patients with NDMM treated with HDT, but practical impediments remain in the routine clinical utilization of this model. The ability to further classify the 17-gene molecular model-based high-risk patients by their translocation (4;14) status indicates the heterogeneity of the disease and suggests that the sole application

TABLE 1
New proposed International Myeloma Working Group molecular cytogenetic classification

	Percentage of Patients	Clinical and Laboratory Features
Hyperdiploid	45	More favorable, IgG-κ, older patients
Nonhyperdiploid	40	Aggressive, IgA-λ, younger individuals
Cyclin D translocation	18	
t(11;14)(q13;q32)	16	Upregulation of CCND1; favorable prognosis; bone lesions. Two subtypes by GEP
t(6;14q)(p21;32)	2	Probably same as CCND1
t(12;14)(p13;q32)	<1	Rare
MMSET translocation	15	
t(4;14)(p16;q32)	15	Upregulation of MMSET; upregulation of FGFR3 in 75% unfavorable prognosis with conventional therapy; bone lesions less frequent
MAF translocation	8	Aggressive
t(14;16)(q32;q23)	5	Confirmed as aggressive by at least two series
t(14;20)(q32;q11)	2	One series shows more aggressive disease
t(8;14)(q24;q32)	1	Unknown effect on outcome but presumed aggressive
Unclassified (other)	15	Various subtypes and some with overlap

Source: From Ref. 88 with permission.

of this molecular model could provide incomplete prognostic information at best. The IMWG recommends adoption of a working genetic classification and has proposed a new molecular cytogenetic classification based on existing data, including considerable overlap between translocation and cyclin classification and University of Arkansas for Medical Sciences-suggested panel (Table 1) (88).

Immunophenotyping

Over the course of the last few decades, a continuous effort to identify diagnosis-, prognosis-, and therapy-related immunophenotypic markers has been instrumental in the recognition of the correlations between certain cellular antigens and the different phenotypic entities of MM. The extramedullary extension of the neoplastic PCs has been associated with a reduced expression or total absence (as in de novo or secondary PC leukemia) of the adhesion molecule, CD56 (89), and upregulation of CD44 on the PCs. CD28 (a T-cell marker) expression correlates with disease progression and is universally expressed in the human myeloma cell lines (89,90). Its association with t(14;16) and del(17p) is notable. The absence of CD45 and CD27 portends a worse outcome. In a multivariate analysis of 95 patients with NDMM who underwent HDT, the lack of CD45 expression was the only significant variable that affected the outcome (median OS of 42 months for CD45– vs. not reached at 4 years for CD45+ MM, $P = 0.004$) (82). A small subset of CD45+ PCs constitutes the proliferative compartment of the BM, and the expression of this antigen is required for IL-6 signaling but prevents insulin growth factor 1 (IGF-1)-mediated AKT pathway activation. Furthermore, a lower degree of angiogenesis, likely due to reduced vascular endothelial growth factor production, was observed with CD45+ expression. CD27 expression is associated with a better OS (92% at 3 years for CD27+ MM vs. 50% in CD27– MM) (91).

CD221 (IGF-1 receptor) overexpression is linked with t(4;14) or t(14;16), whereas CD20 expression is tightly associated with the more favorable t(11;14) and small lymphoplasmacytic morphology. Aberrant CD117 (c-kit) expression is predominant in the MGUS and indolent phases and infrequent (8%) in the relapsed cases (92). It is associated with a superior outcome (3-year OS, 93% for CD117+ vs. 64% for CD117– MM; $P = 0.05$).

The value of immunophenotyping NDMM by multiparametric flow cytometry was clearly established by the Spanish group in a recent prospective analysis of 685 patients treated with HDT (GEM 2000 protocol) (93). A prognostic model, risk stratifying the patients with NDMM into three categories, the poor risk (CD28+/CD117–; 23%), the intermediate risk (CD28–/CD117– or CD28+/CD117+; 56%), and the good risk (CD28–/CD117+, 21%) with OS 45 months, 68 months, and not reached, respectively, was promulgated by this group. The HDT followed by ASCT was not beneficial in approximately one quarter of patients in the high-risk group (93).

Measurement of the Proliferative Capacity

That the rate of clonal PC expansion can affect the disease outcome has been known for a long time, and several methodologies have been used to assess the degree of proliferation. One such test, the PCLI, is a slide-based method that measures the percentage of BM myeloma cells in the S-phase of the cell cycle. The proliferating cells incorporate bromo-2-deoxyuridine, which is detected by BU-1 antibody. A high PCLI (≥ 1) is an independent and powerful predictor of survival in patients treated with conventional chemotherapy or HDT. It serves as a useful adjunct to the chromosomal studies in prognosticating patients. Its incorporation into the ISS enhances the value of the staging system for low (ISS 1) and intermediate (ISS 2) patient groups but not stage 3 patients on conventional therapy or HDT. Even in those in the plateau phase of the disease with apparent stability and less than 10% BMPCs, a distinctive subset of patients with a high PCLI (≥1%) demonstrates short time to disease progression (median, 8 vs. 39 months in the matched control group, with PCLI < 1%; P < 0.0001) and shorter survival (median, 20 vs. 56 months, P < 0.0001) (94). A recent study highlighted the prognostic relevance of PCLI in the patients treated with immunomodulatory agents, thalidomide, and lenalidomide, with high baseline PCLI (≥1) predicting a poorer progression-free survival. However, lenalidomide appeared to negate the adverse impact of high PCLI on OS, an effect not seen in the thalidomide arm. Undoubtedly, a longer follow-up of patients is required to determine the true impact of the PCLI in patients on lenalidomide therapy.

The proliferative activity of PCs can also be determined by flow cytometry, using a DNA/CD38 double-staining technique. A high proportion of PCs in S-phase (>3%) indicated poorer prognosis. A poor correlation between the slide and flow cytometric LI assays has been demonstrated by the Australian group who questioned the sensitivity and accuracy of the less objective slide-based PCLI requiring manual enumeration of the PCs. In the flow cytometric analysis, the PCLI of primitive PCs (CD38++/CD45+) is found to be higher than that of mature myeloma cells (CD38++/CD45) and correlated better with the disease status (mean PCLI of 9.2% in the progressive disease and 2.2% in the plateau, $P ≤ 0.001$).

Ki-67 protein is a marker for proliferation that is expressed by all the cells in the "growth fraction" of the tumor, including the cells in the late G1, S, G2, and mitotic phases of the cell cycle. The Ki-67 proliferative index represents the fraction of myeloma cells expressing Ki-67 antigen as detected by a monoclonal antibody. A higher index indicates poorer prognosis, and a cutoff of 8% could categorize patients with NDMM into two groups with a difference in survival OS (P < 0.07) (95).

Circulating PCs

Monoclonal PCs in the peripheral blood have been an indirect measure of myeloma activity. Circulating PCs are independent prognostic marker for survival in patients with previously untreated myeloma. Patients with 4% or more blood monoclonal plasma cells (BPCs) had a median survival of 2.4 years versus 4.4 years for those with less than 4% BPCs (P < 0.001) (47). A positive correlation between absolute number of circulating PCs and mean MVD, a marker of BM angiogenesis, indirectly suggests angiogenesis-mediated promotion of PC proliferation and circulation (61). A correlation between peripheral blood labeling index and BM labeling index (PCLI) has also been established (96).

Magnetic Resonance Imaging

The superiority of the more sensitive tests, such as the whole-body/spinal magnetic resonance imaging (MRI) and the positron emission tomography (PET) over the conventional radiography is being exploited to accurately prognosticate patients with MM (97). One of the key features of the DS stage I patients is the absence of skeletal involvement detected radiographically. However, 29% to 50% of DS stage I patients demonstrate infiltration of the marrow by MRI. The extent of the BM infiltration influences survival and can be adequately estimated by MRI. Various MRI patterns of the BM infiltration—normal, focal, diffuse, and variegated—have been used to predict the OS (56, 51, 24, and 52 months, respectively). Within each ISS I and II stages, the concomitant detection of diffuse BM infiltration by MRI can segregate the patients into two groups with statistically different survival outcomes suggesting enhancement of the prognostic value of ISS with this test. This finding is similar to the previously described observation noted with the incorporation of PCLI to the ISS. The whole-body multidetector computerized tomography has not been found to be as sensitive as the whole-body MRI for evaluating skeletal involvement in MM.

Positron Emission Tomography

The avidity of metabolically active myeloma cells for 18F fluorodeoxyglucose (FDG), a radiolabeled glucose analog used in conjunction with PET, is well known. Whole-body FDG PET has been shown to detect occult lesions in 4 of 16 previously untreated patients who had negative findings on skeletal survey by standard radiography. Another 25% harbored extramedullary lesions, the detection of which was obviously beyond the realm of conventional radiography. The extramedullary involvement is a marker of poor prognosis in MM. Moreover, the persistence of FDG uptake after the therapy was a predictor of early relapse.

The use of PET scan and MRI overcomes the limitation of conventional radiography in prognosticating patients by the DS staging, and a DS plus staging system that incorporates the findings of PET/MRI to the original DS staging system has been proposed for predicting OS. PET scan can detect both medullary and extramedullary lesion simultaneously and can potentially upstage the patients because of its greater sensitivity (85%) and specificity (92%) (98). A drawback of PET scan is its inability to detect very small lesions (<1 cm). Radiation-induced inflammatory changes can lead to false-positive PET, which should therefore only be performed at the time of diagnosis, or at least 2 months after the therapy (98).

■ RESPONSE TO THERAPY AND RESPONSE DURATION

Although a consistent improvement in the OS of patients with MM has been seen over the course of the last two decades, it is not clear to what extent this is a direct translation of improvement in the overall response rates and an increment in the CR rates, particularly with the use of HDT and novel

agents. It is still debatable whether achievement of CR in and of itself is an indicator of improved survival, and its use as a surrogate marker for OS is falling out of favor because of the inconsistent results in several trials. In the instances where the responders have had a better OS than the nonresponders, the improvement in the results could possibly be attributed to other prognostic factors influencing the outcome. The achievement of similar (40%) CR rates after HDT had previously failed to demonstrate an improvement in the OS in the patients who had cytogenetic abnormalities when compared with the low-risk patients. Furthermore, similar survival outcomes were demonstrated in the Southwest Oncology Group chemotherapy trials in each response category in the 6- and 12-month landmark analyses (99). In contrast, worse outcomes were seen in the patients who developed disease progression because of the persistence and regrowth of the resistant (residual) myeloma cells, indicating that the time to first progression of the disease from the initiation of therapy, that is, the length of stability and not the depth of response, is the best predictor of OS. These data, however, cannot be extrapolated to treatments with novel agents or HDT. In a large cohort of patients (N = 668) who underwent HDT, Barlogie et al. studied the effect of concomitant administration of thalidomide from the time of induction until relapse or the occurrence of adverse events. Notably, an improvement in the CR rate (62% vs. 43% in the control group [HDT without thalidomide]) and the 5-year EFS, but not OS (5-year OS was 65% in both groups; P = 0.90), could be demonstrated. However, after a median follow-up of 8 years, the patients with the karyotypic abnormalities had a distinct improvement in the 8-year OS in the thalidomide arm (46% vs. 27%; P = 0.02). In the GEP-based risk stratification, the high-risk group patients (13%) from the same data set who achieved CR had a superior outcome compared with those who did not (P = 0.001). In the low-risk group, OS was similar, irrespective of the magnitude of response (P = 0.128) (100). Consequently, the attainment of CR should be the goal of therapy in the genetically defined high-risk cohort in which it improves OS.

A study of nearly 500 patients who underwent ASCT within 12 months of diagnosis of MM demonstrated that patients who relapsed early (within 12 months of ASCT; 24%) had a shorter median OS of 26.6.months from diagnosis compared with late relapsers (OS, 90.7 months; $P < 0.001$) (101). Although the traditional prognostic factors such as PCLI of 1 or greater and failure to achieve CR were the predictors of early relapse in this study, patients who required more than one treatment regimen prior to ASCT also had a higher likelihood of relapsing. In a multivariate analysis involving many other prognostic factors, early relapse after ASCT was recognized as an independent predictor of short OS, thereby suggesting that even in the absence of known risk factors (e.g., high-risk cytogenetics, high β_2M, high PCLI) early relapse after ASCT can dictate survival outcomes (101).

■ PREDICTORS OF PROGRESSION OF PREMALIGNANT MONOCLONAL GAMMOPATHIES

The study of the natural history of MGUS has unequivocally established that it may not necessarily follow a stable course (102–104). Indeed, the actuarial probability of progression to MM has been shown to be at 17%, 34%, and 39% at 10, 20, and 25 years of follow-up, respectively, if the competing causes of death are not taken into account (103). The probability of the malignant transformation has been shown to be related to the PC load as calculated by the size of the M component (7% for the M protein of 1 g/dL to 34% for 3 g/dL at 10 years after diagnosis) (104), the degree of BM plasmacytosis (low risk with <5% BMPCs), and an abnormal FLC ratio (105). Furthermore, the involvement of IgA isotype, detectable Bence Jones protein excretion, the presence of circulating PCs, and the reduction of uninvolved immunoglobulins also indicate enhanced risk of evolution to MM (106–110).

Using a simple, four monoclonal antibody-dependent immunophenotypic analysis on the patients with MGUS and SMM, the Spanish Group identified subsets of patients with 95% or more aberrant BMPCs as defined by the absence of CD19 and/or CD45, decreased expression of CD38 and overexpression of CD56. This subset had a 5-year risk of progression to MM at 25% and 64%, respectively, for MGUS and SMM cases (111).

Kyle and colleagues recently proposed a prognostic model to risk stratify patients with SMM after an extensive follow-up of 276 such patients. Their study revealed a 73% cumulative probability of progression to active myeloma or amyloidosis at 15 years and that the serum monoclonal M protein and extent of BM involvement were independent predictors of progression. Their proposed model identified three risk groups of patients: group 1: 10% or more PCs and 3 g/dL or more of monoclonal protein; group 2: 10% or more PCs and less than 3 g/dL of monoclonal protein; and group 3: less than 10% PCs and 3 g/dL or more of monoclonal protein with median time to progression of 2, 8, and 19 years, respectively (112).

■ CLINICAL APPLICATION

A vastly diverse outcome, with an increasing recognition of myeloma as a conglomeration of diseases instead of a single entity, has unequivocally established the need for risk stratification of patients at the time of diagnosis. The mSMART (*Mayo Stratification of Myeloma And Risk*-adapted *Therapy*), an evidence-based consensus statement annunciated by a group of experts at the Mayo Clinic, classifies patients into three distinct subcategories: the high risk (25% of patients), intermediate risk, and standard risk (4,6). The presence of *any* of the following—deletion 17p, t(4;14), t(14;16), cytogenetic deletion of 13q, hypodiploidy, or PCLI 3% or more—confers a poorer prognosis on the patients. The approach to such high-risk patients is based on their transplant eligibility status. Those who are deemed fit to undergo transplant should get the collection of their stem cells adequate for two transplants after a successful induction with three to four cycles of lenalidomide plus low-dose dexamethasone therapy or bortezomib-based regimen (especially if patients have renal failure or lack of response after the initial two cycles of lenalidonide–dexamethasone therapy). After the stem cell banking, a bortezomib-based regimen such as MPV (melphalan, prednisone, and Velcade) or VTD (Velcade, thalidomide, and dexamethasone) should be initiated with the aim of achieving the maximal response, following which reinitiation of lenalidomide and low-dose dexamethasone should be considered. This is one of the few approaches incorporating the current prognostic systems to assist in clinical decision making.

An option of allogeneic transplantation exists in a selected population of younger patients in the high-risk category. The value and the timing of ASCT in the high-risk population are debatable, and the median OS is approximately 2 years, even with double transplantation. Patients with t(4;14) and β_2M 4 mg/L or less plus hemoglobin 10 g/dL or higher are stratified in the intermediate risk category because of the benefit obtained by HDT in such a subset as opposed to other patients belonging to the t(4;14) category. A bortezomib-based regimen such as MPV should be considered in the high-risk patients who are deemed ineligible for transplantation.

■ CONCLUSION AND FUTURE DIRECTIONS

The relevance of the prognostic tools, such as the chromosomal studies and the GEP, in MM is increasingly being recognized. Not only have the cytogenetics and FISH studies supplanted other clinical and laboratory prognostic parameters, they have reinforced the urgent need for an international uniform cytogenetic classification system, a model more reflective of the disease biology and heterogeneity (113). The goal of the current and future therapies is to improve outcome of patients with MM and to blur the line between the high-risk and the standard-risk categories, thereby marginalizing the significance of the prognostic markers. Another challenge for the myeloma community in the rapidly evolving era of novel therapies is to continuously generate viable prognostic models that can definitively predict outcome in all patients.

■ REFERENCES

1. Kyle RA. Prognostic factors in multiple myeloma. *Stem Cells* 1995;13 Suppl 2:56–63.

2. Bergsagel PL. Prognostic factors in multiple myeloma: it's in the genes. *Clin Cancer Res* 2003;9(2):533–534.

3. Dewald GW, Therneau T, Larson D, et al. Relationship of patient survival and chromosome anomalies detected in metaphase and/or interphase cells at diagnosis of myeloma. *Blood* 2005;106(10):3553–3558.

4. Dispenzieri A, Rajkumar SV, Gertz MA, et al. Treatment of newly diagnosed multiple myeloma based on Mayo Stratification of Myeloma and Risk-adapted Therapy (mSMART): consensus statement. *Mayo Clin Proc* 2007;82(3):323–341.

5. Stewart AK, Bergsagel PL, Greipp PR, et al. A practical guide to defining high-risk myeloma for clinical trials, patient counseling and choice of therapy. *Leukemia* 2007;21(3):529–534.

6. Kumar SK, Mikhael JR, Buadi FK, et al. Management of newly diagnosed symptomatic multiple myeloma: updated Mayo Stratification of Myeloma and Risk-Adapted Therapy (mSMART) consensus guidelines. *Mayo Clin Proc* 2009;84(12):1095–1110.

7. Bartl R, Frisch B, Fateh-Moghadam A, Kettner G, Jaeger K, Sommerfeld W. Histologic classification and staging of multiple myeloma. A retrospective and prospective study of 674 cases. *Am J Clin Pathol* 1987;87(3):342–355.

8. Bataille R, Boccadoro M, Klein B, Durie B, Pileri A. C-reactive protein and beta-2 microglobulin produce a simple and powerful myeloma staging system. *Blood* 1992;80(3):733–737.

9. Durie BG, Salmon SE. A clinical staging system for multiple myeloma. Correlation of measured myeloma cell mass with presenting clinical features, response to treatment, and survival. *Cancer* 1975;36(3):842–854.

10. Greipp PR, Katzmann JA, O'Fallon WM, Kyle RA. Value of beta 2-microglobulin level and plasma cell labeling indices as prognostic factors in patients with newly diagnosed myeloma. *Blood* 1988;72(1):219–223.

11. Greipp PR, Lust JA, O'Fallon WM, Katzmann JA, Witzig TE, Kyle RA. Plasma cell labeling index and beta 2-microglobulin predict survival independent of thymidine kinase and C-reactive protein in multiple myeloma. *Blood* 1993;81(12):3382–3387.

12. Greipp PR, San Miguel J, Durie BG, et al. International staging system for multiple myeloma. *J Clin Oncol* 2005;23(15):3412–3420.

13. San Miguel JF, García-Sanz R, González M, et al. A new staging system for multiple myeloma based on the number of S-phase plasma cells. *Blood* 1995;85(2):448–455.

14. San-Miguel J, Harousseau JL, Joshua D, Anderson KC. Individualizing treatment of patients with myeloma in the era of novel agents. *J Clin Oncol* 2008;26(16):2761–2766.

15. Fonseca R, San Miguel J. Prognostic factors and staging in multiple myeloma. *Hematol Oncol Clin North Am* 2007;21(6):1115–40, ix.

16. Rajkumar SV, Greipp PR. Prognostic factors in multiple myeloma. *Hematol Oncol Clin North Am* 1999;13(6):1295–314, xi.

17. San Miguel JF, García-Sanz R. Prognostic features of multiple myeloma. *Best Pract Res Clin Haematol* 2005;18(4):569–583.

18. A predictive model for aggressive non-Hodgkin's lymphoma. The International Non-Hodgkin's Lymphoma Prognostic Factors Project. *N Engl J Med* 1993;329:987–994.

19. Ludwig H, Durie BG, Bolejack V, et al. Myeloma in patients younger than age 50 years presents with more favorable features and shows better survival: an analysis of 10 549 patients from the International Myeloma Working Group. *Blood* 2008;111(8):4039–4047.

20. Nilsson T, Lenhoff S, Turesson I, et al. Cytogenetic features of multiple myeloma: impact of gender, age, disease phase, culture time, and cytokine stimulation. *Eur J Haematol* 2002;68(6):345–353.

21. Sagaster V, Kaufmann H, Odelga V, et al. Chromosomal abnormalities of young multiple myeloma patients (<45 yr) are not different from those of other age groups and are independent of stage according to the International Staging System. *Eur J Haematol* 2007;78(3):227–234.

22. Ross FM, Ibrahim AH, Vilain-Holmes A, et al. UK Myeloma Forum. Age has a profound effect on the incidence and significance of chromosome abnormalities in myeloma. *Leukemia* 2005;19(9):1634–1642.

23. García-Sanz R, González-Fraile MI, Mateo G, et al. Proliferative activity of plasma cells is the most relevant prognostic factor in elderly multiple myeloma patients. *Int J Cancer* 2004;112(5):884–889.

24. Siegel DS, Desikan KR, Mehta J, et al. Age is not a prognostic variable with autotransplants for multiple myeloma. *Blood* 1999;93(1):51–54.

25. Rajkumar SV, Kyle RA. Multiple myeloma: diagnosis and treatment. *Mayo Clin Proc* 2005;80(10):1371–1382.

26. Modiano MR, Villar-Werstler P, Crowley J, Salmon SE. Evaluation of race as a prognostic factor in multiple myeloma. An ancillary of Southwest Oncology Group Study 8229. *J Clin Oncol* 1996;14(3):974–977.

27. Saraf S, Chen YH, Dobogai LC, et al. Prolonged responses after autologous stem cell transplantation in African-American patients with multiple myeloma. *Bone Marrow Transplant* 2006;37(12):1099–1102.

28. Bataille R, Durie BG, Grenier J. Serum beta2 microglobulin and survival duration in multiple myeloma: a simple reliable marker for staging. *Br J Haematol* 1983;55(3):439–447.

29. Kyle RA, Gertz MA, Witzig TE, et al. Review of 1027 patients with newly diagnosed multiple myeloma. *Mayo Clin Proc* 2003;78(1):21–33.

30. Kyle RA. Why better prognostic factors for multiple myeloma are needed. *Blood* 1994;83(7):1713–1716.

31. Kapoor P, Snozek CL, Colby C, et al. Clinical impact of discordance in serum albumin measurements on myeloma international staging system. *J Clin Oncol* 2008;26(24):4051–4052.

32. Merlini G, Perfetti V, Gobbi PG, et al. Acute phase proteins and prognosis in multiple myeloma. *Br J Haematol* 1993;83(4):595–601.

33. Alexandrakis MG, Passam FH, Kyriakou DS, et al. Serum level of interleukin-16 in multiple myeloma patients and its relationship to disease activity. *Am J Hematol* 2004;75(2):101–106.

34. Ballester OF, Moscinski LC, Lyman GH, et al. High levels of interleukin-6 are associated with low tumor burden and low growth fraction in multiple myeloma. *Blood* 1994;83(7):1903–1908.

35. Ludwig H, Nachbaur DM, Fritz E, Krainer M, Huber H. Interleukin-6 is a prognostic factor in multiple myeloma. *Blood* 1991;77(12):2794–2795.

36. Ohtani K, Ninomiya H, Hasegawa Y, et al. Clinical significance of elevated soluble interleukin-6 receptor levels in the sera of patients with plasma cell dyscrasias. *Br J Haematol* 1995;91(1):116–120.

37. Reibnegger G, Krainer M, Herold M, Ludwig H, Wachter H, Huber H. Predictive value of interleukin-6 and neopterin in patients with multiple myeloma. *Cancer Res* 1991;51(23 Pt 1):6250–6253.

38. Rajkumar SV, Buadi F. Multiple myeloma: new staging systems for diagnosis, prognosis and response evaluation. *Best Pract Res Clin Haematol* 2007;20(4):665–680.

39. Snozek CL, Katzmann JA, Kyle RA, et al. Prognostic value of the serum free light chain ratio in newly diagnosed myeloma: proposed incorporation into the international staging system. *Leukemia* 2008;22(10):1933–1937.

40. Dispenzieri A, Zhang L, Katzmann JA, et al. Appraisal of immunoglobulin free light chain as a marker of response. *Blood* 2008;111(10):4908–4915.

41. Ege H, Gertz MA, Markovic SN, et al. Prediction of survival using absolute lymphocyte count for newly diagnosed patients with multiple myeloma: a retrospective study. *Br J Haematol* 2008;141(6):792–798.

42. Kim H, Sohn HJ, Kim S, Lee JS, Kim WK, Suh C. Early lymphocyte recovery predicts longer survival after autologous peripheral blood stem cell transplantation in multiple myeloma. *Bone Marrow Transplant* 2006;37(11):1037–1042.

43. Durie BG, Harousseau JL, Miguel JS, et al; International Myeloma Working Group. International uniform response criteria for multiple myeloma. *Leukemia* 2006;20(9):1467–1473.

44. Kay NE, Leong T, Bone N, et al. T-helper phenotypes in the blood of myeloma patients on ECOG phase III trials E9486/E3A93. *Br J Haematol* 1998;100(3):459–463.

45. Kay NE, Leong TL, Bone N, et al. Blood levels of immune cells predict survival in myeloma patients: results of an Eastern Cooperative Oncology Group phase 3 trial for newly diagnosed multiple myeloma patients. *Blood* 2001;98(1):23–28.

46. San Miguel JF, González M, Gascón A, et al. Lymphoid subsets and prognostic factors in multiple myeloma. Cooperative Group for the Study of Monoclonal Gammopathies. *Br J Haematol* 1992;80(3):305–309.

47. Witzig TE, Gertz MA, Lust JA, Kyle RA, O'Fallon WM, Greipp PR. Peripheral blood monoclonal plasma cells as a predictor of survival in patients with multiple myeloma. *Blood* 1996;88(5):1780–1787.

48. Greipp PR, Leong T, Bennett JM, et al. Plasmablastic morphology—an independent prognostic factor with clinical and laboratory correlates: Eastern Cooperative Oncology Group (ECOG) myeloma trial E9486 report by the ECOG Myeloma Laboratory Group. *Blood* 1998;91(7):2501–2507.

49. Bartl R, Frisch B. Clinical significance of bone marrow biopsy and plasma cell morphology in MM and MGUS. *Pathol Biol* 1999;47(2):158–168.

50. Rajkumar SV, Greipp PR. Angiogenesis in multiple myeloma. *Br J Haematol* 2001;113(3):565.

51. Rajkumar SV, Kyle RA. Angiogenesis in multiple myeloma. *Semin Oncol* 2001;28(6):560–564.

52. Jakob C, Sterz J, Zavrski I, et al. Angiogenesis in multiple myeloma. *Eur J Cancer* 2006;42(11):1581–1590.

53. Vacca A, Ria R, Semeraro F, et al. Endothelial cells in the bone marrow of patients with multiple myeloma. *Blood* 2003;102(9):3340–3348.

54. Vacca A, Ribatti D. Bone marrow angiogenesis in multiple myeloma. *Leukemia* 2006;20(2):193–199.

55. Rajkumar SV, Leong T, Roche PC, et al. Prognostic value of bone marrow angiogenesis in multiple myeloma. *Clin Cancer Res* 2000;6(8):3111–3116.

56. Rajkumar SV, Mesa RA, Fonseca R, et al. Bone marrow angiogenesis in 400 patients with monoclonal gammopathy of undetermined significance, multiple myeloma, and primary amyloidosis. *Clin Cancer Res* 2002;8(7):2210–2216.

57. Sezer O, Niemöller K, Eucker J, et al. Bone marrow microvessel density is a prognostic factor for survival in patients with multiple myeloma. *Ann Hematol* 2000;79(10):574–577.

58. Hanahan D, Folkman J. Patterns and emerging mechanisms of the angiogenic switch during tumorigenesis. *Cell* 1996;86(3):353–364.

59. Kumar S, Witzig TE, Timm M, et al. Bone marrow angiogenic ability and expression of angiogenic cytokines in myeloma: evidence favoring loss of marrow angiogenesis inhibitory activity with disease progression. *Blood* 2004;104(4):1159–1165.

60. Alexandrakis MG, Passam FJ, Ganotakis E, et al. Bone marrow microvascular density and angiogenic growth factors in multiple myeloma. *Clin Chem Lab Med* 2004;42(10):1122–1126.

61. Kumar S, Witzig TE, Greipp PR, Rajkumar SV. Bone marrow angiogenesis and circulating plasma cells in multiple myeloma. *Br J Haematol* 2003;122(2):272–274.

62. Pruneri G, Ponzoni M, Ferreri AJ, et al. Microvessel density, a surrogate marker of angiogenesis, is significantly related to survival in multiple myeloma patients. *Br J Haematol* 2002;118(3):817–820.

63. Schreiber S, Ackermann J, Obermair A, et al. Multiple myeloma with deletion of chromosome 13q is characterized by increased bone marrow neovascularization. *Br J Haematol* 2000;110(3):605–609.

64. Sezer O, Niemöller K, Jakob C, et al. Relationship between bone marrow angiogenesis and plasma cell infiltration and serum beta2-microglobulin levels

in patients with multiple myeloma. *Ann Hematol* 2001;80(10):598–601.

65. Sezer O, Niemöller K, Kaufmann O, et al. Decrease of bone marrow angiogenesis in myeloma patients achieving a remission after chemotherapy. *Eur J Haematol* 2001;66(4):238–244.

66. Andersen NF, Standal T, Nielsen JL, et al. Syndecan-1 and angiogenic cytokines in multiple myeloma: correlation with bone marrow angiogenesis and survival. *Br J Haematol* 2005;128(2):210–217.

67. Iwasaki T, Hamano T, Ogata A, Hashimoto N, Kitano M, Kakishita E. Clinical significance of vascular endothelial growth factor and hepatocyte growth factor in multiple myeloma. *Br J Haematol* 2002;116(4):796–802.

68. Kyrtsonis MC, Vassilakopoulos TP, Siakantaris MP, et al. Serum syndecan-1, basic fibroblast growth factor and osteoprotegerin in myeloma patients at diagnosis and during the course of the disease. *Eur J Haematol* 2004;72(4):252–258.

69. Fonseca R, Barlogie B, Bataille R, et al. Genetics and cytogenetics of multiple myeloma: a workshop report. *Cancer Res* 2004;64(4):1546–1558.

70. Kuehl WM, Bergsagel PL. Multiple myeloma: evolving genetic events and host interactions. *Nat Rev Cancer* 2002;2(3):175–187.

71. Gertz MA, Lacy MQ, Dispenzieri A, et al. Clinical implications of t(11;14)(q13;q32), t(4;14)(p16.3;q32), and -17p13 in myeloma patients treated with high-dose therapy. *Blood* 2005;106(8):2837–2840.

72. Moreau P, Attal M, Garban F, et al; SAKK; IFM Group. Heterogeneity of t(4;14) in multiple myeloma. Long-term follow-up of 100 cases treated with tandem transplantation in IFM99 trials. *Leukemia* 2007;21(9):2020–2024.

73. Lane DP. Cancer. p53, guardian of the genome. *Nature* 1992;358(6381):15–16.

74. Avet-Loiseau H Attal M, Moreau P, et al. Genetic abnormalities and survival in multiple myeloma: the experience of the Intergroupe Francophone du Myelome. *Blood* 2007;109:3489–3495.

75. Chang H, Qi C, Yi QL, Reece D, Stewart AK. p53 gene deletion detected by fluorescence in situ hybridization is an adverse prognostic factor for patients with multiple myeloma following autologous stem cell transplantation. *Blood* 2005;105(1):358–360.

76. Drach J, Ackerman J, Kaufmann H, Königsberg R, Huber H. Deletions of the p53 gene in multiple myeloma. *Br J Haematol* 2000;108(4):886.

77. Drach J, Ackermann J, Fritz E, et al. Presence of a p53 gene deletion in patients with multiple myeloma predicts for short survival after conventional-dose chemotherapy. *Blood* 1998;92(3):802–809.

78. Chang H, Sloan S, Li D, Keith Stewart A. Multiple myeloma involving central nervous system: high frequency of chromosome 17p13.1 (p53) deletions. *Br J Haematol* 2004;127(3):280–284.

79. Pérez-Simón JA, García-Sanz R, Tabernero MD, et al. Prognostic value of numerical chromosome aberrations in multiple myeloma: A FISH analysis of 15 different chromosomes. *Blood* 1998;91(9):3366–3371.

80. Shaughnessy J Jr, Tian E, Sawyer J, et al. Prognostic impact of cytogenetic and interphase fluorescence in situ hybridization-defined chromosome 13 deletion in multiple myeloma: early results of total therapy II. *Br J Haematol* 2003;120(1):44–52.

81. Jagannath S, Richardson PG, Sonneveld P, et al. Bortezomib appears to overcome the poor prognosis conferred by chromosome 13 deletion in phase 2 and 3 trials. *Leukemia* 2007;21(1):151–157.

82. Gutiérrez NC, Castellanos MV, Martín ML, et al; GEM/PETHEMA Spanish Group. Prognostic and biological implications of genetic abnormalities in multiple myeloma undergoing autologous stem cell transplantation: t(4;14) is the most relevant adverse prognostic factor, whereas RB deletion as a unique abnormality is not associated with adverse prognosis. *Leukemia* 2007;21(1):143–150.

83. Moreau P, Facon T, Leleu X, et al; Intergroupe Francophone du Myélome. Recurrent 14q32 translocations determine the prognosis of multiple myeloma, especially in patients receiving intensive chemotherapy. *Blood* 2002;100(5):1579–1583.

84. Chang H, Qi XY, Stewart AK. t(11;14) does not predict long-term survival in myeloma. *Leukemia* 2005;19(6):1078–1079.

85. Avet-Loiseau H, Li C, Magrangeas F, et al. Prognostic significance of copy-number alterations in multiple myeloma. *J Clin Oncol* 2009;27(27):4585–4590.

86. Zhan F, Huang Y, Colla S, et al. The molecular classification of multiple myeloma. *Blood* 2006;108(6):2020–2028.

87. Zhan F, Barlogie B, Mulligan G, Shaughnessy JD Jr, Bryant B. High-risk myeloma: a gene expression based risk-stratification model for newly diagnosed multiple myeloma treated with high-dose therapy is predictive of outcome in relapsed disease treated with single-agent bortezomib or high-dose dexamethasone. *Blood* 2008;111(2):968–969.

88. Fonseca R, Bergsagel PL, Drach J, et al; International Myeloma Working Group. International Myeloma

Working Group molecular classification of multiple myeloma: spotlight review. *Leukemia* 2009; 23(12):2210–2221.

89. Pellat-Deceunynck C, Barillé S, Jego G, et al. The absence of CD56 (NCAM) on malignant plasma cells is a hallmark of plasma cell leukemia and of a special subset of multiple myeloma. *Leukemia* 1998; 12(12):1977–1982.

90. Robillard N, Jego G, Pellat-Deceunynck C, et al. CD28, a marker associated with tumoral expansion in multiple myeloma. *Clin Cancer Res* 1998;4(6):1521–1526.

91. Moreau P, Robillard N, Jégo G, et al. Lack of CD27 in myeloma delineates different presentation and outcome. *Br J Haematol* 2006;132(2):168–170.

92. Bataille R, Pellat-Deceunynck C, Robillard N, Avet-Loiseau H, Harousseau JL, Moreau P. CD117 (c-kit) is aberrantly expressed in a subset of MGUS and multiple myeloma with unexpectedly good prognosis. *Leuk Res* 2008;32(3):379–382.

93. Mateo G, Montalbán MA, Vidriales MB, et al; PETHEMA Study Group; GEM Study Group. Prognostic value of immunophenotyping in multiple myeloma: a study by the PETHEMA/GEM cooperative study groups on patients uniformly treated with high-dose therapy. *J Clin Oncol* 2008; 26(16):2737–2744.

94. Steensma DP, Gertz MA, Greipp PR, et al. A high bone marrow plasma cell labeling index in stable plateau-phase multiple myeloma is a marker for early disease progression and death. *Blood* 2001;97(8):2522–2523.

95. Alexandrakis MG, Passam FH, Kyriakou DS, Dambaki K, Niniraki M, Stathopoulos E. Ki-67 proliferation index: correlation with prognostic parameters and outcome in multiple myeloma. *Am J Clin Oncol* 2004;27(1):8–13.

96. Kumar S, Rajkumar SV, Greipp PR, Witzig TE. Cell proliferation of myeloma plasma cells: comparison of the blood and marrow compartments. *Am J Hematol* 2004;77(1):7–11.

97. D'Sa S, Abildgaard N, Tighe J, Shaw P, Hall-Craggs M. Guidelines for the use of imaging in the management of myeloma. *Br J Haematol* 2007;137(1):49–63.

98. Bredella MA, Steinbach L, Caputo G, Segall G, Hawkins R. Value of FDG PET in the assessment of patients with multiple myeloma. *AJR Am J Roentgenol* 2005;184(4):1199–1204.

99. Durie BG, Jacobson J, Barlogie B, Crowley J. Magnitude of response with myeloma frontline therapy does not predict outcome: importance of time to progression in southwest oncology group chemotherapy trials. *J Clin Oncol* 2004;22(10):1857–1863.

100. Haessler J, Shaughnessy JD Jr, Zhan F, et al. Benefit of complete response in multiple myeloma limited to high-risk subgroup identified by gene expression profiling. *Clin Cancer Res* 2007;13(23):7073–7079.

101. Kumar S, Mahmood ST, Lacy MQ, et al. Impact of early relapse after auto-SCT for multiple myeloma. *Bone Marrow Transplant* 2008;42(6):413–420.

102. Kyle RA. Monoclonal gammopathy of undetermined significance. Natural history in 241 cases. *Am J Med* 1978;64(5):814–826.

103. Kyle RA, Therneau TM, Rajkumar SV, Larson DR, Plevak MF, Melton LJ III. Long-term follow-up of 241 patients with monoclonal gammopathy of undetermined significance: the original Mayo Clinic series 25 years later. *Mayo Clin Proc* 2004;79(7):859–866.

104. Kyle RA, Therneau TM, Rajkumar SV, et al. A long-term study of prognosis in monoclonal gammopathy of undetermined significance. *N Engl J Med* 2002;346(8):564–569.

105. Rajkumar SV, Kyle RA, Therneau TM, et al. Serum free light chain ratio is an independent risk factor for progression in monoclonal gammopathy of undetermined significance. *Blood* 2005;106(3):812–817.

106. Gregersen H, Mellemkjaer L, Ibsen JS, Dahlerup JF, Thomassen L, Sørensen HT. The impact of M-component type and immunoglobulin concentration on the risk of malignant transformation in patients with monoclonal gammopathy of undetermined significance. *Haematologica* 2001;86(11): 1172–1179.

107. Rosiñol L, Cibeira MT, Montoto S, et al. Monoclonal gammopathy of undetermined significance: predictors of malignant transformation and recognition of an evolving type characterized by a progressive increase in M protein size. *Mayo Clin Proc* 2007;82(4):428–434.

108. Cesana C, Klersy C, Barbarano L, et al. Prognostic factors for malignant transformation in monoclonal gammopathy of undetermined significance and smoldering multiple myeloma. *J Clin Oncol* 2002;20(6):1625–1634.

109. Bladé J. Clinical practice. Monoclonal gammopathy of undetermined significance. *N Engl J Med* 2006;355(26):2765–2770.

110. Kumar S, Rajkumar SV, Kyle RA, et al. Prognostic value of circulating plasma cells in monoclonal gammopathy of undetermined significance. *J Clin Oncol* 2005;23(24):5668–5674.

111. Pérez-Persona E, Vidriales MB, Mateo G, et al. New criteria to identify risk of progression in monoclonal gammopathy of uncertain significance

and smoldering multiple myeloma based on multi-parameter flow cytometry analysis of bone marrow plasma cells. *Blood* 2007;110(7):2586–2592.

112. Kyle RA, Remstein ED, Therneau TM, et al. Clinical course and prognosis of smoldering (asymptomatic) multiple myeloma. *N Engl J Med* 2007;356(25):2582–2590.

113. Dispenzieri A. An internationally recognized uniform cytogenetic classification system is needed for multiple myeloma. *Leukemia* 2007;21(1):9–11.

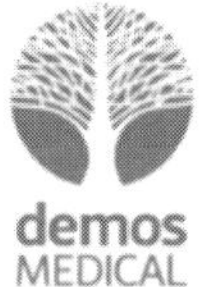

demos
MEDICAL

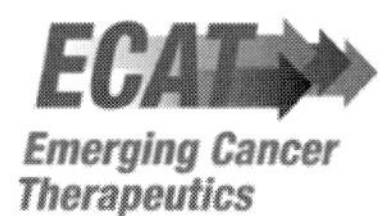

Emerging Cancer
Therapeutics

Initial Treatment of Multiple Myeloma in Transplant-Eligible Patients

Jacob Laubach,* Robert Schlossman, Constantine Mitsiades,
Kenneth Anderson, and Paul Richardson
Harvard Medical School, Boston, MA

■ ABSTRACT

The treatment of multiple myeloma (MM) has changed significantly over the past decade with the introduction of thalidomide, lenalidomide, and bortezomib. These agents are now standard of care for patients with relapsed and newly diagnosed disease. The management of a patient with newly diagnosed multiple myeloma is influenced to a great extent by eligibility for autologous stem cell transplantation (ASCT), which remains a cornerstone of therapy for appropriately selected patients. This chapter focuses on the use of thalidomide, lenalidomide, and bortezomib as part of initial therapy for transplant-eligible MM patients.

■ INTRODUCTION

The management of multiple myeloma (MM) has evolved rapidly over the past decade with the introduction of thalidomide, lenalidomide, and bortezomib, and overall patient outcomes have improved significantly during this period (1). Regimens incorporating these agents now represent the standard of care in relapsed and refractory as well as newly diagnosed disease. Autologous stem cell transplantation (ASCT), meanwhile, remains a cornerstone of MM therapy more than 25 years after its introduction to the field by McElwain and Powles (2). The use of ASCT in MM has evolved over time, and it is now most often utilized as consolidation following induction therapy or at first relapse. The manner in which new approaches to induction therapy are integrated into the overall

---

*Corresponding author, Dana Farber Cancer Institute,
44 Binney St, Boston, MA 02115
E-mail address: jacobp_laubach@dfci.harvard.edu

Emerging Cancer Therapeutics 1:2 (2010) 319–328.
© 2010 Demos Medical Publishing LLC. All rights reserved.
DOI: 10.5003/2151–4194.1.2.319

demosmedpub.com/ecat

management of transplant-eligible MM patients is the focus of this chapter.

■ DIAGNOSIS

As in all cases of suspected MM, the standard diagnostic evaluation for transplant-eligible MM patients includes assessment of electrolytes, cell counts and differential, renal and hepatic function, albumin, $\beta2$-microglobulin, quantitative immunoglobulins, serum free light chains, serum and urine protein electrophoresis with immunofixation, and bone abnormalities based on skeletal survey and, in selected patients, either magnetic resonance imaging or positron emission tomography/computed tomography. The bone marrow aspiration and biopsy are critical and provide information on the degree of bone marrow plasma cell involvement and the presence of cytogenetic abnormalities. Fluorescence in situ hybridization for deletion (del) 13, del 17, translocation (t)(4;14), t(11;14), and t(14;16) is recommended (3). Where available, gene expression profiling may be performed as part of the diagnostic evaluation, and as its role is further defined as part of ongoing clinical research, this modality is likely to play an increasingly important role in the management of MM (4,5).

Overall disease burden and prognosis are estimated on the basis of the initial diagnostic evaluation. The International Staging System (ISS) stage (6) and cytogenetic findings (7) are particularly valuable indicators of prognosis. Moreover, certain high-risk cytogenetic abnormalities such as t(4;14) and del 17 have in the past been associated with poor outcomes following ASCT (8–10), and thus influence decisions regarding the use of high-dose therapy in patients who harbor such gene alterations. Whether this association still applies in the current era of myeloma therapy is uncertain and needs further assessment, as several clinical trials in relapsed MM indicate that bortezomib (11), lenalidomide (12), and combinations of thalidomide/lenalidomide with bortezomib (13–16) overcome the poor prognosis associated with certain high-risk cytogenetic abnormalities.

Concurrent bone marrow processes, such as myelodysplastic syndrome or chronic lymphocytic leukemia, may occur in the setting of MM (17) and influence decisions regarding eligibility for ASCT. In addition, the presence of comorbid conditions and MM-associated organ dysfunction also influences management of patients who may otherwise be eligible for ASCT. Abnormal kidney function (Cr >2 mg/dL), for example, has been associated with an increased risk of transplant-related mortality as well as shortened overall survival (OS) (18). Ultimately, age and the nature as well as severity of comorbid medical conditions are the primary determinants of eligibility for ASCT.

■ GOALS OF THERAPY

The aim of induction therapy is to arrest tumor growth and MM-associated organ dysfunction. In patients who are eligible for ASCT, therapy is administered with the additional aim of preparing the bone marrow for subsequent stem cell harvest. To this end, maximal reduction of tumor burden with induction therapy is desired, as depth of response prior to ASCT appears to correlate with long-term survival following transplant (19,20). Thus, active treatment regimens that result in deep responses and yet are manageable with respect to treatment-associated toxicity are preferred for the transplant-eligible MM patient. With the introduction of thalidomide, lenalidomide, and bortezomib, clinicians can now choose from various options to achieve these aims, including two-, three-, and even four-drug regimens.

■ OPTIONS FOR INITIAL TREATMENT OF ASCT-ELIGIBLE MM PATIENTS

Thalidomide Plus Dexamethasone

The activity of thalidomide plus dexamethasone (thal-dex) as induction therapy was suggested by a retrospective, matched case-control analysis comparing thalidomide plus dexamethasone to the previous standard of care for induction therapy in transplant-eligible patients—the combination of vincristine, doxorubicin, and dexamethasone (VAD) (21). Thal-dex was superior with respect to the rate of very good partial response (VGPR) or better following ASCT (63% vs. 27%, $P < 0.0000$). These two regimens were subsequently compared in a randomized study involving induction in 204 patients with previously untreated MM (22). The rate of ≥ VGPR was higher in the thal-dex group prior to ASCT (35% vs. 13%, $P = 0.0027$), but equivalent in the two groups 6 months after ASCT (44% vs. 42%, $P = 0.87$), indicating that the benefit associated with thal-dex induction was negated following ASCT. In another large randomized study, thal-dex was compared to dexamethasone monotherapy in 470 patients with newly diagnosed, transplant-eligible MM patients (23). Thal-dex was superior to dexamethasone with respect to both overall response rate (63% vs. 46%, $P < 0.001$) and median time to progression (TTP) (23 vs. 6.5 months, $P < 0.01$).

Thal-dex is thus an important option for induction therapy in transplant-eligible MM patients. Extended treatment with thal-dex can be challenging due to side effects associated with thalidomide, particularly peripheral neuropathy (PN) (24), constipation, and fatigue. In addition, thalidomide is associated with an increased incidence of venous thromboembolic events (VTE) (25), and anticoagulation with either warfarin or low molecular weight heparin is generally advised for patients receiving thalidomide as induction therapy (26). Thal-dex can be considered for individuals with renal insufficiency, as it is generally well tolerated and active in patients with mild renal insufficiency (27). In addition, thalidomide is less myelosuppressive than lenalidomide and thus regimens such as thal-dex may benefit patients who present with pronounced cytopenias.

Lenalidomide Plus Dexamethasone

The efficacy of lenalidomide and dexamethasone in newly diagnosed, transplant-eligible MM patients was first demonstrated in a phase II study wherein it produced a partial response (PR) or better in 91% of patients, with a ≥ VGPR rate of 56% (28). Thirteen of 34 patients subsequently underwent ASCT, and in this subgroup the 2-year progression-free survival (PFS) and OS were 83% and 92%, respectively. A low rate of VTE (4%) was observed in this particular single-center trial. This was followed by a phase III study comparing lenalidomide plus high-dose dex (len-Dex) versus lenalidomide plus low-dose dex (len-dex). Lenalidomide was administered in both groups at 25 mg daily for 21 days in each 28 day cycle. Patients in the len-Dex arm received dexamethasone 40 mg on days 1 to 4, 9 to 12, and 17 to 20, whereas those in the len-dex arm received dexamethasone 40 mg weekly. Len-Dex produced higher ORR (81% vs. 70%, $P = 0.009$) and ≥ VGPR (50% vs. 40%, $P = 0.040$) rates, but OS was superior with len-dex (96% vs. 87%, $P = 0.0002$) due to a higher incidence of high-grade toxicities—particularly deep venous vein thrombosis (DVT) and pneumonia—as well as deaths on therapy in the len-Dex group. The rate of VTE even with len-dex was 12% (vs. 25% for len-Dex). The results of this trial highlight the importance of toxicity management in MM management, and support the use of low-dose dex in combination with lenalidomide.

Lenalidomide exhibited a higher level of anti-MM potency in preclinical evaluation (29), and has proven to be a significantly more potent induction agent than thalidomide (30). Lenalidomide is preferred to thalidomide for patients with high-risk cytogenetic abnormalities such as del(13) and t(4;14) on the basis of evidence in relapsed disease that len-dex can overcome the poor prognosis associated with such findings (12). In addition, lenalidomide is associated with minimal PN and is an attractive agent for patients with significant pre-existing neuropathy. Prolonged exposure to lenalidomide prior to or concomitantly at the time of mobilization before ASCT should be avoided, as the agent has been shown to impair stem cell collection (31,32). Aspirin is used in conjunction with lenalidomide to decrease the incidence of therapy-associated VTE. Rash frequently occurs during the course of lenalidomide therapy, but is typically mild and resolves with a short interruption of treatment, antihistamine, and topical corticosteroid (33).

Bortezomib Plus Dexamethasone

Bortezomib is a first-in-class proteasome inhibitor that exerts its anti-MM activity through several mechanisms, including inhibition of nuclear factor-κB (34), induction of caspase-mediated apoptosis, and disruption of IL-6–mediated activation of the pathways involved in MM tumorigenesis (34–36). The efficacy of bortezomib plus dexamethasone (bortez-dex) as induction therapy has been highlighted by an ongoing phase III study in which patients were randomized to receive either bortez-dex or VAD (37). Patients then underwent a second randomization to either consolidation with dexamethasone, cyclophosphamide, etoposide, cisplatin (DCEP) or no consolidation. In a preliminary analysis, bortez-dex was superior with respect to rates of VGPR or better (47% vs. 19%, $P = 0.0001$) and complete response (CR)/near CR (nCR) (21% vs. 8%, $P = 0.0023$). The advantage associated with bortez-dex was especially apparent in patients with advanced ISS stage (β_2M > 3) and those with del(13) by metaphase cytogenetic analysis. Importantly, superior response rates with bortez-dex were also observed following ASCT with respect to rates of both VGPR or better (72% vs. 51%, $P = 0.0001$) and CR/nCr (41% vs. 29%, $P = 0.0089$). DCEP consolidation was not associated with improvement in response in either arm.

As highlighted by these results, bortez-dex is an effective induction regimen in transplant-eligible MM patients. Bortezomib is hepatically metabolized, and can therefore be safely considered for patients with significant renal impairment at the time of diagnosis. In this setting, bortez-dex produces response rates equivalent to those seen in patients with intact renal function and without excess therapy-associated toxicity (38). Bortezomib-containing regimens can also be considered for patients with significant bone disease based on in vitro data demonstrating the ability of botezomib to both inhibit osteoclastogenesis and promote osteoblast differentiation and proliferation (39,40).

PN is a key toxicity associated with bortezomib and can manifest as parasthesias, numbness, temperature dysesthesia, or pain. Bortezomib-associated PN is dose-dependent, and commonly affects long, thinly myelinated sensory nerves to a greater extent than motor nerves, although motor and autonomic dysfunction can also occur in rare occasions. High-grade PN can be prevented by following a standard dose modification algorithm (41). Herpes zoster reactivation has been associated with bortezomib and patients should thus receive antiviral prophylaxis when receiving therapy (42). Thrombocytopenia also occurs frequently in association with bortezomib treatment, but is typically mild in degree among patients with newly diagnosed disease and is very rarely associated with bleeding.

Three- and Four-Drug Regimens for Induction Therapy

Three-drug induction regimens can also be used in the treatment of newly diagnosed, transplant-eligible MM patients. The rationale for these combinations derives from preclinical studies demonstrating synergy between the immunomodulatory drugs, bortezomib, and conventional chemotherapeutic agents (29,43). Such regimens are attractive options for the initial management of MM based on recently published data pointing to the benefit of CR achieved prior to ASCT (19), as they produce higher rates of CR than two-drug regimens. Moreover, they can be particularly useful in patients with high-risk disease characteristics wherein a rapid and deep response to therapy is needed.

Bortezomib, thalidomide, and dexamethasone (bortez-thal-dex) is being compared to thal-dex in an ongoing, randomized phase III study involving transplant-eligible patients with newly diagnosed MM (13). Thalidomide is administered in both arms as a continuous 200-mg dose. Dexamethasone is given in the thal-dex arm as a 40-mg dose on days 1 to 4 and 9 to 12 of each 21-day cycle. Patients in the bortez-thal-dex group receive bortezomib 1.3 mg/m^2 on days 1, 4, 8, and 11 and dexamethasone 20 mg on the day of and the day following bortezomib. The three-drug regimen has exhibited more potent anti-MM activity, producing higher rates of pre-ASCT CR/nCR (33% vs. 12%, $P < 0.001$) and VGPR (61% vs. 30%, $P < 0.001$). Superior responses were seen regardless of disease stage or presence of high-risk cytogenetic abnormalities. Indeed, among patients treated with bortez-thal-dex, response rates were higher in patients with del(13) and t(4;14). A substantial number of patients underwent consolidative ASCT following induction therapy. It is notable that the impressive response to the three-drug induction regimen translated into superior response rates following ASCT, wherein the rate of CR/nCR was 54% with bortez-thal-dex versus 29% with thal-dex ($P < 0.001$). There was a higher rate of high grade PN among patients receiving three-drug induction therapy, but the overall rate of serious adverse events in the two treatment groups was similar and few patients discontinued therapy as a result of treatment-related toxicity. Interestingly, there was a higher rate of DVT with thal-dex, supporting a potential thromboprophylactic effect of bortezomib with this combination. Dose reduction of thalidomide and/or bortezomib for PN can be undertaken as necessary so as to avoid progressive treatment-associated PN.

Lenalidomide, bortezomib, and dexamethasone (len-bortez-dex) has also proven to be highly active in newly diagnosed MM in a multicenter phase I/II study involving newly diagnosed, transplant-eligible MM patients (44). The phase I dose escalation component of the study established the maximum tolerated dose as lenalidomide 25 mg daily on days 1 to 14 of a 21 day cycle; bortezomib 1.3 mg/m^2 on days 1, 4, 8, and 11; and dexamethasone 20 mg on the day of and the day following bortezomib. Thirty-five patients were treated in the phase II portion of the study, wherein the rate of PR was 100%, the rate of VGPR 74%, and the rate of CR/nCR 52%. The median TTP, PFS, and OS have not yet been reached. Although treatment-associated sensory PN occurred in 77% of patients, the majority of cases were grade 1, there was only one instance of grade 3 toxicity, and symptoms were typically reversible with bortezomib dose reduction. With aspirin administered as an adjunct, the regimen was also associated with a low rate of VTE (6%).

Three-drug induction regimens utilizing bortezomib and dexamethasone in conjunction with either an alkylating agent or anthracycline can be considered for transplant-eligible patients as well. Examples of this approach include bortezomib, liposomal doxorubicin, and dexametashone (bortez-dox-dex) and cyclophoshamide, bortezomib, and dexamethasone (cy-bortez-dex). In an ongoing phase III study, patients with newly diagnosed MM are randomized to bortez-dox-dex or VAD, followed by ASCT and maintenance therapy with thalidomide (VAT) arm) or bortezomib 1.3 mg/m^2 every other week (bortez-dox-dex arm) for 2 years (45). Bortez-dox-dex was superior to VAD at interim analysis, producing higher rates of pre-ASCT PR (80% vs. 64%, $P = 0.03$) and VGPR (41% vs. 17%, $P = 0.001$) as well as post-ASCT PR (92% vs. 77%, $P = 0/01$) and CR (15% vs. 4%). Cy-bortez-dex, meanwhile, yielded a VGPR rate of 85% and CR/nCR rate of 64% in a phase II study involving 33 patients with newly diagnosed MM (46).

Several four-drug regimens are currently being evaluated with the aim of further enhancing anti-MM activity. These include bortezomib, cyclophosphamide, thalidomide, and dexamethasone (47); lenalidomide, bortezomib, pegylated liposomal doxorubicin, and dexamethasone (48); and cyclophosphamide, lenalidomide, bortezomib, and dexamethasone (49). Although such combinations are very active as induction therapy, overall response and CR rates have not clearly exceeded those observed with three-drug regimens, and increased toxicity has been seen. Four-drug combinations may be considered for appropriately selected patients with high-risk disease features and are best administered in the context of clinical trials that will ultimately provide greater insight regarding their efficacy and toxicity relative to other induction regimens.

■ CHOICE OF THERAPY

Given the increasingly broad array of induction options available for transplant-eligible MM patients, how does the clinician determine optimal therapy for a given patient? This decision is based on a number of factors, including prognostic factors such as ISS stage and cytogenetic abnormalities; the type and extent of MM-associated organ dysfunction; the presence of extramedullary disease; comorbid conditions such as renal dysfunction and PN; as well as patient preferences regarding the mode of treatment administration. Cost of therapy may also be a consideration in certain circumstances.

Patients with high-risk disease based on ISS stage or cytogenetic analysis are best treated with three-drug therapy containing bortezomib and/or lenalidomide, as combination regimens incorporating these agents have proven to be both active and well tolerated in this setting (13,44). Recent data demonstrating the benefit of pre-ASCT CR also strengthens the argument for regimens that produce higher rates of CR/nCR. Figure 1 highlights the relative efficacy of various induction regimens in terms of depth of response.

Bortez-dex is appropriate for patients who have significant renal impairment at the time of diagnosis as this regimen is effective and well tolerated among such individuals and often leads to improvement in renal function (38). Thal-dex, bortez-thal-dex, and cy-bortez-dex can be considered for patients with renal impairment as well. Len-dex is preferred for patients with pre-existing MM-related PN or other prominent, coexisting neurological disorders. As previously noted, len-dex is associated with a low incidence of treatment-associated PN and, thus, is an ideal choice for such patients. Thal-dex should be considered for patients with significant cytopenias, as it is less myelosuppressive than either len-dex, bortez-dex, or three-drug combinations, but may be less active as a doublet, as compared to either len-dex or bortez-dex.

Extensive extramedullary disease can pose a considerable challenge, and the presence of such involvement generally provides justification for a highly active three-drug combination such as bortez-thal-dex or len-bortez-dex. Several reports have highlighted the effectiveness of bortezomib in the management of extramedullary MM (51,52), although others have described instances of bortezomib resistance (53) in addition to thalidomide or lenalidomide, suggesting that multidrug combinations with cytotoxic chemotherapy may be preferred in this setting.

■ DURATION OF THERAPY

Regardless of the regimen chosen, therapy is typically administered for four to six cycles prior to stem cell harvest, although collection can be undertaken after as few as two or as many as eight cycles of treatment. The actual duration is determined by a given patient's best response to treatment, which is estimated on the basis of laboratory studies such as the serum/urine protein electrophoresis with immunofixation, quantitative immunoglobulin concentration, and serum free light chain assay, as well as results of a postinduction therapy bone marrow evaluation. Ideally, patients undergo stem cell collection at the point of best response to induction therapy. Response is assessed utilizing criteria of the European Group for Blood and

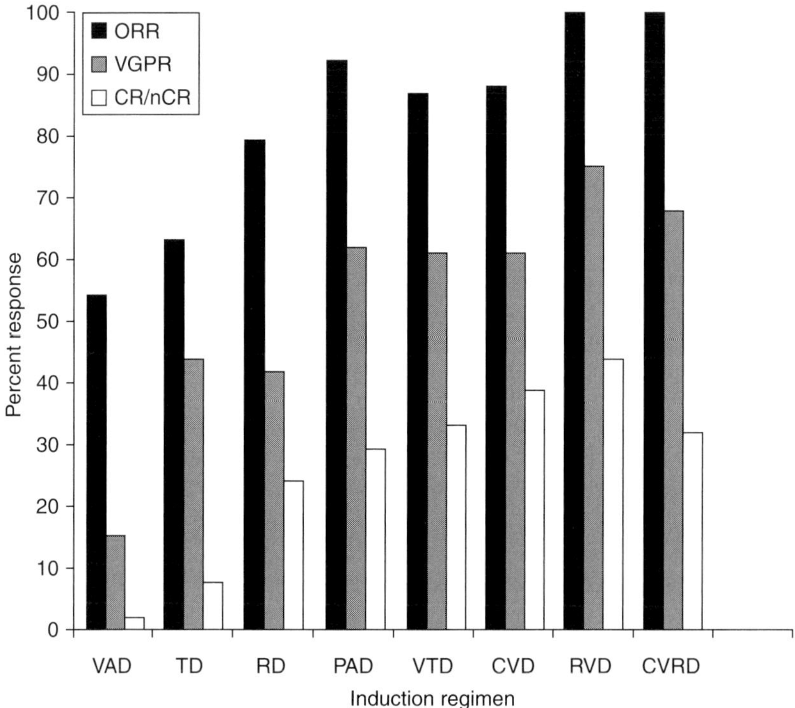

FIGURE 1

Comparison of response rates associated with combination regimens in newly diagnosed multiple myeloma. CR/nCR, complete response/near complete response; CVD, cyclophosphamide-bortezomib-dexamethasone; CVRD, cyclophosphamide-bortezomib-lenalidomide-dexamethasone; ORR, overall response rate; PAD, bortezomib-doxorubicin-dexamethasone; RD, lenalidomide-dexamethasone; RVD, lenalidomide-bortezomib-dexamethasone; TD, thalidomide-dexamethasone; VAD, vincristine-doxorubicin-dexamethasone; VGPR, very good partial response; VTD, bortezomib-thalidomide-dexamethasone. From Ref. 50 with permission.

Marrow Transplantation and/or International Myeloma Working Group (54,55). A 3- to 4-week treatment free interval between induction and stem cell harvest may be beneficial, particularly among patients who received lenalidomide as part of induction (32).

■ SUPPORTIVE CARE

As a final point, the importance of supportive care in the management of MM patients receiving induction therapy prior to ASCT cannot be overemphasized. Treatment outcomes in MM have improved markedly over the past 10 years, with a corresponding increase in median survival following introduction of thalidomide, lenalidomide, and bortezomib (1). Supportive care interventions influence the quality of life a patient experiences while undergoing treatment and managing a long-term chronic illness. Adjunctive therapies such as intravenous bisphosphonate, aspirin for patients treated with immunomodulatory drugs, and acyclovir or equivalent antiviral agent for those receiving bortezomib prevent important disease- and treatment-related toxicities. Analgesics such as Tylenol, opioids, and gabapentin/pregabalin are useful in addressing neuropathic and musculoskeletal pain, whereas nonsteroidal inflammatory drugs should generally be avoided due to the potential nephrotoxic effect of these agents. Integration of specialists in social work and psychology/psychiatry can augment the care of patients as well, and should be considered when circumstances warrant this type of intervention. A comprehensive, integrated approach ensures optimal care from the point of diagnosis and throughout the course of therapy.

■ FUTURE DIRECTIONS

The treatment of newly diagnosed MM will evolve further with ongoing advances in translational and clinical research. Various agents being evaluated in MM have demonstrated promising results in early phase clinical trials and are likely to play a significant role in upfront therapy in the future. These include next-generation immunomodulatory agents and proteasome inhibitors, as well as emerging drug classes such as monoclonal antibodies, histone deacetylase inhibitors, heat-shock protein 90 inhibitors, and others (56). In addition, further study of ASCT will optimize the manner in which this treatment modality is integrated into the overall management of patients with newly diagnosed MM. It is anticipated that advances in these areas will in turn contribute to further improvement in patient outcome.

■ REFERENCES

1. Kumar SK, Rajkumar SV, Dispenzieri A, et al. Improved survival in multiple myeloma and the impact of novel therapies. *Blood* 2008;111:2516–2520.
2. McElwain TJ, Powles RL. High-dose intravenous melphalan for plasma-cell leukemia and myeloma. *Lancet* 1983;2:822–824.
3. National Comprehensive Cancer Network. NCCN clinical practice guidelines in oncology. *Multiple Myeloma* version 3.2010. www.nccn.org.
4. Zhan F, Hardin J, Kordsmeier B, et al. Global gene expression profiling of multiple myeloma, monoclonal gammopathy of undetermined significance, and normal bone marrow plasma cells. *Blood* 2002;99:1745–1757.
5. Zhan F, Huang Y, Colla S, et al. The molecular classification of multiple myeloma. *Blood* 2006;108:2020–2028.
6. Greipp PR, San Miguel J, Durie BG, et al. International staging system for multiple myeloma. *J Clin Oncol* 2005;23:3412–3420.
7. Bergsagel PL, Kuehl WM. Chromosome translocations in multiple myeloma. *Oncogene* 2001;20:5611–5622.
8. Chang H, Sloan S, Li D, et al. The t(4;14) is associated with poor prognosis in myeloma patients undergoing autologous stem cell transplant. *Br J Haematol* 2004;125:64–68.
9. Chang H, Qi C, Yi QL, Reece D, Stewart AK. p53 gene deletion detected by fluorescence in situ hybridization is an adverse prognostic factor for patients with multiple myeloma following autologous stem cell transplantation. *Blood* 2005;105:358–360.
10. Chang H, Qi XY, Samiee S, et al. Genetic risk identifies multiple myeloma patients who do not benefit from autologous stem cell transplantation. *Bone Marrow Transplant* 2005;36:793–796.
11. Jagannath S, Richardson PG, Sonneveld P, et al. Bortezomib appears to overcome the poor prognosis conferred by chromosome 13 deletion in phase 2 and 3 trials. *Leukemia* 2007;21:151–157.
12. Reece D, Song KW, Fu T, et al. Influence of cytogenetics in patients with relapsed or refractory multiple myeloma treated with lenalidomide plus dexamethasone: adverse effect of deletion 17p13. *Blood* 2009;114:522–525.
13. Cavo M, Tacchetti P, Patriarca F, et al. Superior complete response rate and progression-free survival after autologous transplantation with up-front velcade-thalidomide-dexamethasone compared with thalidomide-dexamethasone in newly diagnosed multiple myeloma [Abstract 158]. *Blood* 2008;112.
14. Richardson P, Jagannath S, Jakubowiak A, et al. Lenalidomide, bortezomib, and dexamethasone in patients with relapsed or relapsed/refractory multiple myeloma (MM): encouraging response rates and tolerability with correlation of outcome and adverse cytogenetics in a phase II study [Abstract 1742]. *Blood* 2008;112.
15. Anderson KC, Jagannath S, Jakubowiak A, et al. Phase II study of lenalidomide, bortezomib, and

dexamethasone in patients with relapsed or relapsed and refractory multiple myeloma [Abstract 8545]. *J Clin Oncol* 2008;26:15S.

16. Richardson PG, Weller E, Jagannath S, et al. Multicenter, phase I, dose-escalation trial of lenalidomide plus bortezomib for relapsed and relapsed/refractory multiple myeloma. *J Clin Oncol* 2009;27: 5713–5719.

17. Shibata K, Shimamoto Y, Nakazato S, Matsuzaki M, Tadano J. Refractory anaemia with ringed sideroblasts concurrent with multiple myeloma—a brief review of the recent literature. *Haematologia* (Budap) 1997; 28:199–205.

18. Gertz MA, Lacy MQ, Dispenzieri A, et al. Impact of age and serum creatinine value on outcome after autologous blood stem cell transplantation for patients with multiple myeloma. *Bone Marrow Transplant* 2007;39:605–611.

19. Kim JS, Kim K, Cheong JW, et al. Complete remission status before autologous stem cell transplantation is an important prognostic factor in patients with multiple myeloma undergoing upfront single autologous transplantation. *Biol Blood Marrow Transplant* 2009;15:463–470.

20. Gertz MA, Kumar S, Lacy MQ, et al. Stem cell transplantation in multiple myeloma: impact of response failure with thalidomide or lenalidomide induction. *Blood* 2010;115:2348–2353.

21. Cavo M, Zamagni E, Tosi P, et al. Superiority of thalidomide and dexamethasone over vincristine-doxorubicindexamethasone (VAD) as primary therapy in preparation for autologous transplantation for multiple myeloma. *Blood* 2005;106:35–39.

22. Macro M, Divine M, Yuzunhan Y, et al. Dexamethasone+thalidomide (dex/thal) compared to VAD as a pre-transplant treatment in newly diagnosed multiple myeloma (MM): a randomized trial [Abstract 57]. *Blood* 2006;108:22a.

23. Rajkumar SV, Rosinol L, Hussein M, et al. Multicenter, randomized, double-blind, placebo-controlled study of thalidomide plus dexamethasone compared with dexamethasone as initial therapy for newly diagnosed multiple myeloma. *J Clin Oncol* 2008;26: 2171–2177.

24. Mileshkin L, Stark R, Day B, Seymour JF, Zeldis JB, Prince HM. Development of neuropathy in patients with myeloma treated with thalidomide: patterns of occurrence and the role of electrophysiologic monitoring. *J Clin Oncol* 2006;24:4507–4514.

25. Zangari M, Anaissie E, Barlogie B, et al. Increased risk of deep-vein thrombosis in patients with multiple myeloma receiving thalidomide and chemotherapy. *Blood* 2001;98:1614–1615.

26. Zangari M, Barlogie B, Anaissie E, et al. Deep vein thrombosis in patients with multiple myeloma treated with thalidomide and chemotherapy: effects of prophylactic and therapeutic anticoagulation. *Br J Haematol* 2004;126:715–721.

27. Tosi P, Zamagni E, Tacchetti P, et al. Thalidomidedexamethasone as induction therapy prior to autologous stem-cell transplantation in patients with newly diagnosed multiple myeloma and renal insufficiency. *Biol Blood Marrow Transplant* 2010;16:1115–1121.

28. Lacy MQ, Gertz MA, Dispenzieri A, et al. Long-term results of response to therapy, time to progression, and survival with lenalidomide plus dexamethasone in newly diagnosed myeloma. *Mayo Clin Proc* 2007;82:1179–1184.

29. Hideshima T, Chauhan D, Shima Y, et al. Thalidomide and its analogues overcome drug resistance of human multiple myeloma cells to conventional therapy. *Blood* 2000;96:2943–2950.

30. Gay F, Hayman SR, Lacy MQ, et al. Lenalidomide plus dexamethasone versus thalidomide plus dexamethasone in newly diagnosed multiple myeloma: a comparative analysis of 411 patients. *Blood* 2010;115: 1343–1350.

31. Kumar S, Dispenzieri A, Lacy MQ, et al. Impact of lenalidomide therapy on stem cell mobilization and engraftment post-peripheral blood stem cell transplantation in patients with newly diagnosed myeloma. *Leukemia* 2007;21:2035–2042.

32. Paripati H, Stewart AK, Cabou S, et al. Compromised stem cell mobilization following induction therapy with lenalidomide in myeloma. *Leukemia* 2008;22: 1282–1284.

33. Sviggum HP, Davis MD, Rajkumar SV, Dispenzieri A. Dermatologic adverse effects of lenalidomide therapy for amyloidosis and multiple myeloma. *Arch Dermatol* 2006;142:1298–1302.

34. Hideshima T, Chauhan D, Richardson P, et al. NF-κB as a therapeutic target in multiple myeloma. *J Biol Chem* 2002;277:16639–16647.

35. Hideshima T, Chauhan D, Hayashi T, et al. Proteasome inhibitor PS-341 abrogates IL-6 triggered signaling cascades via caspase-dependent downregulation of gp130 in multiple myeloma. *Oncogene* 2003;22:8386–8393.

36. Hideshima T, Mitsiades C, Akiyama M, et al. Molecular mechanisms mediating antimyeloma activity of proteasome inhibitor PS-341. *Blood* 2003;101: 1530–1534.

37. Harousseau JL, Mathiot C, Attal M, et al. Bortezomib/ dexamethasone versus VAD as induction prior to autologous stem cell transplantation (ASCT) in previously untreated multiple myeloma (MM): updated data from IFM2005/01 trial [Abstract 8505]. *J Clin Oncol* 2008;26:8547.

38. Chanan-Khan AA, Kaufman JL, Mehta J, et al. Activity and safety of bortezomib in multiple myeloma patients with advanced renal failure: a multicenter retrospective study. *Blood* 2007;109:2604–2606.

39. von Metzler I, Krebbel H, Hecht M, et al. Bortezomib inhibits human osteoclastogenesis. *Leukemia* 2007;21: 2025–2034.

40. Mukherjee S, Raje N, Schoonmaker JA, et al. Pharmacologic targeting of a stem/progenitor population in vivo is associated with enhanced bone regeneration in mice. *J Clin Invest* 2008;118:491–504.

41. Richardson PG, Sonneveld P, Schuster MW, et al. Reversibility of symptomatic peripheral neuropathy with bortezomib in the phase III APEX trial in relapsed multiple myeloma: impact of a dose-modification guideline. *Br J Haematol* 2009;144:895–903.

42. Richardson PG, Sonneveld P, Schuster MW, et al. Bortezomib or high-dose dexamethasone for relapsed multiple myeloma. *N Engl J Med* 2005;352: 2487–2498.

43. Mitsiades N, Mitsiades CS, Richardson PG, et al. The proteasome inhibitor PS-341 potentiates sensitivity of multiple myeloma cells to conventional chemotherapeutic agents: therapeutic applications. *Blood* 2003;101:2377–2380.

44. Richardson PG, Lonial S, Jakubowiak AJ, et al. High response rates and encouraging time-to-event data with lenalidomide, bortezomib, and dexamethasone in newly diagnosed multiple myeloma: final results of a phase I/II study [Abstract 1218]. *Blood* 2009;114:501–502.

45. Sonneveld P, Van der Holt B, Schmidt-Wolf I, et al. First analysis of HOVON-65/GMMG-HD4 randomized phase III trial comparing bortezomib, adriamycine, dexamethasone (PAD) vs VAD as induction treatment prior to high dose melphalan (HDM) in patients with newly diagnosed multiple myeloma (MM) [Abstract 653]. *Blood* 2008;112.

46. Reeder CB, Stewart AK, Hentz JG, et al. Efficacy of induction with cybord in newly diagnosed multiple myeloma [Abstract 8517]. *J Clin Oncol* 2008;26.

47. Bensinger W, Jagannath S, Vescio R, et al. A phase II study of bortezomib (Velcade), cyclophosphamide (Cytoxan), thalidomide (Thalomid), and dexamethasone as first-line therapy for multiple myeloma [Abstract 94]. *Blood* 2008;112.

48. Jakubowiak AJ, Reece DE, Hofmeister CC, et al. Lenalidomide, bortezomib, pegylated liposomal doxorubicin, and dexamethasone in newly diagnosed multiple myeloma: updated results of phase I/II MMRC trial [Abstract 132]. *Blood* 2009;114.

49. Kumar S, Flinn IW, Hari PN, et al. Novel three- and four-drug combinations of bortezomib, dexamethasone, cyclophosphamide, and lenalidomide for newly diagnosed multiple myeloma: encouraging results from the multi-center, randomized, phase 2 EVOLUTION study [Abstract 127]. *Blood* 2009;114.

50. Stewart AK, Richardson, PG, San Miguel JF. How I treat multiple myeloma in younger patients. *Blood* 2009;114:5436.

51. Laura R, Cibeira MT, Uriburu C, et al. Bortezomib: an effective agent in extramedullary disease in multiple myeloma. *Eur J Haematol* 2006;76:405–408.

52. Hughes M, Micallef-Eynaud P. Bortezomib in relapsed multiple myeloma complicated by extramedullary plasmacytomas. *Clin Lab Haematol* 2006;28: 267–269.

53. Ali R, Ozkalemkas F, Ozkan A, et al. Bortezomib and extramedullary disease in multiple myeloma: the shine and dark side of the moon. *Leuk Res* 2007;31:1153–1155.

54. Blade J, Samson D, Reece D, et al. Criteria for evaluating disease response and progression in patients with multiple myeloma treated by high-dose therapy and haemopoietic stem cell transplantation. Myeloma Subcommittee of the EBMT. European Group for Blood and Marrow Transplant. *Br J Haematol* 1998;102:1115–1123.

55. Durie BG, Harousseau JL, Miguel JS, et al. International uniform response criteria for multiple myeloma. *Leukemia* 2006;20:1467–1473.

56. Richardson PG, Mitsiades C, Schlossman R, Munshi N, Anderson K. New drugs for myeloma. *Oncologist* 2007;12:664–689.

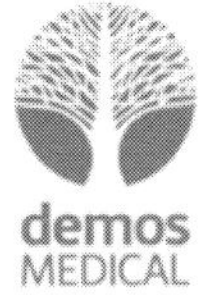

demos
MEDICAL

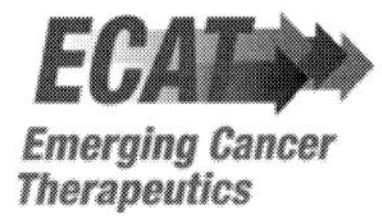

ECAT
Emerging Cancer
Therapeutics

Current Trends in Hematopoietic Stem Cell Transplantation for Multiple Myeloma

Hari Parameswaran and Ayman Saad

Medical College of Wisconsin, Milwaukee, WI

■ ABSTRACT

The first decade of the 21st century has seen more progress in the treatment of multiple myeloma (MM) than ever before. The advent of novel multitargeted drugs has extended the survival of patients with MM. Although the role of planned up-front autologous hematopoietic stem cell transplantation (ASCT) is increasingly questioned, MM still remains the commonest indication for ASCT in North America. The conceptual basis for ASCT, that is, achievement of a complete remission, is a highly desirable albeit somewhat controversial end point. In contrast, subgroups of patients with unfavorable biologic risk factors do not seem to benefit as much even from ASCT or currently available new drugs, and no plateau in survival curves has been demonstrated even in approaches that integrate novel drugs and ASCT followed by maintenance. New pretransplant conditioning regimens and routine posttransplant consolidation followed by maintenance/extended therapy are emerging as new trends in ASCT. Allogeneic hematopoietic stem cell transplantation (alloSCT) is not widely applicable or recommended for MM despite one randomized study suggesting superiority over tandem ASCT. The existence of a graft-versus-MM effect is supported by evidence, but the early promise of reduced intensity conditioning alloSCT inducing sustained "cures" has not been fulfilled. Because MM remains an incurable disease, the scope for improvement in therapy is tremendous. Strategies in current clinical trials integrating transplantation with novel drug therapy prior to or after transplant and in conditioning are likely to change established treatment paradigms. This review examines the changing role of autologous and allogeneic transplantation in MM in the era of novel drugs.

---

*Corresponding author, Medical College of Wisconsin, Milwaukee, WI

E-mail address: phari@mcw.edu

Emerging Cancer Therapeutics 1:2 (2010) 329–362.
© 2010 Demos Medical Publishing LLC. All rights reserved.
DOI: 10.5003/2151–4194.1.2.329   demosmedpub.com/ecat

■ INTRODUCTION

The incidence of multiple myeloma (MM) is increasing in the United States, with approximately 20,000 patients diagnosed every year and approximately 60,000 persons living with MM (1). Two major prospective randomized clinical trials (2,3) and several nonrandomized comparisons (4–7) demonstrated that high-dose therapy with autologous hematopoietic stem cell transplantation (ASCT) is superior to conventional chemotherapy (CC) in prolonging event-free survival (EFS) and overall survival (OS). In several other randomized studies, a superior EFS was shown and no OS benefit could be established (8–10), whereas in another study, even an EFS advantage was not shown (11). A large meta-analysis also suggested benefit in EFS but not OS (12), whereas previous expert panels and evidence-based reviews recommended up-front ASCT as a means of extending survival (13,14). MM is the most common indication for hematopoietic stem cell transplantation in North America, with more than 6,000 transplants performed yearly based on most recent Center for International Blood and Marrow Transplant Research (CIBMTR) registration data (15).

Nontransplant options available to patients with MM have expanded with novel antineoplastic agents such as thalidomide, lenalidomide, and bortezomib. The advent of these agents seems to have improved the survival of newly diagnosed patients and those relapsing after ASCT (16). However, MM is incurable, with almost all patients eventually relapsing and succumbing to MM even after achieving complete remission (CR). Newer strategies aimed at improving the outcomes of transplantation have focused on posttransplant consolidation with a second ASCT (tandem ASCT) or chemotherapy, novel conditioning regimens, sequential ASCT followed by allogeneic hematopoietic stem cell transplantation (alloSCT) (tandem alloSCT) using reduced intensity conditioning (RIC), and extended posttransplant therapy (maintenance) after transplant. We discuss the current state of transplant-based treatment strategies, the impact of novel antimyeloma agents in altering the need for and the timing of ASCT, the role of alloSCT, and the use of extended posttransplant therapy.

■ AUTOLOGOUS TRANSPLANTATION IN THE CC ERA

High-dose melphalan (MEL) followed by autologous bone marrow stem cell rescue was shown to produce meaningful remissions even in patients with relapsed and/or refractory MM (17) in the 1980s. In this period, preceding the advent of novel antimyeloma drugs such as immunomodulatory drugs (IMIDs) and proteasome inhibitors, survival of newly diagnosed patients was significantly shorter than in the modern era where initial novel agent therapy is standard (16,18). Several randomized trials in the 1990s compared ASCT to CC in newly diagnosed patients. The Intergroupe Francophone Myeloma (IFM) group (2) and the Medical Research Council, United Kingdom (MRC) (3) led national clinical trials in France and the United Kingdom, respectively, demonstrating that patients randomized to high-dose therapy with ASCT had significantly higher CR rates, CR duration, EFS, and OS. Palumbo et al. showed survival benefit in the 50- to 70-year age group, whereas the upper age limit was 64 to 65 years in the IFM and MRC studies. Other randomized studies have not been uniformly positive for a survival benefit (9–11,19,20), as summarized in Table 1. Interestingly, all of these studies except the US Intergroup study (19) showed superior CR rates for the ASCT arm, which translated into an improvement in EFS. The PETHEMA study led by Blade et al. (11) and the US Intergroup study are unique in not showing an EFS benefit for ASCT recipients.

Lessons from Early Randomized Studies

The US Intergroup study and the Spanish PETHEMA study (11,19) are the two major studies

TABLE 1

Selected randomized trials of conventional chemotherapy compared with single ASCT as up-front therapy

Study	Transplant Arm	N Age (years)	CR % CC vs. SCT	Comments
Attal (2) IFM90	MEL 140 + TBI 8 Gy and marrow graft	200 ≤65	5 vs. 22*	OS and EFS superior for transplant
Child (3) MRC7	MEL 200 and autologous PBSCT	401 ≤64	8 vs. 44*	OS and EFS superior for ASCT
Blade (11) PETHEMA	MEL 200 or MEL 140 + 12 Gy TBI and autologous PBSCT	164 ≤65	11 vs. 30*	Only initial responders randomized OS and EFS similar for ASCT vs. CC
Palumbo (8) IMMSG	MEL 100 x2 with autologous PBSCT	194; 50–70	6 vs. 25*	EFS and OS superior for ASCT
Barlogie (19) SWOG S9321	MEL 140 + TBI 12 Gy with autologous PBSCT	899 <70	15 vs. 17	OS and EFS similar for ASCT vs. CC. 55% of patients relapsing after CC received salvage ASCT
Fermand (9)	CCNU + etoposide + cyclophosphamide + melphalan & TBI	185 <56	20 vs. 57	EFS superior for ASCT. No OS difference as patients in CC randomized to ASCT at relapse. QOL superior for ASCT
Fermand (10)	MEL 200 or MEL 140 + BU	55–65	20 vs. 36	EFS and OS similar to CC. QOL superior for early ASCT

Long-term survival data (21):

IFM 90—10-year OS 19% and EFS 6% when both arms combined. ASCT arm continued to be superior over CC for OS and EFS.

S9321—10-year OS 22% and EFS 18% when arms combined.

CC, conventional chemotherapy; PBSC, peripheral blood stem cell.

Definitions of response were based on non-uniform criteria.

* Statistically significant difference ($P < 0.05$)

that are discordant in that they did not provide similar benefit for patients receiving ASCT. In the PETHEMA trial, only those patients responding to initial chemotherapy were randomized to ASCT versus continuing CC, thus excluding initial nonresponders. A higher CR rate in the ASCT arm of this study did not translate into superior EFS. This study thus provides the valuable insight that the benefit of up-front ASCT is limited in patients who are good responders to initial induction therapy. The US Intergroup Study (S9321) was the largest comparison of CC to ASCT. After initial induction therapy (vincristine–adriamycin–dexamethasone [VAD]), patients were randomized to receive ASCT or vincristine–BCNU–melphalan–cyclophosphamide–prednisone (VBMCP) chemotherapy for 1 year. Responding patients in each arm were later rerandomized to observation versus interferon (IFN) maintenance. The VBMCP and early ASCT groups were similar in terms of EFS (21 vs. 25 months P = 0.14). Median OS (53 vs. 62 months P = 0.87) was also similar, most likely because 52% of patients in the VBMCP arm had a late (salvage) transplant at relapse/progression. The CR rates were also not significantly different between CC versus ASCT (15% vs. 17%), which is unique to this study among all the randomized CC versus ASCT studies. The failure to achieve a substantial increase in CR rates with ASCT is possibly due to the suboptimal conditioning therapy employed (MEL plus total body irradiation [TBI]) (22) and also likely due to the superiority of VBMCP maintenance for 1 year over CC regimens used in other studies. Importantly, the S9321 trial showed that upfront ASCT and salvage ASCT (received by 52% of subjects in the CC arm) at the time of relapse or progression were comparable. This in fact confirms earlier observations from another French study (MAG 95) that survival was comparable between early versus delayed ASCT (9).

Another study that showed superior CR rates for ASCT but no EFS or OS advantage was the HOVON (20) study which again used an unconventional cyclophosphamide and TBI-based conditioning regimen in the ASCT arm and sequential intermediate-dose MEL in the conventional therapy arm. The heterogeneity in patient selection, differing treatment regimens used in the CC arm, and the variety in conditioning regimens in up-front ASCT studies mean that they do not readily yield to cross comparison or data collation. With this caveat, a detailed meta-analysis (12) found that there was an advantage in EFS or freedom from progression (hazard ratio = 0.75, 95% confidence interval = 0.59–0.96) but not a survival benefit. The EFS benefit was significant even in patients not responding to initial chemotherapy.

In summary, these studies indicate the value of ASCT in establishing CR and providing an EFS advantage in the prenovel agent era. Survival benefit was more difficult to prove especially in studies that permitted or planned for delayed ASCT

at relapse as well as studies conducted in later time periods when novel agents were available as salvage option for relapsing patients. A long-term analysis of the US Intergroup study and some of the French studies suggests that the OS benefit for ASCT recipients in the IFM90 study has held up over 10 years of follow-up (21). It is important to note that, with one exception, these studies were restricted to patients aged 65 or younger, and among classic conditioning regimens, MEL with or without TBI was used in the two studies that showed OS benefit.

CR after Autologous Transplantation

CC for MM resulted in very low CR rates (23), with ASCT being the most powerful tool to induce better CR rates. In the pre-ASCT era, therefore, it was difficult to show a survival advantage based on degree of response (24–26). Similarly, the quality of response or the depth of disease reduction achieved with ASCT was critical to longer EFS or OS in the majority of CC versus ASCT trials noted earlier. Because the overall goal of therapy is long-term survival, it has been debated whether achievement of a CR is a necessary or practical end point for prolonged survival (27). Many studies in the MM literature investigating the role of CR after transplant have not employed statistical methods such as landmark analysis or treatment of response status as a time-dependent covariate. The statistical flaws underlying "survival by tumor response" analyses are beyond the scope of the current discussion but need to be kept in mind when interpreting the following results (28).

A large meta analysis (29) of nearly 5,000 patients suggested highly significant correlation between maximal depth of response during or after ASCT and long-term survival outcomes. These findings have been replicated in other analyses in patients receiving ASCT (30). In a recent retrospective analysis of prospectively enrolled IFM studies (31), it was shown that the achievement of CR or very good partial response (VGPR) (by the European Group for Blood and Marrow Transplantation [EBMT]/International Bone Marrow Transplant Registry [IBMTR] criteria [32]) after ASCT was a simple but critical prognostic factor even more informative than a CR. Newer response criteria (33) with even more stringently defined remissions have been proposed, but these higher grades of CR have not yet been validated in large prospective series (34). The goal of VGPR + CR rates (≥VGPR response) as a treatment objective is thus justified, but not enough data exist to substitute this as a surrogate for superior overall efficacy or clinical benefit when comparing therapies wherein a survival endpoint is still necessary. However, it is also clear that current remission criteria could be refined further and additional elimination of minimal residual disease can be shown by more sensitive techniques such as multicolor flow cytometry. Such immunophenotypic remissions may prove even more predictive of outcomes as suggested by a Spanish group (35).

It is also notable that some studies even in the novel agent setting fail to show an absolute survival or EFS benefit for patients achieving higher response rate (36,37), with treatment-related toxicity being a significant driver of overall success. Rajkumar et al. (38) reported the Mayo Clinic experience wherein patients who underwent ASCT had a similar EFS and OS whether they achieved CR or not following ASCT. The Arkansas group report showed that achieving a strictly defined CR after tandem ASCT may be predictive of survival only in patients with high-risk disease (39). The Arkansas group also found that in patients who had preceding MGUS or smoldering MM, stringently defined CR was significantly lower compared with de novo MM, but these lower CR rates did not translate into inferior survival after tandem ASCT (40). A recent analysis by the same group using CR as a time-dependent covariate indicated that the sustenance of CR over time rather than its mere achievement after ASCT was prognostically more significant in the context of high-risk disease (41). Thus, although achieving CR status

may not be a prerequisite for long-term survival in some patients, for those with genetically defined high-risk disease, achievement and sustenance of CR are key (42).

■ IMPACT OF THE ASCT ERA ON SURVIVAL OF PATIENTS WITH MM

Comparison of population-based myeloma survival data from recent time periods to the pre-ASCT era have shown that 5- and 10-year survival rates for all patients with MM have increased, with the most dramatic survival improvement in the younger "transplant eligible" cohort (18,43). These improvements predated the novel agent era and started in the mid-1990s when ASCT was established as a treatment option in MM. Similar data have been reported in a large single-institution cohort spanning 35 years by Kumar et al., who also found a dramatic increase in median survival correlating with increased use of ASCT from the mid-1990s and from the use of novel agents in the 2000s (16).

Choice of Conditioning Therapy for Autologous Transplantation

CIBMTR registration data indicate that the vast majority (>80%) of ASCT for MM use high-dose MEL as conditioning therapy. Several combinations of other agents as well as MEL and TBI have been tried. The early trials used a variety of different regimens in conditioning, as noted in Table 1. The only randomized trial of high-dose MEL (200 mg/m²) also known as MEL200 compared with a combination of MEL (140 mg/m²) and 8-Gy TBI was done by the IFM group (22). The MEL–TBI regimen was associated with significantly worse mucositis, whereas hematologic recovery, transfusion requirements, and the duration of hospitalization were superior with MEL200. Survival and progression-free survival (PFS) were similar in both arms, although the trend (P = 0.05) for OS favored MEL200.

Some groups have attempted to reduce the toxicity from ASCT by reducing the dose of MEL. Palumbo et al. randomized patients to tandem ASCT after MEL200 versus intermediate-dose MEL at 100 mg/m^2 (MEL100) (44). Surprisingly, the rates of completion of tandem ASCT, hospitalization rates, as well as transplant-related mortality (TRM) at 3.1% versus 2.9%, respectively, were similar in both groups. Similarly, ≥VGPR rates and OS were no different between the groups, but MEL200 had a superior EFS (31.4 vs. 26.2 months) and time to progression, with a more pronounced advantage in those younger than 60 years. MEL200 is thus considered the standard of care for conditioning before ASCT in MM in patients who can tolerate the procedure (e.g., younger and with acceptable renal function). In older patients, intermediate-dose MEL100 has been tried in various studies in Europe. The IFM 99–06 trial in patients aged 65 to 75 years showed no superiority for MEL100 versus CC of MEL–prednisone (MP) and in fact inferiority for both approaches compared with the MP and thalidomide combination (45). The GIMEMA study arrived at the opposite conclusion in patients aged 50 to 70 years, showing superiority for MEL100 over MP (8).

Because relapse is the most important cause of treatment failure after ASCT, other groups have attempted to increase the dose intensity of conditioning. Higher doses of MEL (higher than 200 mg/m^2) have been tried in dose-escalation studies (46) based on the dose–response relationship of MEL in MM. Limited experience suggests a maximum tolerated dose of 280 mg/m^2 and significant cardiac and gastrointestinal toxicity. The interindividual variability in clinical response to MEL has been shown to correlate with both the rate of formation of and the rate of repair of DNA damage in the *p53* gene in peripheral blood lymphocytes (47). Some of the other conditioning approaches analyzed in comparative studies have been the combinations of busulfan and MEL (48,49), busulfan and cyclophosphamide (50), idarubicin and MEL (with or without other agents such as cyclophosphamide or busulfan) (51–53),

thiotepa, busulfan, and cyclophosphamide (54). At this time, these regimens appear to be either more toxic or without mature results to recommend as an acceptable alternative to MEL200 (55). The use of novel agents in conditioning is also being explored. Newer approaches at delivering higher doses of radiation therapy to the marrow prior to ASCT without increasing overall toxicity are also being explored with the use of helical tomotherapy or bone-seeking radioisotopes (56,57).

A recent phase II study from the IFM group compared patients receiving bortezomib and high-dose MEL (MEL200) conditioning prior to ASCT with matched historical controls receiving MEL200 (58). Superior ≥VGPR rates (70%) were observed with the combination without any increase in toxicity or TRM. Compared with matched controls, the addition of bortezomib resulted in higher CR rates without additional toxicity. In a current clinical trial at the University of Arkansas, tandem ASCTs are administered after conditioning, incorporating both classes of approved novel agents. This regimen (TT3-Lite) uses fractionated MEL200 in four successive daily fractions (MEL50 × 4) with the addition of bortezomib, thalidomide, and dexamethasone (VTD).

■ TANDEM AUTOLOGOUS TRANSPLANTS

After the feasibility of double intensification with ASCT had been reported (59–61), the Arkansas group pioneered the planned tandem autologous transplant approach in their Total Therapy program with non-cross-resistant induction chemotherapy regimens culminating in tandem ASCT (7,62). They reported impressive EFS and OS of 43 months and 68 months, respectively, superior to historical controls. In the next version of Total Therapy (TT2) trial, thalidomide was incorporated into a tandem ASCT approach, with even higher 7-year continuous CR rates(45%) and improved overall median EFS (5.1 years) and OS (8 years) reported. Subsequent Total Therapy 3 (TT3) trial from this group additionally included bortezomib in the induction regimen and posttransplant consolidation. With a median follow-up of 20 months, 2-year estimates of EFS and OS were 84% and 86%, respectively (63). In a matched comparison of 300 patients, TT3 resulted in superior EFS and CR duration compared with TT2 (64,65). Although these are excellent outcomes, these data are unfortunately not randomized and represent prospective single-center outcomes from a highly specialized team.

Randomized Trials of Tandem Autologous Transplantation

The French Intergroup trial (IFM94) was the first published randomized trial (66) comparing single to double ASCT. Patients with previously untreated MM were randomized to undergo either a single ASCT (using MEL 140 mg/m^2 + TBI 8 Gy) or planned tandem ASCTs (MEL 140 mg/m^2 followed by MEL 140 mg/m^2 + TBI 8 Gy) followed by IFN-2α maintenance therapy. The projected 7-year EFS and OS benefits were significantly better for the double ASCT arm (10% vs. 20% for EFS and 21% vs. 42% for OS). In a non-preplanned subgroup analysis, the benefit of the second ASCT was not significant for patients in a good remission status (≥VGPR) 3 months after the first ASCT. Another randomized study (Bologna 96) has confirmed the observation that the second ASCT does not benefit patients in CR after the first transplant (67). However, this and the HOVON 24 study of single versus tandem ASCT failed to show an OS benefit for the tandem procedure, although CR rate and EFS were superior in the tandem group.

Here again, the heterogeneity of the trials in terms of induction therapy and conditioning regimen (MEL/busulfan in Bologna 96, cyclophosphamide/TBI in HOVON) indicates that the trial data cannot be easily merged in meta-analysis. These results are summarized in Table 2 (7,66–71). Yet another study comparing single ASCT with thalidomide maintenance versus tandem ASCT has now been retracted but contributed to a published meta-analysis. In addition, the availability of novel agents for treatment of relapse post-ASCT means that OS differences are unlikely to be shown (72,73). Thus, tandem ASCT in randomized studies has shown to produce higher CR rates on per protocol analyses and superior EFS overall but not OS benefit (with the notable exception of IFM94). These benefits are most marked and statistically significant in patients who are not in a good response state (≥VGPR) after the first ASCT. The authors of the IFM94 trial suggest that the difference in projected survival with tandem ASCT does not correlate with improved response rates but longer duration of responses.

The potential shortcomings of the tandem approach are an increase in morbidity and overall health care costs, the lack of additional benefit in patients who have already achieved CR with a first ASCT, unrealistic expectations of a cure, and the lack of any impact on early mortality in the first 4 years. In addition for patients not in an excellent remission status after an ASCT, extended therapy with novel agents might offer similar benefit as a second ASCT. Also CR + VGPR rates of more than 50% to 70% are achievable now, with novel agent induction and single ASCT reducing the benefit of a second ASCT. A second ASCT is often feasible in patients (74) who relapse after the first ASCT, provided stem cells are available or can be harvested. There are no randomized studies that compare a salvage second transplant at relapse to a planned up-front tandem second transplant. A retrospective analysis by the EBMT suggested that the completion of a second ASCT before relapse and within 6 to 12 months of the first transplant resulted in superior outcomes (75).

Autologous Transplantation After Novel Agent Induction—Is There Additional Benefit?

The novel agent era in MM was heralded by the use of thalidomide in the late 1990s, followed by lenalidomide and bortezomib. Innovation and

TABLE 2

Trials of tandem autologous stem cell transplant

Author	N	Age	Conditioning Regimen First → Second	CR % Single vs. Double	Median EFS mo Single vs. Double	Median OS mo Single vs. Double	Follow-Up
IFM94 (66)	399	60	MEL 140 +TBI → MEL 140	42 vs. 50	25 vs. 30*	48 vs. 58*	75 M
GMMG HD2 (68)	261	65	MEL 200 → MEL 200	NR	23 vs. 29*	No difference	NR
MAG 95 (69,70)	227	55	MEL 140 → MEL 140 + Etoposide + TBI	39 vs. 37	31 vs. 33	49 vs. 73*	53 M
Bologna 96 (67)	321	60	MEL 200 → MEL 120 + BU 12	33 vs. 47	23 vs. 35*	65 vs. 71	55 M
Hovon 24 (71)	303	<65	MEL 70 x2 → CY + TBI 9Gy	13 vs. 32*	24 vs. 27*	50 vs. 55	50 M
Arkansas TTI (7)	123	<70	Total therapy I	40%	49	62	Historical Controls

Abbreviations: BU, busulfan; CY, cyclophosphamide; MEL, melphalan (doses in mg/m²); NR, not reported; TBI, total body irradiation.

* Statistically significant difference (P < 0.05)

controversy in the role of transplant for MM center on the integration of these agents in the therapy of newly diagnosed MM either with or without ASCT. Until the introduction of the new drugs, response status before ASCT had minimal impact on the eventual outcome of ASCT, with patients refractory to initial therapy obtaining as much or perhaps greater additional benefit from the procedure compared with responders (76–78). Incorporation of the new drugs into the initial treatment of myeloma has resulted in increased response rates including higher CR rates compared with those seen with the previous CC/steroid-based regimens and similar to post-ASCT CR rates from the past.

Thalidomide, the earliest novel drug, when combined with dexamethasone for induction resulted in superior overall response rates compared with dexamethasone alone or VAD. However, the CR rates before ASCT were still low (79), and the CR rates post-ASCT were similar to dexamethasone-based induction (80,81). In another randomized study, thalidomide-based combination therapy with adriamycin–dexamethasone resulted in greater pretransplant responses, but posttransplant CR rates were again similar (82). The gains in using thalidomide for an extended period in combination with tandem ASCT have been compared in two studies (83,84). Cavo et al. described a retrospective experience wherein ≥VGPR rates were better in patients receiving thalidomide from induction and continued until a second ASCT in a tandem approach. This resulted in superior EFS of 51% at 4 years compared with non-thalidomide induction and tandem ASCT. In the Arkansas TT2 study, the use of thalidomide in all phases of an intense program of induction, followed by tandem ASCT and chemotherapy consolidation with maintenance therapy, was associated with superior response rates and EFS but not OS. For patients with cytogenetic abnormalities (a high-risk subgroup), there was a survival benefit to receiving thalidomide. The lack of clear survival benefit, the equalization of CR rates after ASCT, and high discontinuation rates (21–39%) (85,86) associated with extended use of thalidomide suggest at best a modest overall clinical benefit for this agent over CC.

In contrast to the data described earlier, the use of bortezomib and lenalidomide and their combinations in initial therapy produce pretransplant CR + VGPR ($\geq$VGPR) rates matching those after ASCT from the prenovel agent era. In addition, compared with CC induction, the superior pre-ASCT responses seem to be sustained after ASCT. Bortezomib–dexamethasone combination compared with VAD by the IFM group (IFM 2005–01 trial) resulted in significantly superior $\geq$VGPR rates pre-ASCT as well as post-ASCT (87). The superior induction did not result in superior EFS overall, although there was a trend (P = 0.06). The authors suggest that this was due to baseline imbalances in the treatment arms with regard to high-risk patients as well as the effect of consolidative and maintenance treatments used in the trial. Interestingly, bortezomib induction was shown to provide an EFS benefit in patients with higher stage MM and overcome high genetic risk subgroups (t(4:14) and del17p). Similarly, the GIMEMA group showed that patients receiving induction therapy with VTD versus thalidomide–dexamethasone (TD) regimen had significant superiority in $\geq$VGPR rates both before (61% vs. 30%) and sustained after ASCT (75% vs. 53%), respectively. At relatively short follow-up, EFS was significantly superior with VTD compared with TD (20-month estimate: 93% vs. 86%, P = 0.04) but not OS (88). Another European study showed that bortezomib in combination with adriamycin and dexamethasone induced significantly more partial response + VGPR + CR as compared with VAD and that this difference is also sustained after ASCT (89).

Lenalidomide also induces outstanding CR + VGPR rates in combination with high-dose pulsed dexamethasone (51%) or low-dose weekly dexamethasone (40%) as shown in the randomized ECOG 4A03 trial. In this trial, despite high $\geq$VGPR rates rivaling those of standard ASCT, a landmark analysis of 4-month survivors indicated that those pursuing ASCT had a 3-year survival of 92% versus 79% in those continuing lenalidomide. Similar data from the Mayo clinic on patients treated with lenalidomide induction and maintenance suggest a median EFS of 32 months, with a superior EFS in patients proceeding to ASCT versus those who did not (83% vs. 59% at 2 years) (90). In the ECOG trial described earlier, ASCT versus continuing lenalidomide therapy was not a study question per se or even a predefined endpoint. However, data from this trial caution us against abandoning the up-front ASCT strategy for MM too soon. A recent single-center analysis of transplant-eligible patients receiving thalidomide or lenalidomide induction followed by early ASCT versus continuing induction therapy was presented by the Mayo clinic group. Median time to ASCT in the delayed group was 39 months, and the approach of continued initial therapy with delayed transplant at the time of first relapse was comparable in outcomes to up-front transplant (91).

Is It Time to Abandon Autologous Transplantation?

The IFM group randomized patients aged 65 to 75 years to MP versus MEL–prednisone–thalidomide (MPT) versus intermediate-dose (100 mg/m^2) MEL-based ASCT (45). The MPT regimen was associated with a significantly superior OS of 51.6 months versus 33.2 months for MP and 38.3 months for the "reduced intensity ASCT." This study is the only randomized mature comparison of a novel agent regimen against ASCT but suffers from the flaw that ASCT was preceded by nonstandard conditioning regimen likely of lower antineoplastic efficacy (44). In a recent analysis, Palumbo et al. (92) reported that after lenalidomide induction, consolidative therapy with the combination of MEL–prednisone–lenalidomide

(MPR) versus standard MEL (200 mg/m^2)-based ASCT were statistically equivalent in terms of CR rates, OS, and EFS. These data and the absence of other randomized trials comparing novel induction versus ASCT have led to the controversial suggestion that up-front ASCT is no longer necessary in MM because superior CR rates are possible with novel induction regimens.

Clearly, the combinations of novel agent triplets and quadruplets have resulted in CR + VGPR rates similar or superior (reaching 70%) to those after conventional induction followed by ASCT (93–97) (summarized in Table 3 (36,87,88,92,94,96–106)). Time to progression in the absence of subsequent ASCT is not available for most of these novel induction combinations at this time. Where data are available, the combinations alone do not seem to provide freedom from progression of more than 22 to 32 months (90,97,104). However, incremental increases in CR for recipients of ASCT following novel induction and the superior survival of the nonrandomized upfront ASCT group in the ECOG4A03 trial point to the continuing efficacy of upfront ASCT. Similarly, the outstanding long-term survival from the Arkansas group integrating tandem ASCT and novel agents argues for additive strategies incorporating novel drugs in induction, consolidation, and maintenance. In contrast, the randomized trial of MPT versus intermediate-dose MEL ASCT data from IFM 99–06, the lack of response rate, or EFS advantage in the MPR versus ASCT study could argue against an additional benefit with transplant for patients already in a good remission. The need for an up-front ASCT in the novel agent induction era is thus an area of controversy not likely to be settled until a randomized trial.

Given the incurable nature of MM despite novel agents, the role of ASCT can be reformulated as an up-front versus delayed ASCT question. Even in the prenovel agent era, delayed ASCT at relapse was shown to be similar in overall outcomes to upfront ASCT (9,19), with only a quality-of-life benefit for ASCT shown in the French MAG-95 trial (9). One approach would be to harvest peripheral blood stem cells (PBSCs) for any potential transplant candidate early after established response to novel agent induction but defer ASCT to relapse or progression. However, continuing therapy with novel agents is also with significant financial and quality-of-life costs. The toxicity of extended therapy in terms of peripheral neuropathy, risk of venous thromboembolism, and viral reactivation among other potential risks need to be considered (107) against the temporary decrement in quality of life with ASCT. In the modern era, nonrelapse mortality for ASCT is less than 5% (108), with experienced centers performing transplants in the outpatient setting with close to 1% TRM at 100 days (109). On the other hand, novel agent induction could be associated with significant mortality. In addition, the feasibility of ASCT at relapse or progression could be negatively impacted by the cost of stem cell storage, decline in performance status, or development of comorbid illnesses in the patient. The timing of stem cell collection for ASCT, the long-term storage costs of products, the toxicities of extended novel agent therapy, the ultimate utilization of salvage transplant at relapse versus up-front transplant, and pharmacoeconomic as well as quality-of-life comparisons with either of these strategies are issues that need to be addressed in prospective trials. In this context, clinical trials randomizing patients to ongoing novel agent therapy versus ASCT after initial induction have now been designed. The end points reported for such trials should include quality-of-life endpoints as well as pharmacoeconomic measurements in addition to traditional survival and response criteria.

The only randomized study where ASCT was inferior to a novel agent regimen has been the IFM 99–06 discussed earlier. At the same time, a strategy integrating ASCT after bortezomib-based induction and followed by consolidation and long-term extended therapy with lenalidomide has been shown to induce incremental CR benefit at each step and excellent EFS at 2 years (69%) with a low TRM even in patients aged 65 to 75 years (110). In the United States, the BMT Clinical Trials

TABLE 3

Comparison of very good partial remission rates with novel induction regimens

Study	N	Regimen	≥VGPR* Rate After Induction	Comment
Rajkumar et al. (36)	445	Rd/RD	45%*	Median EFS 19–24 months for high- or low-dose dexamethasone arms respectively. Subset of 90 patients received ASCT after 4 cycles had superior 2-year EFS 63–65%.
IFM 2005–01 (87,98)	240	VD → ASCT	47%*	ISS stage 2/3 patients and those with high-risk disease benefited most from superior induction even after ASCT in both the control (VAD) and VD arms
Cavo et al. (88)	199	VTD	61%*	PFS benefit for VTD over TD control arm even after ASCT in both arms
Richardson et a.l (99)	35	VRD	69%*	Estimated 1-year EFS 76% & OS 100%
Kumar et al. (100)	33	CRD	40%*	Weekly cyclophosphamide at 300 mg/m^2
Jakubowiak et al. (101)	68	VRDoxD	58%*	Successful autologous PBSC harvest
Reeder et al. (94)	33	CyBorD	61%*	23 patients underwent ASCT with 74% in >VGPR at day 100
San Miguel et al. (97)	344	VMP	41%*	Median time to progression 24 months. VMP with superior OS compared with MP
Mateos et al. (102)	260	VMP vs. VTP	32 vs. 37% CR/nCR	Included subsequent VT or VP maintenance. Median PFS 33 months for whole cohort but not reached for VMP → VT or VTP → VT subsets.
Kumar et al. (96,103)	43	CVRD	57%*	Overall response rate 94%, but CR+VGPR rate equal to VRD arm
Palumbo et al. (104)	167	MPT	29%*	Median time to progression 24.7 months and superior to MP but OS similar
Palumbo et al. (92)	202	Rd → MPR	51%*	EFS at 1 year 96%, MPR improved depth of response after Rd
Palumbo et al. (105)	254	VMPT → VT	55%*	Excellent 2-year PFS of 70% superior to VMP control arm
Palumbo et al. (106)	459	MPR → R vs. MPR vs. MP	32%* for MPR	PFS was superior for MPR with R maintenance but similar for MPR and MP suggesting possible lack of correlation with response depth and clinical benefit

C/Cy, cyclophosphamide; D, high-dose dexamethasone; d, low-dose dexamethasone; Dox, pegylated doxorubicin; M, melphalan; P, prednisone; R, lenalidomide; T, thalidomide; V/Bor, bortezomib.

Network (BMT CTN) proposes to test a similar approach in a national ASCT-based clinical trial in patients younger than 70 years. Such aggressive strategies also need to be tested in future trials against non-ASCT-based extended treatment approaches.

Role of Autologous Transplantation in High-Risk Disease

Myeloma is now recognized as a biologically heterogeneous disease (111,112), and the efficacy of therapies vary based on genetically defined risk (113,114). In a large retrospective analysis, the IFM group analyzed cytogenetic and interphase fluorescence in situ hybridization data from more than 1,000 patients undergoing transplant-based therapies. In multivariate analysis, the genomic aberrations t(4;14) or del(17p), along with a high β-2-microglobulin level, were predictive of inferior survival, with a median OS of 19 months (115). Several other studies have established metaphase cytogenetic abnormalities of chromosome 13 in addition to t(14:16), t(4;14), and del(17p) (116–119) as predictive of high-risk MM. The Arkansas group have pioneered the use of gene expression profiling to develop a model that predicts outcomes in patients undergoing Total Therapy (120), but practical clinical experience at other institutions is scant for this approach.

Autologous transplant has yielded inferior survival in high-risk MM (121), and the benefit of ASCT has been questioned in these patients (122) because the expected benefit was not commensurate with transplant-related morbidity. Subgroup analyses from several trials (97,114) suggest that bortezomib is equally effective in patients with del(13), t(4;14), or t(14;16) or 17p deletion status as in those without. The Arkansas TT3 experience with the use of bortezomib in induction, consolidation, and maintenance in the setting of tandem ASCT has provided evidence that sustained CR can be achieved and correlates with superior OS in high-risk patients (65). Although randomized data

are not available, establishing a CR and sustaining it seems to be of much greater importance in the high-risk patient subset compared with standard-risk MM (41,123). These patients should therefore be ideally treated with bortezomib containing novel agent regimens with the goal of establishing a CR and then maintained on additional therapy aimed at sustaining the response. Autologous transplant thus remains an integral element in achieving the deepest possible response in high-risk patients.

■ ADVANCES IN STEM CELL MOBILIZATION

After the initial use of bone marrow as a source of the hematopoietic graft in ASCT for MM, PBSCs became the standard of care because they led to faster engraftment and hematologic reconstitution. Guidelines for induction therapy have therefore emphasized the importance of identifying patients eligible for ASCT and avoiding MEL-based induction in "transplant eligible" patients (124). Radiation therapy to significant volume of hematopoietic marrow was also discouraged in transplant-eligible patients as another factor leading to poor PBSC collections (125). The optimum PBSC dose in current clinical practice is a minimal dose of 2 million CD34 cells/kg and an "optimal" dose of 4 to 6 million CD34 cells/kg or greater. This is based on data showing that infusion of less than 2 million CD34 cells/kg was associated with slower hematologic recovery and infusion of more than 5 million CD34 cells/kg led to faster robust platelet recovery (126).

Granulocyte colony stimulating factor (GCSF) or chemotherapy followed by GCSF are the most common strategies for PBSC collection (127). Recent availability of a new agent, plerixafor, for PBSC mobilization has improved mobilization strategies (128). This agent inhibits the binding of stem cells to the marrow stroma, resulting in the release of CD34-positive cells into peripheral blood, thus facilitating their mobilization. Plerixafor in combination with GCSF was effective in mobilizing PBSC in patients who failed traditional mobilization, decreased the number of apheresis procedures needed to reach optimal cell dose, and was more effective as an initial mobilizing regimen than GCSF alone (129–131). Use of plerixafor will likely make mobilization of PBSC feasible in difficult-to-mobilize patients (up to 15%) (132)) who may not have been considered for ASCT previously. The International Myeloma Working Group has published a consensus statement regarding the status of PBSC harvest and ASCT in MM. Early and optimal PBSC harvest was recommended as an integral component of MM treatment planning. It was also recommended to evaluate plerixafor using pharmacoeconomic and resource utilization end points.

Maintenance Therapy

Maintenance is based on the concept of ongoing therapy after transplant to further suppress the malignant clone and thus delay progression/relapse of MM. Attempts at using maintenance after achievement of a stable remission started even in the pre-ASCT era but failed to provide any benefit (133) or sometimes a marginal survival benefit (134). Following ASCT, maintenance therapy with IFN, although initially promising (135), was eventually shown to be ineffective by the US intergroup study when no EFS or OS differences could be shown between patients randomized to IFN versus observation after a response to CC or ASCT (19). Ideally, maintenance treatment should be with minimal side effects, be effective against myeloma, be easy to administer, and, ultimately, improve EFS and OS.

Novel antimyeloma agents have shown superior results as maintenance therapy. Thalidomide maintenance after tandem ASCT has been studied in several major randomized studies (84,86,136,137). Another trial has unfortunately been retracted (138). These data are summarized in Table 4. The randomized phase III French (IFM-99 02) trial assessed the impact of randomization to

thalidomide maintenance (2 months after ASCT) on duration of response. Patients randomized to thalidomide demonstrated superior 3-year EFS compared with those randomized to no treatment or to pamidronate alone (52% vs. 36% vs. 37%, respectively). Survival at 4 years was superior for patients randomized to receive maintenance thalidomide (87%) compared with the other arms (74–77%). Patients who at least had a VGPR after ASCT did not benefit from thalidomide in subgroup analysis. Thalidomide was discontinued because of toxicity in 39% of patients. The results of the Arkansas tandem approach randomizing patients to thalidomide or no thalidomide during induction and as maintenance in combination with dexamethasone and IFN following tandem ASCT initially suggested a higher CR rate and EFS benefit for thalidomide despite increased toxicity (136). When initially reported, survival was not superior in the thalidomide arm secondary to short postrelapse survival. In longer term follow-up analysis, thalidomide was shown to improve survival in patients, especially those with abnormal cytogenetics (84). Both trials described earlier have benefited from a combined long-term reappraisal of their benefits (21). The survival benefit of the IFM 9902 trial has not held up with 5-year survival estimates of 70% for the no-thalidomide arm and 74% for thalidomide maintenance ($P = 0.53$). The OS benefit for thalidomide in TT2 is still statistically significant, with 5-year estimates of 68% versus 65% for no thalidomide ($P = 0.04$). One important observation was the short postrelapse survival of patients receiving extended duration thalidomide, which also explains the loss of survival benefit on longer term follow-up.

Spencer et al. randomized 269 patients after a single ASCT to receive indefinite prednisolone maintenance versus 114 patients receiving prednisolone + thalidomide (thalidomide group) (137). Three-year EFS rates (23% vs. 42%) and OS rates (75% vs. 86%) were significantly in favor of thalidomide. Importantly, in this study, the EFS benefits were observed even in patients achieving a CR or VGPR after ASCT. In the NCIC-MY9 study from

TABLE 4
Selected trials of maintenance therapy post-ASCT

Study	Agent	Duration of Therapy	Comments
Barlogie (136) TT2	Thalidomide vs. no thalidomide	Until progression/AE after tandem ASCT	Higher CR rates and EFS in thalidomide arm and on longer term follow-up for OS (21)
Attal et al. (86) IFM 9902	Thalidomide + pamidronate vs. observation	Until progression/AE after tandem ASCT	CR rate, 4-year OS superior for thalidomide but high discontinuation rate. Also OS advantage lost in longer term follow-up (21).
Spencer et al. (137)	Thalidomide + prednisolone vs. prednisolone	For 12 months after single ASCT	CR rates and 3-year OS superior for thalidomide/ prednisone arm
Hovon 50 (139)	Thalidomide vs. interferon A	Until progression/AE after single or tandem ASCT	CR/VGPR rates and EFS significantly superior for thalidomide. OS similar and lower post relapse survival in thalidomide arm
BMT CTN 0102 (140)	Thalidomide + dexamethasone vs observation	For 12 months after tandem ASCT	Results awaited
CALGB 100104 (141)	Lenalidomide vs. placebo	Till progression after single ASCT	Study terminated and unblinded in December 2009 after interim assessment indicated superior EFS for lenalidomide arm
GMMG HD4 (89)	Thalidomide vs. bortezomib	For 2 years after single or tandem ASCT	Higher CR rates in bortezomib arm but impact of maintenance unknown

Canada that randomized patients to 200 mg or 400 mg of thalidomide combined with alternate-day 50-mg prednisone, the 400-mg arm was prematurely stopped because of excessive toxicity, and 31% of patients in the 200-mg thalidomide arm required dose reductions (142). Thus, three separate phase III studies found thalidomide maintenance to improve EFS and possibly OS. However, the use of thalidomide is associated with significant side effects, and the risk of toxicity may outweigh benefits especially in patients who are in a VGPR after ASCT. Also, optimum duration of maintenance is unknown, and the risk of overtreatment should be considered especially if post-ASCT maintenance acts similar to consolidation in patients who have

greater residual burden. The possible risks of overtreatment could be higher cumulative toxicity and lower postrelapse survival caused by the evolution of resistant clones due to selection pressure.

Several completed and ongoing trials include immunomodulator (IMIDs) or proteasome inhibitor maintenance therapies (Table 4). The BMT CTN 0102 trial randomized patients after tandem ASCT to 1 year of thalidomide 200 mg/day plus dexamethasone or observation. Lenalidomide was evaluated in the CALGB 100104 post-ASCT maintenance trial. This trial utilized lenalidomide at a dose of 10/15 mg versus placebo after a single ASCT and was prematurely terminated in December 2009 after interim results suggested attainment of the primary end point of superior EFS in the lenalidomide arm. Bortezomib added as consolidation and maintenance along with TD in the Arkansas TT3 program has yielded superior early results compared with historical data from previous versions of Total Therapy. A German–Dutch consortium evaluating bortezomib (every 2 weeks for 2 years) versus thalidomide (50 mg daily) in maintenance after ASCT consolidation is also expected to report mature results soon (89).

"Salvage" Second Transplants at Relapse

It has been shown that a salvage ASCT at relapse after prior transplant showed benefit for patients with more than 12 months remission duration and normal β-2-microglobulin (74,143,144). However, patients relapsing within 12 to 18 months of their first ASCT have a poor prognosis, and a second ASCT is of much less benefit (145,146). Novel therapies, salvage ASCT, or salvage alloSCT are all options in the setting of relapsed disease. Limited comparisons suggest that although autografting and allografting are both feasible, disease progression remains the major cause of failure. Median EFS and OS in the salvage ASCT versus alloSCT setting were 6.8 months versus 7.3 months and 29 months versus 13 months, respectively, in a series from the MD Anderson Cancer Center (144). An earlier series with myeloablative allografts versus salvage ASCT from the Arkansas group showed similar CR rates but prohibitively higher TRM after alloSCT albeit with a lower risk of disease progression (147). These studies also suggest that the outcomes of salvage ASCT are determined by the number of prior lines of therapy (possibly a surrogate for chemotherapy resistance or toxicities of therapy) and the time from first ASCT to relapse in addition to biologic prognostic factors. In the tandem ASCT setting, a (third) salvage ASCT at relapse while associated with acceptable CR rates (29%) resulted in a disappointing 19% OS at 2 years (148). It is unknown whether novel agents after relapse prior to salvage ASCT or in

maintenance after salvage ASCT can improve the outcomes of the salvage transplants.

■ ALLOGENEIC TRANSPLANTATION

Allogeneic transplantation is not performed commonly for MM, with only an estimated less than 2% of patients annually receiving this modality. There are certain clear advantages such as a tumor-free graft source, strong evidence for graft-versus-myeloma (GVM) effect (149,150), durable molecular CRs (148,151–153), and a significantly reduced risk of relapse after alloSCT compared with ASCT (154). The advanced age of patients with MM at diagnosis, significant TRM and morbidity after alloSCT, and the lack of sustained cure in most patients after alloSCT have on the other hand reduced enthusiasm for alloSCT (155).

GVM—Fact or Fiction

Multiple lines of observation have confirmed the existence of a clinically beneficial immune-mediated graft-versus-tumor (GVT) effect after alloSCT in many cancers. The induction of sustained antineoplastic effect by the infusion of donor lymphocytes (DLI) (156,157), the association of graft-versus-host disease (GVHD) with disease responses or protection from relapse (158–160), and lower relapse rates in recipients of unmanipulated (T cell replete) allografts compared with those receiving T cell-depleted grafts or syngeneic grafts (161) are considered key findings proving the existence of a clinically beneficial GVT phenomenon in a specific disease state. All of the above can be shown in the setting of alloSCT for MM.

Myeloma (idiotype)-specific CD4 T cell response could be transferred from an immunized marrow donor to patient in early studies by Kwak (162). The success of DLI in patients with (163–167) residual or progressive MM after alloSCT is also evidence for GVM. Although the durability of responses after DLI is modest, the occurrence of GVHD (acute or chronic) after DLI seems to be the most powerful predictor of a response (164,166,168). Recently, a large registry study also found that the occurrence of chronic GVHD after alloSCT correlated with freedom from progression (169). In vitro or in vivo (using alemtuzumab or antithymocyte globulin [ATG]) T cell depletion has been associated with higher relapse rates and the need for DLI after alloSCT in MM (170–172). Thus, there is clear scientific evidence for a clinically relevant GVM effect.

TRM after Allogeneic Transplantation

Despite these immunologic benefits, conventional myeloablative allogeneic transplantation in MM was associated with a significantly inferior EFS and OS compared with ASCT (173,174). In an analysis of unrelated donor allotransplants facilitated by the National Marrow Donor Program, the 5-year OS was dismal at 9% (175). These inferior outcomes stemming from a significant (up to or >50%) TRM (147) dampened enthusiasm for alloSCT until the development of less intense conditioning regimens defined as RIC and nonmyeloablative stem cell transplantation (NST) conditioning (176). Even with myeloablative alloSCT, some patients surviving the risk of TRM enjoyed prolonged disease-free survival. The allogeneic arm of US Intergroup S9321 study was aborted after an early TRM of 53% was observed. However, survivors of alloSCT had a plateau in the survival curve at 22%, with no late events indicating a likely cure (19). TRM related to disease stage, remission status pretransplant, donor recipient sex mismatch, prior therapies, and severe GVHD (177,178) has decreased significantly over the past decade to approximately 30% to 35% (179,180) even with myeloablative transplants. A single-center analysis by Arora et al. (181) described an encouraging 4-year survival of 64% in their ablative alloSCT patients compared with 50% (*P* = 0.04) in the autologous transplant setting. For patients surviving beyond 1 year after transplant, OS and EFS were significantly superior in the allogeneic setting.

RIC Allogeneic Transplantation

Reduced intensity regimens (RIC/NST) are designed to cause less host tissue damage and less inflammatory cytokine secretion, with the intent of lowering the risk of TRM and, possibly, severe GVHD (182,183). Conceptually, they utilize the GVT effect for disease control while reducing TRM and regimens because of age or concurrent medical conditions (184–187). The intensity of these regimens varies, ranging from low (2 Gy) doses of TBI that do not induce cytopenia to combinations of fludarabine with busulfan and/or MEL that induce significant (though reversible) cytopenia (188–194). In early studies, this approach proved feasible both in the up-front and salvage settings in MM. The Seattle group who pioneered the NST approach initially reported on their results in three groups of patients—relapsed patients who had failed prior ASCT (*n* = 14); relapsed patients who had not received prior ASCT (*n* = 19); and a third group who were candidates for a sequential ASCT followed by NST (*n* = 84). The predicted 4-year OS were 40%, 35%, and 70% in the corresponding groups, whereas TRM was 2% at day 100 and 17% overall (195). A comparison between RIC/NST and myeloablative alloSCT from the EBMT group suggested that although patients receiving RIC were older and more likely to have advanced disease including prior autologous transplants, TRM was significantly lower in this group (24% vs. 37% at 2 years in the ablative cohort) (180). However, there was a significantly higher risk of relapse in the RIC cohort, although OS and EFS were similar in both groups. A recent CIBMTR analysis demonstrated a major practice switch to RIC/NST alloSCT in clinical practice with concomitant reduction in the numbers of myeloablative allografts (196) performed in the years 2001–2005 compared with the two preceding 5-year blocks. The switch to RIC has also resulted in older patients with MM receiving alloSCT and increasing numbers of alloSCT performed after prior autoSCT. There was no change in OS over time because the decline in TRM was negated by an increase in relapse risk in later years. Outcomes after NST/RIC alloSCT need to be interpreted in the context of the conditioning regimen used (T cell depletion vs. not), the setting of the transplant (salvage vs. up-front), the type of donor (related vs. unrelated), and the approach (planned sequential tandem vs. not).

In patients with high-risk or relapsed MM, the Arkansas group, using an RIC approach with MEL100 mg/m^2, had impressive response rates but high 1-year TRM of 38% (197). The OS results remained poor in the salvage setting compared with the up-front tandem approach, and no true plateau has yet been documented in EFS. In patient groups composed mainly of progressive/relapsed MM, the 2-year OS and EFS have been reported to be 25% and 22%, respectively, by Einsele et al. (198) and 30% and 19% by Giralt et al. (199) using RIC approaches. The 1-year TRM has been in the 23% to 40% range in these studies. Other series (summarized in Table 5 (190,198–209)) were also with disappointing EFS. Therefore, in the salvage setting, unless TRM can be reduced or a significant plateau in survival can be shown on follow-up, the RIC/NST approach has a limited role outside of clinical trials.

Planned Sequential Autologous Followed by NST/RIC Allogeneic Transplantation

The existence of GVM effect after DLI independent of chemotherapy suggested that RIC/NST allogeneic transplantation strategies might be useful in patients with MM who have minimal disease at the time of allogeneic transplant. This led to the use of initial ASCT for steep tumor reduction followed by a planned (tandem) NST/RIC allotransplant aimed at using the GVM effect to eradicate minimal residual disease with a goal of long-term disease control. Early studies indicated

(200,201,210) that in a tandem setting where an NST or RIC allograft followed an ASCT, the approach yielded excellent short-term (24 month) EFS and OS, with TRM ranging from 11% in the matched related setting to 26% in the unrelated setting. Maloney et al. described the initial sequential ASCT/NST data from the Seattle consortium in 54 patients, median age 52 years, half of them with refractory or relapsed disease. CR was reported in 57%, and overall TRM was 22%. At a median follow-up of 60 months, OS and EFS were 69% and 38%, respectively. Sensitive disease prior to transplant predicted lower TRM (7% vs. 27%) (200).

Long-term results of up-front tandem ASCT–alloSCT protocol from the Seattle group are now available (207). After a high-dose MEL-based ASCT, 102 patients received 2-Gy TBI with or without fludarabine, followed by alloSCT from human leukocyte antigen (HLA)-matched sibling donors. The majority of patients received the tandem transplants with 10 months of diagnosis. Although 60% of patients with detectable disease achieved CR and TRM that was low at 18% at 5 years, median EFS was a disappointing 3 years and median time to progression was 5 years. Five-year OS and EFS were 64% and 36%, respectively, with patients transplanted within 10 months of initial therapy having 5-year OS of 69% and EFS of 37%. Delay of more than 10 months and a β-2-microglobulin of more than 3.5 µg/mL at diagnosis correlated with shorter OS and EFS, whereas Karnofsky scores less than 90% at alloSCT correlated with shorter EFS. Bruno et al. described Gruppo Italiano Trapianti di Midollo experience of 100 newly diagnosed patients who received induction therapy followed by ASCT followed by TBI-based NST and sibling allografts (209). Although CR rates increased to 53% after alloSCT, median EFS was only 37 months. Profound cytoreduction (CR/VGPR) before alloSCT was associated with longer EFS, but chronic GVHD was not correlated with CR or response duration. The lack of an apparent cure with ongoing late relapses was disappointing in both studies.

TABLE 5
Selected phase 2 data in reduced intensity allogeneic transplantation for MM

Study	N	URD	Setting	Conditioning	Acute GVHD%	Chronic GVHD%	CR %	TRM%	OS	EFS % or Median	Comment/Survival Estimate
Giralt 2002 (199)	22	9	Salvage	FLU 120 + MEL 140	46	30	32	40	30%	19%	24 months
Maloney (200) 2003	54	NA	Tandem	TBI 2 GY	38	46	57	15	78%	55%	18 months
Einsele 2003 (198)	22	15	Salvage	FLU 150+Cy 40 TBI 2 GY + ATG	5	6	27	23	25%	22%	24 months
Kroger 2002 (201)	21	21	Tandem	Flu 180 + MEL 100 + ATG	38	37	40	26	74%	53%	24 months
Badros & Lee 2002–2003 (202,203)	45	11	Salvage	MEL 100	78	58	64	38	36%	13%	36 months
Perez-Simon 2003 (204)	29	0	Salvage	FLU 150 + MEL 140	52	21	28	21	60%	33%	24 months
Gerull 2004 (205)	56	NR	Salvage	TBI +/- FLU 90 Some MEL based	36	61	NA	20	40%	25%	OS & EFS 18 months Median follow-up 21 months
Kroger 2004 (190)	120	35	Both	FLU + MEL	46	47	49	18	59%	39%	2-year OS and EFS
Vesole 2009 (206)	23	0	Tandem	FLU + CY	17	57	30	8.7	78%	3.6 years	2-year OS
Rotta 2009 (207)	102	0	Tandem	TBI 2 Gy ± FLU	42	74	60	18	NR	3 years	Median TTP—5 years OS median not reached
Kroger 2010 (208)	49	49	Salvage	FLU + MEL	25	35	46	25	26%	20%	5-year follow-up. TRM at 1 year 53% for mismatched
Bruno (209)	100	0	Tandem	TBI 2 Gy	38	50	53	11	NR	3.1 years	5-year follow-up with median OS not reached

MEL, melphalan (doses in mg/m^2); ATG, antithymocyte globulin; FLU, fludarabine (in mg/m^2); BU, busulfan; TBI, total body irradiation; NA, not available; NR, not reached; CY, cyclophosphamide (in mg/m^2).

Randomized Studies of Tandem alloSCT with RIC/NST

Bruno et al. described the outcomes of 245 patients, younger than 65 years, genetically assigned to (based on availability of) a matched sibling alloSCT versus a second ASCT after initial induction and a first autotransplant (154). Eighty patients with an HLA-identical sibling were offered TBI-based NST allotransplant, whereas 82 patients without an HLA-identical sibling were assigned to receive a second ASCT. In a donor versus no donor analysis, at a median follow-up of 45 months, OS and EFS were significantly longer in patients with sibling donors (80 vs. 54 months and 35 vs. 29 months, respectively). Overall, 58 and 46 patients completed the tandem autologous–allogeneic and the tandem autologous programs, with CR rates of 55% versus 26%, respectively, and TRM of 10% and 2%, respectively. In an update of this study after follow-up of nearly 5 years, OS was not reached for the 80 patients with an HLA-identical sibling and was 56 months for those without (P = 0.009)(211). This was the first randomized study showing an advantage for alloSCT over ASCT in MM.

Other prospective studies have not described similar superiority for alloSCT. The IFM99–03/99–04 clinical trials were parallel prospective risk adapted trials of tandem ASCT (IFM9904) or sequential ASCT followed by NST (IFM9903) in high-risk MM defined by a β-2-microglobulin less than 3 mg/L and chromosome 13 deletion (212). Sixty-five patients were randomized to receive alloSCT, with RIC consisting of busulfan, fludarabine, and high-dose ATG. Patients without sibling donors (N = 219) were assigned to tandem ASCT, and 166 patients completed this. Compared with the 46 patients out of 65 who underwent the entire ASCT/RIC alloSCT program, no difference was observed regarding EFS (median 25 vs. 21 months, P = 0.88). Survival was similar (median OS 57 vs. 41 months, P = 0.08), but a longer postrelapse survival was noticed in the tandem ASCT arm. A third study by the Spanish PETHEMA group

(213) enrolled patients who were not in at least a near CR after an initial ASCT to a second tandem ASCT versus a biologically assigned RIC based on sibling donor availability. An increase in CR rate (40% vs. 11%, P = 0.001) and a trend toward a longer EFS (median 31 months vs. not reached, P = 0.08) in favor of alloSCT was observed. Around 60% of patients did not undergo assigned therapy in this study, thus reducing the ability of the trial to show statistical superiority.

Two other randomized studies of alloSCT have been presented but not yet published. The EBMT conducted a study where patients were randomized to tandem ASCT followed by RIC (fludarabine + TBI) allografting versus ASCT based on the availability of an HLA-identical sibling donor (214). One hundred and seven patients were allocated to tandem ASCT–RIC, and 251 patients without a donor to the ASCT arm. The 2-year TRM was 13% in the tandem alloSCT and 5% in the ASCT arm (P = 0.014). The CR rates (43% vs. 38%), relapse/progression rates (49% vs. 75%), EFS (35% vs. 18%), and OS (65% vs. 57%) at 60 months were all in favor of the tandem alloSCT arm. A prospective German study compared tandem ASCT with an RIC alloSCT following ASCT for high-risk MM with 13q-MM. Patients with an HLA-matched sibling or unrelated donors were allocated to the tandem alloSCT arm (fludarabine + MEL RIC). AlloSCT was performed in 126 patients, with 60% receiving unrelated grafts. AlloSCT resulted in higher CR rates (59 vs. 32%; P = 0.003) and acceptable TRM of 12% at 2 years. The projected 3-year survival was 72% for ASCT versus 60% for alloSCT (P = NS). Table 6 (140,154,212–215) summarizes the available randomized NST/RIC data in the up-front tandem setting.

The continuing risk of relapse with no plateau in relapse curves and a 50% to 60% PFS at 3 years detracts considerably from the early promise of RIC/NST alloSCT. Thus, the GVM effect alone may not be sufficient to maintain responses after alloSCT. For the present, mature results of randomized trials of tandem alloSCT approaches

TABLE 6

Randomized studies of allogeneic HLA matched transplants vs. tandem autologous transplants

Author	N allo	Trial Setting	Conditioning for AlloSCT vs. ASCT	CGVHD allo	TRM allo	OS	EFS	Conclusion
Bruno (154)	245/58	Post induction biological assignment based on sibling match donor	MEL ASCT followed by TBI 2 Gy vs. MEL doses 100–200 mg/m²	32%	10%	Median 80 vs. 54 months $P = 0.01$	Median 35 vs. 29 months $P = 0.02$	Only study with clear benefit for alloSCT in intention to treat, sibling vs. no sibling analysis
Garban (212) IFM 9903–04	284/65	Parallel prospective studies limited to high-risk disease (β2M & del 13 by FISH)	MEL 200 ASCT followed by FLU-EU + ATG alloSCT vs. MEL 200 ASCT	42%	11%	Median 34 vs. 48 months $P = 0.07$	Median 19 vs. 22 months $P = 0.58$	30% did not complete AlloSCT. No benefit to AlloSCT in this study
Rosinol (213)	110/25	Limited to patients not in CR after a first ASCT	FLU-MEL alloSCT vs. CVB or MEL 200 ASCT	66%	16%	Median NR vs. 58 months $P = 0.9$	Median 20 vs. 26 months $P = 0.4$	Higher CR rate after alloSCT but no survival benefit
Knop (215)	199/126	Limited to patients with 13q- by FISH, Unrelated donor grafts in 60%	MEL 200 ASCT followed by FLU-MEL vs. MEL 200 ASCT	N/R	13%	3-year OS 60% vs. 72% $P = 0.22$	N/R	Largest trial in high-risk patients and with unrelated donors

Garhton (214)	358/107	Post induction biological assignment based on sibling match donor	MEL 200 ASCT followed by FLU—TBI2 Gy vs. MEL 200 ASCT	N/R	13%	5-year OS 65% vs. 57 % P = NS	5-year PFS 35% vs. 19% $P < 0.05$	AlloSCT with lower risk of relapse and with improved PFS with benefit for del 13 subset
BMTCTN 0102 (140)	710/226	Post induction assignment based on availability of matched sibling donor	MEL 200 ASCT followed by TBI 2Gy alloSCT vs. MEL 200 ASCT	Results awaited in 2010. This is the largest trial of tandem ASCT vs. autologous followed by RIC alloSCT approach				

Allo, allogeneic; SCT, arm; FLU, fludarabine; BU, busulfan; MEL, melphalan (dose in mg/m^2); CVB, cyclophosphamide/etoposide/BCNU.

are awaited (BMT Clinical Trials Network 0102). Because acute GVHD and relapse impact survival negatively after RIC/NST, several strategies such as T cell-depleted grafts, augmented immunosuppression with ATG (198) or alemtuzumab (216), preemptive DLI (216), and posttransplant novel agent maintenance therapies have all been proposed to improve the results of allogeneic transplantation in MM (217). These approaches as well as attempts to increase the intensity of conditioning therapy to achieve superior antineoplastic activity are still in clinical trials. Given general advances in HLA typing, antifungal therapy, and supportive care, future efforts at improving outcomes after allogeneic transplant should also focus on strategies to make myeloablative regimens safer.

■ SUMMARY

ASCT is still a crucial component of the overall treatment strategy for MM in patients who are medically eligible to undergo this procedure. Despite improvements in induction therapy and availability of novel drugs, MM continues to be characterized by a relapsing clinical course. Retaining the ASCT option by facilitating optimal PBSC collection is important because therapeutic efficacy of high-dose therapy is well established even in the delayed or salvage setting. Novel agent combination therapy will no doubt change the current treatment paradigms, but at this time, it is still unclear whether ASCT is better performed as consolidation following induction versus as later therapy in the delayed relapsed setting. Improvements in mobilization therapy, integration of novel agents in induction, conditioning and maintenance, as well as improvements in supportive care will significantly improve the gains made in the last decade. Allogeneic transplants remain challenging, but the vision of utilizing graft versus MM effect to effect a cure without compromising mortality and morbidity needs to be explored in carefully designed trials incorporating novel therapies and immunosuppression strategies.

■ REFERENCES

1. Horner M, Ries LA, Krapcho M, et al. *SEER Cancer Statistics Review, 1975–2006.* Bethesda, MD: National Cancer Institute; 2009. http://seer.cancer.gov/csr/1975_2006/, based on November 2008 SEER data submission, posted to the SEER web site, 2009.

2. Attal M, Harousseau JL, Stoppa AM, et al. A prospective, randomized trial of autologous bone marrow transplantation and chemotherapy in multiple myeloma. Intergroupe Français du Myélome. *N Engl J Med* 1996;335(2):91–97.

3. Child JA, Morgan GJ, Davies FE, et al.; Medical Research Council Adult Leukaemia Working Party. High-dose chemotherapy with hematopoietic stem-cell rescue for multiple myeloma. *N Engl J Med* 2003;348(19):1875–1883.

4. Lenhoff S, Hjorth M, Holmberg E, et al. Impact on survival of high-dose therapy with autologous stem cell support in patients younger than 60 years with newly diagnosed multiple myeloma: a population-based study. Nordic Myeloma Study Group. *Blood* 2000;95(1):7–11.

5. Palumbo A, Triolo S, Argentino C, et al. Dose-intensive melphalan with stem cell support (MEL100) is superior to standard treatment in elderly myeloma patients. *Blood* 1999;94(4):1248–1253.

6. Gianni AM, Tarella C, Bregni M, et al. High-dose sequential chemoradiotherapy, a widely applicable regimen, confers survival benefit to patients with high-risk multiple myeloma. *J Clin Oncol* 1994;12(3):503–509.

7. Barlogie B, Jagannath S, Vesole DH, et al. Superiority of tandem autologous transplantation over standard therapy for previously untreated multiple myeloma. *Blood* 1997;89(3):789–793.

8. Palumbo A, Bringhen S, Petrucci MT, et al. Intermediate-dose melphalan improves survival of myeloma patients aged 50 to 70: results of a randomized controlled trial. *Blood* 2004;104(10):3052–3057.

9. Fermand JP, Ravaud P, Chevret S, et al. High-dose therapy and autologous peripheral blood stem cell transplantation in multiple myeloma: up-front or rescue treatment? Results of a multicenter sequential randomized clinical trial. *Blood* 1998;92(9):3131–3136.

10. Fermand JP, Katsahian S, Divine M, et al.; Group Myelome-Autogreffe. High-dose therapy and autologous blood stem-cell transplantation compared with conventional treatment in myeloma patients aged 55 to 65 years: long-term results of a randomized control

trial from the Group Myelome-Autogreffe. *J Clin Oncol* 2005;23(36):9227–9233.

11. Bladé J, Rosiñol L, Sureda A, et al.; Programa para el Estudio de la Terapéutica en Hemopatía Maligna (PETHEMA). High-dose therapy intensification compared with continued standard chemotherapy in multiple myeloma patients responding to the initial chemotherapy: long-term results from a prospective randomized trial from the Spanish cooperative group PETHEMA. *Blood* 2005;106(12):3755–3759.

12. Koreth J, Cutler CS, Djulbegovic B, et al. High-dose therapy with single autologous transplantation versus chemotherapy for newly diagnosed multiple myeloma: A systematic review and meta-analysis of randomized controlled trials. *Biol Blood Marrow Transplant* 2007;13(2):183–196.

13. Imrie K, Esmail R, Meyer RM; Members of the Hematology Disease Site Group of the Cancer Care Ontario Practice Guidelines Initiative. The role of high-dose chemotherapy and stem-cell transplantation in patients with multiple myeloma: a practice guideline of the Cancer Care Ontario Practice Guidelines Initiative. *Ann Intern Med* 2002;136(8):619–629.

14. Hahn T, Wingard JR, Anderson KC, et al. The role of cytotoxic therapy with hematopoietic stem cell transplantation in the therapy of multiple myeloma: an evidence-based review. *Biol Blood Marrow Transplant* 2003;9(1):4–37.

15. Pasquini M, Wang Z. Current use and outcome of hematopoietic stem cell transplantation: Part I CIBMTR summary slides. *CIBMTR Newsletter* 2009; 15(1):7–11. http://www.cibmtr.org/publications/Newsletter/index.html. Accessed March 30, 2010.

16. Kumar SK, Rajkumar SV, Dispenzieri A, et al. Improved survival in multiple myeloma and the impact of novel therapies. *Blood* 2008;111(5):2516–2520.

17. McElwain TJ, Powles RL. High-dose intravenous melphalan for plasma-cell leukaemia and myeloma. *Lancet* 1983;2(8354):822–824.

18. Turesson I, Velez R, Kristinsson SY, Landgren O. Patterns of improved survival in patients with multiple myeloma in the twenty-first century: a population-based study. *J Clin Oncol* 2010;28(5):830–834.

19. Barlogie B, Kyle RA, Anderson KC, et al. Standard chemotherapy compared with high-dose chemoradiotherapy for multiple myeloma: final results of phase III US Intergroup Trial S9321. *J Clin Oncol* 2006;24(6):929–936.

20. Segeren CM, Sonneveld P, van der Holt B, et al.; Dutch-Belgian Hemato-Oncology Cooperative Study Group. Overall and event-free survival are not improved by the use of myeloablative therapy following intensified chemotherapy in previously untreated patients with multiple myeloma: a prospective randomized phase 3 study. *Blood* 2003;101(6):2144–2151.

21. Barlogie B, Attal M, Crowley J, et al. Long-term follow-up of autotransplantation trials for multiple myeloma: update of protocols conducted by the intergroupe francophone du myelome, southwest oncology group, and university of arkansas for medical sciences. *J Clin Oncol* 2010;28(7):1209–1214.

22. Moreau P, Facon T, Attal M, et al.; Intergroupe Francophone du Myélome. Comparison of 200 mg/m(2) melphalan and 8 Gy total body irradiation plus 140 mg/m(2) melphalan as conditioning regimens for peripheral blood stem cell transplantation in patients with newly diagnosed multiple myeloma: final analysis of the Intergroupe Francophone du Myélome 9502 randomized trial. *Blood* 2002;99(3):731–735.

23. Kyle RA, Leong T, Li S, et al. Complete response in multiple myeloma: clinical trial E9486, an Eastern Cooperative Oncology Group study not involving stem cell transplantation. *Cancer* 2006;106(9):1958–1966.

24. Durie BG, Jacobson J, Barlogie B, Crowley J. Magnitude of response with myeloma frontline therapy does not predict outcome: importance of time to progression in southwest oncology group chemotherapy trials. *J Clin Oncol* 2004;22(10):1857–1863.

25. Oivanen TM, Kellokumpu-Lehtinen P, Koivisto AM, Koivunen E, Palva I. Response level and survival after conventional chemotherapy for multiple myeloma: a Finnish Leukaemia Group study. *Eur J Haematol* 1999;62(2):109–116.

26. Facon T, Mary JY, Pégourie B, et al.; Intergroupe Francophone du Myélome (IFM) group. Dexamethasone-based regimens versus melphalan-prednisone for elderly multiple myeloma patients ineligible for high-dose therapy. *Blood* 2006;107(4):1292–1298.

27. Rajkumar SV. Treatment of myeloma: cure vs control. *Mayo Clin Proc* 2008;83(10):1142–1145.

28. Anderson JR, Cain KC, Gelber RD. Analysis of survival by tumor response. *J Clin Oncol* 1983; 1(11):710–719.

29. van de Velde HJK, Liu X, Chen G, Cakana A, Deraedt W, Bayssas M. Complete response correlates with long-term survival and progression-free survival in high-dose therapy in multiple myeloma. *Haematologica* 2007;92(10):1399–1406.

30. Lahuerta JJ, Mateos MV, Martínez-López J, et al. Influence of pre- and post-transplantation responses on outcome of patients with multiple myeloma: sequential improvement of response and achievement

of complete response are associated with longer survival. *J Clin Oncol* 2008;26(35):5775–5782.

31. Harousseau JL, Avet-Loiseau H, Attal M, et al. Achievement of at least very good partial response is a simple and robust prognostic factor in patients with multiple myeloma treated with high-dose therapy: long-term analysis of the IFM 99–02 and 99–04 Trials. *J Clin Oncol* 2009;27(34):5720–5726.

32. Bladé J, Samson D, Reece D, et al. Criteria for evaluating disease response and progression in patients with multiple myeloma treated by high-dose therapy and haemopoietic stem cell transplantation. Myeloma Subcommittee of the EBMT. European Group for Blood and Marrow Transplant. *Br J Haematol* 1998;102(5):1115–1123.

33. Durie BG, Harousseau JL, Miguel JS, et al.; International Myeloma Working Group. International uniform response criteria for multiple myeloma. *Leukemia* 2006;20(9):1467–1473.

34. Giarin MM, Giaccone L, Sorasio R, et al. Serum free light chain ratio, total kappa/lambda ratio, and immunofixation results are not prognostic factors after stem cell transplantation for newly diagnosed multiple myeloma. *Clin Chem* 2009;55(8):1510–1516.

35. Paiva B, Vidriales MB, Cerveró J, et al.; GEM (Grupo Español de MM)/PETHEMA (Programa para el Estudio de la Terapéutica en Hemopatías Malignas) Cooperative Study Groups. Multiparameter flow cytometric remission is the most relevant prognostic factor for multiple myeloma patients who undergo autologous stem cell transplantation. *Blood* 2008;112(10):4017–4023.

36. Rajkumar SV, Jacobus S, Callander NS, et al.; Eastern Cooperative Oncology Group. Lenalidomide plus high-dose dexamethasone versus lenalidomide plus low-dose dexamethasone as initial therapy for newly diagnosed multiple myeloma: an open-label randomised controlled trial. *Lancet Oncol* 2010;11(1):29–37.

37. Ludwig H, Hajek R, Tóthová E, et al. Thalidomide-dexamethasone compared with melphalan-prednisolone in elderly patients with multiple myeloma. *Blood* 2009;113(15):3435–3442.

38. Rajkumar SV, Fonseca R, Dispenzieri A, et al. Effect of complete response on outcome following autologous stem cell transplantation for myeloma. *Bone Marrow Transplant* 2000;26(9):979–983.

39. Haessler J, Shaughnessy JD Jr, Zhan F, et al. Benefit of complete response in multiple myeloma limited to high-risk subgroup identified by gene expression profiling. *Clin Cancer Res* 2007;13(23):7073–7079.

40. Pineda-Roman M, Bolejack V, Arzoumanian V, et al. Complete response in myeloma extends survival without, but not with history of prior monoclonal gammopathy of undetermined significance or smouldering disease. *Br J Haematol* 2007;136(3):393–399.

41. Hoering A, Crowley J, Shaughnessy JD Jr, et al. Complete remission in multiple myeloma examined as time-dependent variable in terms of both onset and duration in Total Therapy protocols. *Blood* 2009;114(7):1299–1305.

42. Harousseau JL, Attal M, Avet-Loiseau H. The role of complete response in multiple myeloma. *Blood* 2009;114(15):3139–3146.

43. Brenner H, Gondos A, Pulte D. Recent major improvement in long-term survival of younger patients with multiple myeloma. *Blood* 2008;111(5):2521–2526.

44. Palumbo A, Bringhen S, Bruno B, et al. Melphalan 200 mg/m(2) versus melphalan 100 mg/m(2) in newly diagnosed myeloma patients: a prospective, multicenter phase 3 study. *Blood* 2010;115(10):1873–1879.

45. Facon T, Mary JY, Hulin C, et al.; Intergroupe Francophone du Myélome. Melphalan and prednisone plus thalidomide versus melphalan and prednisone alone or reduced-intensity autologous stem cell transplantation in elderly patients with multiple myeloma (IFM 99–06): a randomised trial. *Lancet* 2007;370(9594):1209–1218.

46. Phillips GL, Meisenberg B, Reece DE, et al. Amifostine and autologous hematopoietic stem cell support of escalating-dose melphalan: a phase I study. *Biol Blood Marrow Transplant* 2004;10(7):473–483.

47. Dimopoulos MA, Souliotis VL, Anagnostopoulos A, Papadimitriou C, Sfikakis PP. Extent of damage and repair in the p53 tumor-suppressor gene after treatment of myeloma patients with high-dose melphalan and autologous blood stem-cell transplantation is individualized and may predict clinical outcome. *J Clin Oncol* 2005;23(19):4381–4389.

48. Ria R, Falzetti F, Ballanti S, et al. Melphalan versus melphalan plus busulphan in conditioning to autologous stem cell transplantation for low-risk multiple myeloma. *Hematol J* 2004;5(2):118–122.

49. Blanes M, de la Rubia J, Lahuerta JJ, et al. Single daily dose of intravenous busulfan and melphalan as a conditioning regimen for patients with multiple myeloma undergoing autologous stem cell transplantation: a phase II trial. *Leuk Lymphoma* 2009;50(2):216–222.

50. Talamo G, Claxton DF, Dougherty DW, et al. BU and CY as conditioning regimen for autologous transplant in patients with multiple myeloma. *Bone Marrow Transplant* 2009;44(3):157–161.

51. Heyll A, Söhngen D, Kobbe G, et al. Idarubicin, melphalan and cyclophosphamide: an intensified high-dose regimen for the treatment of myeloma patients. *Leukemia* 1997;11 (suppl 5):S32–S34.

52. Fenk R, Schneider P, Kropff M, et al.; West German Myeloma Study Group. High-dose idarubicin, cyclophosphamide and melphalan as conditioning for autologous stem cell transplantation increases treatment-related mortality in patients with multiple myeloma: results of a randomised study. *Br J Haematol* 2005;130(4):588–594.

53. Meloni G, Capria S, Trasarti S, et al. High-dose idarubicine, busulphan and melphalan as conditioning for autologous blood stem cell transplantation in multiple myeloma. A feasibility study. *Bone Marrow Transplant* 2000;26(10):1045–1049.

54. Anagnostopoulos A, Aleman A, Ayers G, et al. Comparison of high-dose melphalan with a more intensive regimen of thiotepa, busulfan, and cyclophosphamide for patients with multiple myeloma. *Cancer* 2004;100(12):2607–2612.

55. Lahuerta JJ, Grande C, Blade J, et al.; Spanish Multiple Myeloma Group. Myeloablative treatments for multiple myeloma: update of a comparative study of different regimens used in patients from the Spanish registry for transplantation in multiple myeloma. *Leuk Lymphoma* 2002;43(1): 67–74.

56. Christoforidou AV, Saliba RM, Williams P, et al. Results of a retrospective single institution analysis of targeted skeletal radiotherapy with (166)Holmium-DOTMP as conditioning regimen for autologous stem cell transplant for patients with multiple myeloma. Impact on transplant outcomes. *Biol Blood Marrow Transplant* 2007;13(5):543–549.

57. Wong JY, Rosenthal J, Liu A, Schultheiss T, Forman S, Somlo G. Image-guided total-marrow irradiation using helical tomotherapy in patients with multiple myeloma and acute leukemia undergoing hematopoietic cell transplantation. *Int J Radiat Oncol Biol Phys* 2009;73(1):273–279.

58. Roussel M, Moreau P, Huynh A, et al.; Intergroupe Francophone du Myélome (IFM). Bortezomib and high-dose melphalan as conditioning regimen before autologous stem cell transplantation in patients with de novo multiple myeloma: a phase 2 study of the Intergroupe Francophone du Myelome (IFM). *Blood* 2010;115(1):32–37.

59. Björkstrand B, Ljungman P, Bird JM, Samson D, Gahrton G. Double high-dose chemoradiotherapy with autologous stem cell transplantation can induce molecular remissions in multiple myeloma. *Bone Marrow Transplant* 1995;15(3):367–371.

60. Harousseau JL, Milpied N, Laporte JP, et al. Double-intensive therapy in high-risk multiple myeloma. *Blood* 1992;79(11):2827–2833.

61. Jagannath S, Vesole DH, Glenn L, Crowley J, Barlogie B. Low-risk intensive therapy for multiple myeloma with combined autologous bone marrow and blood stem cell support. *Blood* 1992;80(7):1666–1672.

62. Barlogie B, Jagannath S, Desikan KR, et al. Total therapy with tandem transplants for newly diagnosed multiple myeloma. *Blood* 1999;93(1):55–65.

63. Barlogie B, Anaissie E, van Rhee F, et al. Incorporating bortezomib into upfront treatment for multiple myeloma: early results of total therapy 3. *Br J Haematol* 2007;138(2):176–185.

64. Barlogie B, Haessler J, Pineda-Roman M, et al. Completion of premaintenance phases in total therapies 2 and 3 improves clinical outcomes in multiple myeloma: an important variable to be considered in clinical trial designs. *Cancer* 2008;112(12): 2720–2725.

65. Pineda-Roman M, Zangari M, Haessler J, et al. Sustained complete remissions in multiple myeloma linked to bortezomib in total therapy 3: comparison with total therapy 2. *Br J Haematol* 2008;140(6):625–634.

66. Attal M, Harousseau JL, Facon T, et al.; InterGroupe Francophone du Myélome. Single versus double autologous stem-cell transplantation for multiple myeloma. *N Engl J Med* 2003;349(26):2495–2502.

67. Cavo M, Tosi P, Zamagni E, et al. Prospective, randomized study of single compared with double autologous stem-cell transplantation for multiple myeloma: Bologna 96 clinical study. *J Clin Oncol* 2007;25(17):2434–2441.

68. Goldschmidt H. Single vs. double high-dose therapy in multiple myeloma: Second analysis of the GMMG-HD2 Trial. *Haematologica* 2005;90(suppl 1 Presented at the 10th International Myeloma Workshop): 38 PL 8.02.

69. Fermand JP, Alberti C, Marolleau JP. Single versus double high dose therapy supported with autologous blood stem cell transplantation using unselected or CD34 enriched ABSC: results of a two by two designed randomized trial in 230 young patients with multiple myeloma (abstract). *Hematol J* 2003;4 (suppl 1):S59.

70. Fermand JP. High dose therapy supported with autologous blood stem cell transplantation multiple myeloma: long term follow up of the prospective

studies of the MAG group. *Haematologica* 2005;90 (suppl 1 Presented at the 10th International Myeloma Workshop):40 PL 8.05.

71. Sonneveld P, van der Holt B, Segeren CM, et al.; Dutch-Belgian Hemato-Oncology Cooperative Group (HOVON). Intermediate-dose melphalan compared with myeloablative treatment in multiple myeloma: long-term follow-up of the Dutch Cooperative Group HOVON 24 trial. *Haematologica* 2007;92(7):928–935.

72. Kumar A, Kharfan-Dabaja MA, Glasmacher A, Djulbegovic B. Tandem versus single autologous hematopoietic cell transplantation for the treatment of multiple myeloma: a systematic review and meta-analysis. *J Natl Cancer Inst* 2009;101(2):100–106.

73. Giralt S, Vesole DH, Somlo G, et al.; Blood and Marrow Transplant Clinical Trials Network Multiple Myeloma Working Group. Re: Tandem vs single autologous hematopoietic cell transplantation for the treatment of multiple myeloma: a systematic review and meta-analysis. *J Natl Cancer Inst* 2009;101(13):964; author reply 966–964; author reply 967.

74. Tricot G, Jagannath S, Vesole DH, Crowley J, Barlogie B. Relapse of multiple myeloma after autologous transplantation: survival after salvage therapy. *Bone Marrow Transplant* 1995;16(1):7–11.

75. Morris C, Iacobelli S, Brand R, et al.; Chronic Leukaemia Working Party Myeloma Subcommittee, European Group for Blood and Marrow Transplantation. Benefit and timing of second transplantations in multiple myeloma: clinical findings and methodological limitations in a European Group for Blood and Marrow Transplantation registry study. *J Clin Oncol* 2004;22(9):1674–1681.

76. Singhal S, Powles R, Sirohi B, Treleaven J, Kulkarni S, Mehta J. Response to induction chemotherapy is not essential to obtain survival benefit from high-dose melphalan and autotransplantation in myeloma. *Bone Marrow Transplant* 2002;30(10):673–679.

77. Alexanian R, Weber D, Delasalle K, Handy B, Champlin R, Giralt S. Clinical outcomes with intensive therapy for patients with primary resistant multiple myeloma. *Bone Marrow Transplant* 2004;34(3):229–234.

78. Kumar S, Lacy MQ, Dispenzieri A, et al. High-dose therapy and autologous stem cell transplantation for multiple myeloma poorly responsive to initial therapy. *Bone Marrow Transplant* 2004;34(2):161–167.

79. Cavo M, Zamagni E, Tosi P, et al.; Bologna 2002 study. Superiority of thalidomide and dexamethasone over vincristine-doxorubicindexamethasone (VAD) as primary therapy in preparation for autologous transplantation for multiple myeloma. *Blood* 2005;106(1):35–39.

80. Macro M, Divine M, Uzunhan Y, et al. Dexamethasone+Thalidomide (Dex/Thal) Compared to VAD as a Pre-Transplant Treatment in Newly Diagnosed Multiple Myeloma (MM): a randomized trial. *ASH Annual Meeting Abstracts* 2006;108(11): Abstract 57.

81. Kumar S, Dingli D, Dispenzieri A, et al. Impact of additional cytoreduction following autologous SCT in multiple myeloma. *Bone Marrow Transplant* 2008;42(4):259–264.

82. Lokhorst HM, Schmidt-Wolf I, Sonneveld P, et al.; Dutch-Belgian HOVON; German GMMG. Thalidomide in induction treatment increases the very good partial response rate before and after high-dose therapy in previously untreated multiple myeloma. *Haematologica* 2008;93(1):124–127.

83. Cavo M, Di Raimondo F, Zamagni E, et al. Short-term thalidomide incorporated into double autologous stem-cell transplantation improves outcomes in comparison with double autotransplantation for multiple myeloma. *J Clin Oncol* 2009;27(30):5001–5007.

84. Barlogie B, Pineda-Roman M, van Rhee F, et al. Thalidomide arm of Total Therapy 2 improves complete remission duration and survival in myeloma patients with metaphase cytogenetic abnormalities. *Blood* 2008;112(8):3115–3121.

85. Offidani M, Corvatta L, Polloni C, et al. Thalidomide-dexamethasone versus interferon-alpha-dexamethasone as maintenance treatment after ThaDD induction for multiple myeloma: a prospective, multicentre, randomised study. *Br J Haematol* 2009;144(5):653–659.

86. Attal M, Harousseau JL, Leyvraz S, et al.; Inter-Groupe Francophone du Myélome (IFM). Maintenance therapy with thalidomide improves survival in patients with multiple myeloma. *Blood* 2006;108(10):3289–3294.

87. Harousseau J-L, Avet-Loiseau H, Attal M, et al. High complete and very good partial response rates with bortezomib—dexamethasone as induction prior to ASCT in newly diagnosed patients with high-risk myeloma: results of the IFM2005–01 Phase 3 trial. *ASH Annual Meeting Abstracts* 2009;114(22): Abstract 353.

88. Cavo M, Tacchetti P, Patriarca F, et al. Superior complete response rate and progression-free survival after autologous transplantation with up-front velcade-thalidomide- dexamethasone compared with

thalidomide-dexamethasone in newly diagnosed multiple myeloma. *ASH Annual Meeting Abstracts* 2008;112(11):Abstract 158.

89. Sonneveld P, van der Holt B, Schmidt-Wolf IGH, et al. First analysis of HOVON-65/GMMG-HD4 randomized phase III trial comparing bortezomib, adriamycine, dexamethasone (PAD) vs VAD as induction treatment prior to high dose melphalan (HDM) in patients with newly diagnosed multiple myeloma (MM). *ASH Annual Meeting Abstracts* 2008;112(11):Abstract 653.

90. Lacy MQ, Gertz MA, Dispenzieri A, et al. Long-term results of response to therapy, time to progression, and survival with lenalidomide plus dexamethasone in newly diagnosed myeloma. *Mayo Clin Proc* 2007;82(10):1179–1184.

91. Kumar S, Lacy MQ, Dispenzieri A, et al. Novel agents for initial therapy of multiple myeloma: comparable results with continued initial therapy and delayed transplantation at relapse versus early transplantation. *Blood (ASH Annual Meeting Abstracts)* 2009;114(22):Abstract 956.

92. Palumbo A, Cavallo F, Yehuda DB, et al. A prospective, randomized study of melphalan, prednisone, lenalidomide (MPR) versus melphalan (200 mg/ m²) and autologous transplantation (Mel200) in newly diagnosed myeloma patients: an interim analysis. *ASH Annual Meeting Abstracts* 2009;114(22): Abstract 350.

93. Wang M, Giralt S, Delasalle K, Handy B, Alexanian R. Bortezomib in combination with thalidomide-dexamethasone for previously untreated multiple myeloma. *Hematology* 2007;12(3):235–239.

94. Reeder CB, Reece DE, Kukreti V, et al. Cyclophosphamide, bortezomib and dexamethasone induction for newly diagnosed multiple myeloma: high response rates in a phase II clinical trial. *Leukemia* 2009; 23(7):1337–1341.

95. Popat R, Oakervee HE, Hallam S, et al. Bortezomib, doxorubicin and dexamethasone (PAD) front-line treatment of multiple myeloma: updated results after long-term follow-up. *Br J Haematol* 2008;141(4): 512–516.

96. Kumar S, Flinn IW, Noga SJ, et al. Safety and efficacy of novel combination therapy with bortezomib, dexamethasone, cyclophosphamide, and lenalidomide in newly diagnosed multiple myeloma: initial results from the phase I/II multi-center EVOLUTION study. *ASH Annual Meeting Abstracts* 2008;112(11): Abstract 93.

97. San Miguel JF, Schlag R, Khuageva NK, et al.; VISTA Trial Investigators. Bortezomib plus melphalan and prednisone for initial treatment of multiple myeloma. *N Engl J Med* 2008;359(9): 906–917.

98. Harousseau JL. Bortezomib/dexamethasone versus VAD as induction prior to autologous stem cell transplantion (ASCT) in previously untreated multiple myeloma (MM): Updated data from IFM 2005/01 trial. *J Clin Oncol* 2008;26(suppl):Abstract 8505.

99. Richardson PG, Lonial S, Jakubowiak AJ, et al. High response rates and encouraging time-to-event data with lenalidomide, bortezomib, and dexamethasone in newly diagnosed multiple myeloma: final results of a phase I/II study. *ASH Annual Meeting Abstracts* 2009;114(22):Abstract 1218.

100. Kumar S, Hayman S, Buadi F, et al. Phase II trial of lenalidomide (Revlimid™) with cyclophosphamide and dexamethasone (RCd) for newly diagnosed myeloma. *ASH Annual Meeting Abstracts* 2008;112(11):Abstract 91.

101. Jakubowiak AJ, Reece DE, Hofmeister CC, et al. Lenalidomide, bortezomib, pegylated liposomal doxorubicin, and dexamethasone in newly diagnosed multiple myeloma: updated results of phase I/II MMRC trial. *ASH Annual Meeting Abstracts* 2009;114(22):Abstract 132.

102. Mateos M-V, Oriol A, Martinez J, et al. A prospective, multicenter, randomized, trial of bortezomib/melphalan/prednisone (VMP) versus bortezomib/thalidomide/prednisone (VTP) as induction therapy followed by maintenance treatment with bortezomib/thalidomide (VT) versus bortezomib/prednisone (VP) in elderly untreated patients with multiple myeloma older than 65 years. *ASH Annual Meeting Abstracts* 2009;114(22):Abstract 3.

103. Kumar S, Flinn IW, Hari PN, et al. Novel three- and four-drug combinations of bortezomib, dexamethasone, cyclophosphamide, and lenalidomide, for newly diagnosed multiple myeloma: encouraging results from the multi-center, randomized, phase 2 EVOLUTION study. *ASH Annual Meeting Abstracts* 2009;114(22):Abstract 127.

104. Palumbo A, Bringhen S, Liberati AM, et al. Oral melphalan, prednisone, and thalidomide in elderly patients with multiple myeloma: updated results of a randomized controlled trial. *Blood* 2008;112(8):3107–3114.

105. Palumbo A, Bringhen S, Rossi D, et al. Bortezomib, melphalan, prednisone and thalidomide (VMPT)

followed by maintenance with bortezomib and thalidomide for initial treatment of elderly multiple myeloma patients. *ASH Annual Meeting Abstracts* 2009;114(22):Abstract 128.

106. Palumbo A, Dimopoulos MA, Delforge M, et al. A phase III study to determine the efficacy and safety of lenalidomide in combination with melphalan and prednisone (MPR) in elderly patients with newly diagnosed multiple myeloma. *ASH Annual Meeting Abstracts* 2009;114(22):Abstract 613.

107. Gleason C, Nooka A, Lonial S. Supportive therapies in multiple myeloma. *J Natl Compr Canc Netw* 2009;7(9):971–979.

108. Hari PN, Majhail NS, Zhang MJ, et al. Race and outcomes of autologous hematopoietic cell transplantation for multiple myeloma. *Biol Blood Marrow Transplant* 2010;16(3):395–402.

109. Gertz MA, Ansell SM, Dingli D, et al. Autologous stem cell transplant in 716 patients with multiple myeloma: low treatment-related mortality, feasibility of outpatient transplant, and effect of a multidisciplinary quality initiative. *Mayo Clin Proc* 2008;83(10):1131–1138.

110. Palumbo A, Gay F, Falco P, et al. Bortezomib as induction before autologous transplantation, followed by lenalidomide as consolidation-maintenance in untreated multiple myeloma patients. *J Clin Oncol* 2010;28(5):800–807.

111. Stewart AK, Fonseca R. Review of molecular diagnostics in multiple myeloma. *Expert Rev Mol Diagn* 2007;7(4):453–459.

112. Fonseca R, Bergsagel PL, Drach J, et al.; International Myeloma Working Group. International Myeloma Working Group molecular classification of multiple myeloma: spotlight review. *Leukemia* 2009;23(12):2210–2221.

113. Kapoor P, Kumar S, Fonseca R, et al. Impact of risk stratification on outcome among patients with multiple myeloma receiving initial therapy with lenalidomide and dexamethasone. *Blood* 2009;114(3):518–521.

114. Jagannath S, Richardson PG, Sonneveld P, et al. Bortezomib appears to overcome the poor prognosis conferred by chromosome 13 deletion in phase 2 and 3 trials. *Leukemia* 2007;21(1):151–157.

115. Avet-Loiseau H, Attal M, Moreau P, et al. Genetic abnormalities and survival in multiple myeloma: the experience of the Intergroupe Francophone du Myélome. *Blood* 2007;109(8):3489–3495.

116. Fassas AB, Spencer T, Sawyer J, et al. Both hypodiploidy and deletion of chromosome 13 independently confer poor prognosis in multiple myeloma. *Br J Haematol* 2002;118(4):1041–1047.

117. Fonseca R, Barlogie B, Bataille R, et al. Genetics and cytogenetics of multiple myeloma: a workshop report. *Cancer Res* 2004;64(4):1546–1558.

118. Fonseca R, Blood E, Rue M, et al. Clinical and biologic implications of recurrent genomic aberrations in myeloma. *Blood* 2003;101(11):4569–4575.

119. Fonseca R, Harrington D, Oken MM, et al. Biological and prognostic significance of interphase fluorescence in situ hybridization detection of chromosome 13 abnormalities (delta13) in multiple myeloma: an eastern cooperative oncology group study. *Cancer Res* 2002;62(3):715–720.

120. Shaughnessy JD Jr, Zhan F, Burington BE, et al. A validated gene expression model of high-risk multiple myeloma is defined by deregulated expression of genes mapping to chromosome 1. *Blood* 2007;109(6):2276–2284.

121. Gertz MA, Lacy MQ, Dispenzieri A, et al. Clinical implications of t(11;14)(q13;q32), t(4;14)(p16.3;q32), and -17p13 in myeloma patients treated with high-dose therapy. *Blood* 2005;106(8):2837–2840.

122. Dispenzieri A, Rajkumar SV, Gertz MA, et al. Treatment of newly diagnosed multiple myeloma based on Mayo Stratification of Myeloma and Risk-adapted Therapy (mSMART): consensus statement. *Mayo Clin Proc* 2007;82(3):323–341.

123. Barlogie B, Anaissie E, Haessler J, et al. Complete remission sustained 3 years from treatment initiation is a powerful surrogate for extended survival in multiple myeloma. *Cancer* 2008;113(2):355–359.

124. Boccadoro M, Palumbo A, Bringhen S, et al. Oral melphalan at diagnosis hampers adequate collection of peripheral blood progenitor cells in multiple myeloma. *Haematologica* 2002;87(8):846–850.

125. Perea G, Sureda A, Martino R, et al. Predictive factors for a successful mobilization of peripheral blood CD34+ cells in multiple myeloma. *Ann Hematol* 2001;80(10):592–597.

126. Bensinger W, Appelbaum F, Rowley S, et al. Factors that influence collection and engraftment of autologous peripheral-blood stem cells. *J Clin Oncol* 1995;13(10):2547–2555.

127. Giralt S, Stadtmauer EA, Harousseau JL, et al.; IMWG. International myeloma working group (IMWG) consensus statement and guidelines regarding the current status of stem cell collection and high-dose therapy for multiple myeloma and the role of plerixafor (AMD 3100). *Leukemia* 2009;23(10):1904–1912.

128. Cashen AF. Plerixafor hydrochloride: a novel agent for the mobilization of peripheral blood stem cells. *Drugs Today* 2009;45(7):497–505.

129. Flomenberg N, Devine SM, Dipersio JF, et al. The use of AMD3100 plus G-CSF for autologous hematopoietic progenitor cell mobilization is superior to G-CSF alone. *Blood* 2005;106(5):1867–1874.

130. Devine SM, Flomenberg N, Vesole DH, et al. Rapid mobilization of CD34+ cells following administration of the CXCR4 antagonist AMD3100 to patients with multiple myeloma and non-Hodgkin's lymphoma. *J Clin Oncol* 2004;22(6):1095–1102.

131. DiPersio JF, Micallef IN, Stiff PJ, et al.; 3101 Investigators. Phase III prospective randomized double-blind placebo-controlled trial of plerixafor plus granulocyte colony-stimulating factor compared with placebo plus granulocyte colony-stimulating factor for autologous stem-cell mobilization and transplantation for patients with non-Hodgkin's lymphoma. *J Clin Oncol* 2009;27(28):4767–4773.

132. Wuchter P, Ran D, Bruckner T, et al. Poor mobilization of hematopoietic stem cells-definitions, incidence, risk factors, and impact on outcome of autologous transplantation. *Biol Blood Marrow Transplant* 2010;16(4):490–499.

133. Belch A, Shelley W, Bergsagel D, et al. A randomized trial of maintenance versus no maintenance melphalan and prednisone in responding multiple myeloma patients. *Br J Cancer* 1988;57(1):94–99.

134. Browman GP, Bergsagel D, Sicheri D, et al. Randomized trial of interferon maintenance in multiple myeloma: a study of the National Cancer Institute of Canada Clinical Trials Group. *J Clin Oncol* 1995;13(9):2354–2360.

135. Cunningham D, Powles R, Malpas J, et al. A randomized trial of maintenance interferon following high-dose chemotherapy in multiple myeloma: long-term follow-up results. *Br J Haematol* 1998; 102(2):495–502.

136. Barlogie B, Tricot G, Anaissie E, et al. Thalidomide and hematopoietic-cell transplantation for multiple myeloma. *N Engl J Med* 2006;354(10):1021–1030.

137. Spencer A, Prince HM, Roberts AW, et al. Consolidation therapy with low-dose thalidomide and prednisolone prolongs the survival of multiple myeloma patients undergoing a single autologous stem-cell transplantation procedure. *J Clin Oncol* 2009;27(11):1788–1793.

138. Abdelkefi A, Ladeb S, Torjman L, et al.; Tunisian Multiple Myeloma Study Group. Single autologous stem-cell transplantation followed by maintenance therapy with thalidomide is superior to double autologous transplantation in multiple myeloma: results of a multicenter randomized clinical trial. *Blood* 2008;111(4):1805–1810.

139. Lokhorst HM, van der Holt B, Zweegman S, et al.; Dutch-Belgian Hemato-Oncology Group (HOVON). A randomized phase 3 study on the effect of thalidomide combined with adriamycin, dexamethasone, and high-dose melphalan, followed by thalidomide maintenance in patients with multiple myeloma. *Blood* 2010;115(6):1113–1120.

140. Pasquini MC, Ewell M, Stadtmauer EA, et al. Biologic assignment clinical trials in hematopoietic stem cell transplantation (HSCT) for multiple myeloma: baseline characteristics by treatment allocation from BMT CTN 0102 according to availability of an HLA-matched sibling donor. *Blood (ASH Annual Meeting Abstracts)* 2007;110(11): Abstract 3028.

141. McCarthy PL, Owzar K, Stadtmauer EA, et al. Phase III intergroup study of lenalidomide (CC-5013) versus placebo maintenance therapy following single autologous stem cell transplant for multiple myeloma (CALGB 100104): initial report of patient accrual and adverse events. *Blood (ASH Annual Meeting Abstracts)* 2009;114(22): Abstract 3416.

142. Stewart AK, Chen CI, Howson-Jan K, et al. Results of a multicenter randomized phase II trial of thalidomide and prednisone maintenance therapy for multiple myeloma after autologous stem cell transplant. *Clin Cancer Res* 2004;10(24):8170–8176.

143. Olin RL, Vogl DT, Porter DL, et al. Second auto-SCT is safe and effective salvage therapy for relapsed multiple myeloma. *Bone Marrow Transplant* 2009; 43(5):417–422.

144. Qazilbash MH, Saliba R, De Lima M, et al. Second autologous or allogeneic transplantation after the failure of first autograft in patients with multiple myeloma. *Cancer* 2006;106(5):1084–1089.

145. Kumar SK, Dingli D, Dispenzieri A, et al. Impact of pretransplant therapy in patients with newly diagnosed myeloma undergoing autologous SCT. *Bone Marrow Transplant* 2008;41(12):1013–1019.

146. Alvares CL, Davies FE, Horton C, Patel G, Powles R, Morgan GJ. The role of second autografts in the management of myeloma at first relapse. *Haematologica* 2006;91(1):141–142.

147. Mehta J, Tricot G, Jagannath S, et al. Salvage autologous or allogeneic transplantation for multiple myeloma refractory to or relapsing after

a first-line autograft? *Bone Marrow Transplant* 1998;21(9):887–892.

148. Lee CK, Barlogie B, Zangari M, et al. Transplantation as salvage therapy for high-risk patients with myeloma in relapse. *Bone Marrow Transplant* 2002;30(12):873–878.

149. Gahrton G, Tura S, Flesch M, et al. Allogeneic bone marrow transplantation in 24 patients with multiple myeloma reported to the EBMT registry. *Hematol Oncol* 1988;6(2):181–186.

150. Gahrton G, Tura S, Ljungman P, et al. Allogeneic bone marrow transplantation in multiple myeloma. European Group for Bone Marrow Transplantation. *N Engl J Med* 1991;325(18):1267–1273.

151. Corradini P, Cavo M, Lokhorst H, et al.; Chronic Leukemia Working Party of the European Group for Blood and Marrow Transplantation (EBMT). Molecular remission after myeloablative allogeneic stem cell transplantation predicts a better relapse-free survival in patients with multiple myeloma. *Blood* 2003;102(5):1927–1929.

152. Cavo M, Terragna C, Martinelli G, et al. Molecular monitoring of minimal residual disease in patients in long-term complete remission after allogeneic stem cell transplantation for multiple myeloma. *Blood* 2000;96(1):355–357.

153. Martinelli G, Terragna C, Zamagni E, et al. Polymerase chain reaction-based detection of minimal residual disease in multiple myeloma patients receiving allogeneic stem cell transplantation. *Haematologica* 2000;85(9):930–934.

154. Bruno B, Rotta M, Patriarca F, et al. A comparison of allografting with autografting for newly diagnosed myeloma. *N Engl J Med* 2007;356(11):1110–1120.

155. Stewart AK. Reduced-intensity allogeneic transplantation for myeloma: reality bites. *Blood* 2009; 113(14):3135–3136.

156. Drobyski WR, Keever CA, Roth MS, et al. Salvage immunotherapy using donor leukocyte infusions as treatment for relapsed chronic myelogenous leukemia after allogeneic bone marrow transplantation: efficacy and toxicity of a defined T-cell dose. *Blood* 1993;82(8):2310–2318.

157. Kolb HJ, Schattenberg A, Goldman JM, et al.; European Group for Blood and Marrow Transplantation Working Party Chronic Leukemia. Graft-versus-leukemia effect of donor lymphocyte transfusions in marrow grafted patients. *Blood* 1995;86(5):2041–2050.

158. Sullivan KM, Fefer A, Witherspoon R, et al. Graft-versus-leukemia in man: relationship of acute and chronic graft-versus-host disease to relapse of acute leukemia following allogeneic bone marrow transplantation. *Prog Clin Biol Res* 1987;244:391–399.

159. Weiden PL, Flournoy N, Thomas ED, et al. Antileukemic effect of graft-versus-host disease in human recipients of allogeneic-marrow grafts. *N Engl J Med* 1979;300(19):1068–1073.

160. Weiden PL, Sullivan KM, Flournoy N, Storb R, Thomas ED. Antileukemic effect of chronic graft-versus-host disease: contribution to improved survival after allogeneic marrow transplantation. *N Engl J Med* 1981;304(25):1529–1533.

161. Horowitz MM, Gale RP, Sondel PM, et al. Graft-versus-leukemia reactions after bone marrow transplantation. *Blood* 1990;75(3):555–562.

162. Kwak LW, Taub DD, Duffey PL, et al. Transfer of myeloma idiotype-specific immunity from an actively immunised marrow donor. *Lancet* 1995;345(8956):1016–1020.

163. Tricot G, Vesole DH, Jagannath S, Hilton J, Munshi N, Barlogie B. Graft-versus-myeloma effect: proof of principle. *Blood* 1996;87(3):1196–1198.

164. Lokhorst HM, Schattenberg A, Cornelissen JJ, et al. Donor lymphocyte infusions for relapsed multiple myeloma after allogeneic stem-cell transplantation: predictive factors for response and long-term outcome. *J Clin Oncol* 2000;18(16):3031–3037.

165. Salama M, Nevill T, Marcellus D, et al. Donor leukocyte infusions for multiple myeloma. *Bone Marrow Transplant* 2000;26(11):1179–1184.

166. Lokhorst HM, Wu K, Verdonck LF, et al. The occurrence of graft-versus-host disease is the major predictive factor for response to donor lymphocyte infusions in multiple myeloma. *Blood* 2004;103(11):4362–4364.

167. Verdonck LF, Lokhorst HM, Dekker AW, Nieuwenhuis HK, Petersen EJ. Graft-versus-myeloma effect in two cases. *Lancet* 1996;347(9004): 800–801.

168. van de Donk NW, Kröger N, Hegenbart U, et al. Prognostic factors for donor lymphocyte infusions following non-myeloablative allogeneic stem cell transplantation in multiple myeloma. *Bone Marrow Transplant* 2006;37(12):1135–1141.

169. Hari PN, Barret JA, Shrestha S, et al. Reduced intensity allogeneic hematopoietic stem cell transplant (HSCT) for myeloma (MM)—chronic graft versus host disease (GVHD) is associated with lower risk of relapse and superior progression free survival (PFS)—a CIBMTR analysis. *Blood (ASH Annual Meeting Abstracts)* 2009;114:Abstract 53.

170. Alyea E, Weller E, Schlossman R, et al. T-cell–depleted allogeneic bone marrow transplantation followed by donor lymphocyte infusion in patients with multiple myeloma: induction of graft-versus-myeloma effect. *Blood* 2001;98(4):934–939.

171. Lokhorst HM, Segeren CM, Verdonck LF, et al.; Dutch-Belgian Hemato-Oncology Cooperative Group. Partially T-cell-depleted allogeneic stem-cell transplantation for first-line treatment of multiple myeloma: a prospective evaluation of patients treated in the phase III study HOVON 24 MM. *J Clin Oncol* 2003;21(9):1728–1733.

172. Moreau P, Garban F, Attal M, et al.; IFM Group. Long-term follow-up results of IFM99–03 and IFM99–04 trials comparing nonmyeloablative allotransplantation with autologous transplantation in high-risk de novo multiple myeloma. *Blood* 2008;112(9):3914–3915.

173. Björkstrand BB, Ljungman P, Svensson H, et al. Allogeneic bone marrow transplantation versus autologous stem cell transplantation in multiple myeloma: a retrospective case-matched study from the European Group for Blood and Marrow Transplantation. *Blood* 1996;88(12):4711–4718.

174. Alyea E, Weller E, Schlossman R, et al. Outcome after autologous and allogeneic stem cell transplantation for patients with multiple myeloma: impact of graft-versus-myeloma effect. *Bone Marrow Transplant* 2003;32(12):1145–1151.

175. Ballen KK, King R, Carston M, et al. Outcome of unrelated transplants in patients with multiple myeloma. *Bone Marrow Transplant* 2005;35(7):675–681.

176. Bacigalupo A, Ballen K, Rizzo D, et al. Defining the intensity of conditioning regimens: working definitions. *Biol Blood Marrow Transplant* 2009;15(12):1628–1633.

177. Gahrton G, Tura S, Ljungman P, et al. Prognostic factors in allogeneic bone marrow transplantation for multiple myeloma. *J Clin Oncol* 1995;13(6):1312–1322.

178. Bensinger WI, Buckner CD, Anasetti C, et al. Allogeneic marrow transplantation for multiple myeloma: an analysis of risk factors on outcome. *Blood* 1996;88(7):2787–2793.

179. Gahrton G, Svensson H, Cavo M, et al.; European Group for Blood and Marrow Transplantation. Progress in allogenic bone marrow and peripheral blood stem cell transplantation for multiple myeloma: a comparison between transplants performed 1983–93 and 1994–8 at European Group for Blood and Marrow Transplantation centres. *Br J Haematol* 2001;113(1):209–216.

180. Crawley C, Iacobelli S, Björkstrand B, Apperley JF, Niederwieser D, Gahrton G. Reduced-intensity conditioning for myeloma: lower nonrelapse mortality but higher relapse rates compared with myeloablative conditioning. *Blood* 2007;109(8):3588–3594.

181. Arora M, McGlave PB, Burns LJ, et al. Results of autologous and allogeneic hematopoietic cell transplant therapy for multiple myeloma. *Bone Marrow Transplant* 2005;35(12):1133–1140.

182. Tsai T, Goodman S, Saez R, et al. Allogeneic bone marrow transplantation in patients who relapse after autologous transplantation. *Bone Marrow Transplant* 1997;20(10):859–863.

183. Storb R, Yu C, Wagner JL, et al. Stable mixed hematopoietic chimerism in DLA-identical littermate dogs given sublethal total body irradiation before and pharmacological immunosuppression after marrow transplantation. *Blood* 1997;89(8):3048–3054.

184. Giralt S, Estey E, Albitar M, et al. Engraftment of allogeneic hematopoietic progenitor cells with purine analog-containing chemotherapy: harnessing graft-versus-leukemia without myeloablative therapy. *Blood* 1997;89(12):4531–4536.

185. Khouri IF, Keating M, Körbling M, et al. Transplant-lite: induction of graft-versus-malignancy using fludarabine-based nonablative chemotherapy and allogeneic blood progenitor-cell transplantation as treatment for lymphoid malignancies. *J Clin Oncol* 1998;16(8):2817–2824.

186. Slavin S, Nagler A, Naparstek E, et al. Non-myeloablative stem cell transplantation and cell therapy as an alternative to conventional bone marrow transplantation with lethal cytoreduction for the treatment of malignant and nonmalignant hematologic diseases. *Blood* 1998;91(3):756–763.

187. Spitzer TR, McAfee S, Sackstein R, et al. Intentional induction of mixed chimerism and achievement of antitumor responses after nonmyeloablative conditioning therapy and HLA-matched donor bone marrow transplantation for refractory hematologic malignancies. *Biol Blood Marrow Transplant* 2000;6(3A):309–320.

188. de Lima M, Couriel D, Thall PF, et al. Once-daily intravenous busulfan and fludarabine: clinical and pharmacokinetic results of a myeloablative, reduced-toxicity conditioning regimen for allogeneic stem cell transplantation in AML and MDS. *Blood* 2004;104(3):857–864.

189. Khouri IF, Lee MS, Saliba RM, et al. Nonablative allogeneic stem cell transplantation for chronic lymphocytic leukemia: impact of rituximab on immunomodulation and survival. *Exp Hematol* 2004;32(1):28–35.

190. Kröger N, Perez-Simon JA, Myint H, et al. Relapse to prior autograft and chronic graft-versus-host disease are the strongest prognostic factors for outcome of melphalan/fludarabine-based dose-reduced allogeneic stem cell transplantation in patients with multiple myeloma. *Biol Blood Marrow Transplant* 2004;10(10):698–708.

191. Maris MB, Sandmaier BM, Storer BE, et al. Allogeneic hematopoietic cell transplantation after fludarabine and 2 Gy total body irradiation for relapsed and refractory mantle cell lymphoma. *Blood* 2004;104(12):3535–3542.

192. McSweeney PA, Niederwieser D, Shizuru JA, et al. Hematopoietic cell transplantation in older patients with hematologic malignancies: replacing high-dose cytotoxic therapy with graft-versus-tumor effects. *Blood* 2001;97(11):3390–3400.

193. Niederwieser D, Maris M, Shizuru JA, et al. Low-dose total body irradiation (TBI) and fludarabine followed by hematopoietic cell transplantation (HCT) from HLA-matched or mismatched unrelated donors and postgrafting immunosuppression with cyclosporine and mycophenolate mofetil (MMF) can induce durable complete chimerism and sustained remissions in patients with hematological diseases. *Blood* 2003;101(4):1620–1629.

194. Russell JA, Savoie ML, Balogh A, et al. Allogeneic transplantation for adult acute leukemia in first and second remission with a novel regimen incorporating daily intravenous busulfan, fludarabine, 400 CGY total-body irradiation, and thymoglobulin. *Biol Blood Marrow Transplant* 2007;13(7):814–821.

195. Storb R. From myeloablative to nonmyeloablawtive conditioning regimens in multiple myeloma. In: Boccadero M, Pileri A, eds. *Multiple Myeloma 2004*. Turin, Italy: International Myeloma Foundation; 2004:148.

196. Kumar S, Shrestha S, Zhang M-J, et al. Allogeneic stem cell transplantation (SCT) for multiple myeloma (MM)—what has changed?: a CIBMTR analysis from 1989—2005. *ASH Annual Meeting Abstracts* 2009;114(22):Abstract 54.

197. Tricot G. Allogeneic transplantation. In: Boccadero M, Pileri A, eds. *Multiple Myeloma 2004*. Turin, Italy;2004:143.

198. Einsele H, Schäfer HJ, Hebart H, et al. Follow-up of patients with progressive multiple myeloma undergoing allografts after reduced-intensity conditioning. *Br J Haematol* 2003;121(3):411–418.

199. Giralt S, Aleman A, Anagnostopoulos A, et al. Fludarabine/melphalan conditioning for allogeneic transplantation in patients with multiple myeloma. *Bone Marrow Transplant* 2002;30(6):367–373.

200. Maloney DG, Molina AJ, Sahebi F, et al. Allografting with nonmyeloablative conditioning following cytoreductive autografts for the treatment of patients with multiple myeloma. *Blood* 2003;102(9):3447–3454.

201. Kröger N, Sayer HG, Schwerdtfeger R, et al. Unrelated stem cell transplantation in multiple myeloma after a reduced-intensity conditioning with pretransplantation antithymocyte globulin is highly effective with low transplantation-related mortality. *Blood* 2002;100(12):3919–3924.

202. Badros A, Barlogie B, Siegel E, et al. Improved outcome of allogeneic transplantation in high-risk multiple myeloma patients after nonmyeloablative conditioning. *J Clin Oncol* 2002;20(5):1295–1303.

203. Lee CK, Badros A, Barlogie B, et al. Prognostic factors in allogeneic transplantation for patients with high-risk multiple myeloma after reduced intensity conditioning. *Exp Hematol* 2003;31(1):73–80.

204. Pérez-Simón JA, Martino R, Alegre A, et al. Chronic but not acute graft-versus-host disease improves outcome in multiple myeloma patients after non-myeloablative allogeneic transplantation. *Br J Haematol* 2003;121(1):104–108.

205. Gerull S, Hegenbart U, Goerner M. Non-myeloablative allogeneic transplantation in patients with relapsed or refractory multiple myeloma. *Blood* 2004;104(11):[Abstract 2759].

206. Vesole DH, Zhang L, Flomenberg N, Greipp PR, Lazarus HM, Huff CA; ECOG Myeloma and BMT Committees. A Phase II trial of autologous stem cell transplantation followed by mini-allogeneic stem cell transplantation for the treatment of multiple myeloma: an analysis of Eastern Cooperative Oncology Group ECOG E4A98 and E1A97. *Biol Blood Marrow Transplant* 2009;15(1):83–91.

207. Rotta M, Storer BE, Sahebi F, et al. Long-term outcome of patients with multiple myeloma after autologous hematopoietic cell transplantation and nonmyeloablative allografting. *Blood* 2009;113(14):3383–3391.

208. Kröger N, Shimoni A, Schilling G, et al. Unrelated stem cell transplantation after reduced intensity conditioning for patients with multiple myeloma

relapsing after autologous transplantation. *Br J Haematol* 2010;148(2):323–331.

209. Bruno B, Rotta M, Patriarca F, et al. Nonmyeloablative allografting for newly diagnosed multiple myeloma: the experience of the Gruppo Italiano Trapianti di Midollo. *Blood* 2009;113(14):3375–3382.

210. Kröger N, Schwerdtfeger R, Kiehl M, et al. Autologous stem cell transplantation followed by a dose-reduced allograft induces high complete remission rate in multiple myeloma. *Blood* 2002;100(3):755–760.

211. Bruno B, Sorasio R, Patriarca F, et al. An update of a comparison of nonmyeloablative allografting with autografting for newly diagnosed myeloma. *ASH Annual Meeting Abstracts* 2007;110(11): Abstract 482.

212. Garban F, Attal M, Michallet M, et al. Prospective comparison of autologous stem cell transplantation followed by dose-reduced allograft (IFM99–03 trial) with tandem autologous stem cell transplantation (IFM99–04 trial) in high-risk de novo multiple myeloma. *Blood* 2006;107(9):3474–3480.

213. Rosiñol L, Pérez-Simón JA, Sureda A, et al.; Programa para el Estudio y la Terapéutica de las Hemopatías Malignas y Grupo Español de Mieloma (PETHEMA/GEM). A prospective PETHEMA study of tandem autologous transplantation versus autograft followed by reduced-intensity conditioning allogeneic transplantation in newly diagnosed multiple myeloma. *Blood* 2008;112(9):3591–3593.

214. Gahrton G, Bjorkstrand B, Iacobelli S, et al. Tandem autologous (ASCT)/allogeneic reduced intensity conditioning transplantation (RIC) with identical sibling donor versus ASCT in previously untreated multiple myeloma (MM): long term follow up of a prospective controlled trial by the EBMT. *ASH Annual Meeting Abstracts* 2009;114(22): Abstract 52.

215. Knop S, Liebisch P, Hebart H, et al. Allogeneic stem cell transplant versus tandem high-dose melphalan for front-line treatment of deletion 13q14 myeloma—an interim analysis of the German DSMM V trial. *ASH Annual Meeting Abstracts* 2009;114(22):Abstract 51.

216. Peggs K, Mackinnon S. Graft-versus-myeloma: are durable responses a clinical reality following donor lymphocyte infusion? *Leukemia* 2004;18(9):1541–1542; author reply 1542.

217. Lokhorst H, Mutis T, Bloem A, et al. Strategies to improve the graft-versus-myeloma effect of allogeneic stem cell transplantation and donor lymphocyte infusions in multiple myeloma. *Haematologica* 2005;90(suppl 1 Presented at the 10th International Myeloma Workshop):49 PL 9.04.

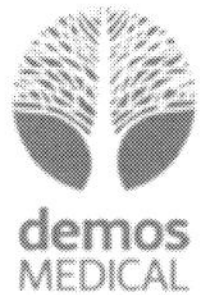

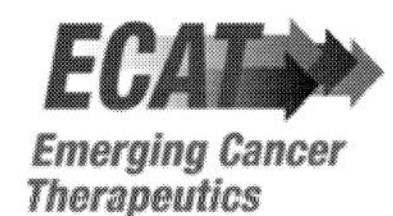

Treatment of Myeloma in Transplant-Ineligible Patients

Francesca Gay, Stefania Oliva, and Antonio Palumbo*

Azienda Ospedaliero-Universitaria San Giovanni Battista, Torino, Italy

■ ABSTRACT

Patients with multiple myeloma (MM) not eligible for autologous stem cell transplantation (ASCT) have traditionally been treated with the oral combination melphalan-prednisone (MP). The introduction of novel agents, such as immunomodulatory drugs and proteasome inhibitors, has substantially changed the treatment paradigm of this disease. The addition of new drugs to the traditional MP regimen has led to three-drug combinations that are now considered new standards of care for elderly patients ineligible for ASCT. Five randomized phase III studies, comparing MP plus thalidomide (MPT) versus MP, have all shown prolonged time to progression (TTP) with MPT; however, only in two of these studies, the improvement in TTP translated into an improvement in overall survival (OS). In one randomized study, treatment with MP plus bortezomib was correlated with an increase in both TTP and OS compared with MP. Preliminary data on melphalan-prednisone-lenalidomide combinations have shown the superiority of this three-drug regimen to MP. Promising results have also been reported with the combination of lenalidomide plus low-dose dexamethasone. These regimens may be considered all valuable options for patients with MM, and they may help tailor specific treatment approaches, based on patient comorbidities and biological age, taking into account the toxicity profiles of treatment regimens. Accurate management of therapy-related adverse events and a gentler approach with appropriate dose reductions for patients older than 75 years can greatly increase treatment efficacy.

*Corresponding author, Divisione di Ematologia dell'Università di Torino, Azienda Ospedaliero-Universitaria San Giovanni Battista, Via Genova 3, 10126 Torino, Italy
   E-mail addresses: appalumbo@yahoo.com

Emerging Cancer Therapeutics 1:2 (2010) 363–382.
© 2010 Demos Medical Publishing LLC. All rights reserved.
DOI: 10.5003/2151–4194.1.2.363

INTRODUCTION

Multiple myeloma (MM) is the second most common hematological malignancy (1). The median age at diagnosis is 71 years, with around 65% of patients older than 65 years. The annual age-specific incidence increased considerably with age, till up to more than 40% of patients older than 80 years (2). The number of older patients is expected to rise over time as a consequence of the increased life expectancy of the normal population.

Recognition of organ damage and its correlation with MM is the first step to correctly identify either symptomatic newly diagnosed or relapsed MM. Patients with symptomatic MM should be treated immediately (3).

THERAPEUTIC CONSIDERATIONS

Despite age 65 being usually considered the upper limit for transplant in many European countries, it is worth noting that biological age and chronological age do not always correspond. In the light of this, transplant eligibility may be evaluated on the basis of the former rather than the latter. This is actually what happens in some countries, like in the United States, where a greater emphasis is placed on biological age. There are various factors, other than age, to determine whether patients can be considered eligible for autologous stem cell transplantation (ASCT) or not, such as performance status, impaired renal failure, and comorbidities. In particular, patients are generally considered eligible for ASCT if they have normal cardiac function (normal electrocardiogram and echocardiography or multiple-gated acquisition evaluation and New York Heart Association class I/II), normal pulmonary function (normal chest X-ray, normal spirometry, and normal diffusion capacity), and normal liver and renal function.

Different treatment options are now available for transplant-ineligible patients: standard treatment should always be supported by evidence of improved progression-free survival (PFS) provided by at least one randomized trial, and although phase II trials should be considered as important scientific evidence, they need to be confirmed by randomized trials before deciding the standards of care. Therefore, this paper focuses on the results of the most recent phase III studies in transplant-ineligible patients. Patients with MM not eligible for ASCT have traditionally been treated with the oral combination melphalan-prednisone (MP). The introduction of novel agents, such as immunomodulatory drugs (IMIDs) (thalidomide and lenalidomide) and proteasome inhibitors (bortezomib), has substantially changed the treatment paradigm of this disease. The addition of these new drugs to the traditional oral combination MP regimen has led to three-drug combinations that are now considered new standards of care for elderly patients ineligible for ASCT.

TREATMENT OF NEWLY DIAGNOSED PATIENTS

The "Old" Standard of Care: Melphalan and Prednisone

For more than 40 years, the oral combination MP has been considered the conventional treatment for elderly patients (older than 65 years) or young patients ineligible for high-dose therapy. In a meta-analysis of 27 randomized trials comparing different chemotherapy-regimens with MP, higher response rates were reported with the former, but this did not translate into an improved survival benefit (4). The partial response (PR) rate with MP is approximately 50%, and the median survival is about 3 to 4 years. MP is a well-tolerated treatment, but responses can sometimes take up to 6 months to occur (5). In a randomized trial comparing MP with melphalan plus dexamethasone (MD), high-dose dexamethasone (HD), and HD plus interferon-α, the improvement reported in PFS in patients receiving melphalan as part of the induction treatment (both MP and MD) did not translate into a survival advantage. Moreover, the morbidity associated with dexamethasone-based regimens (in particular, severe pyogenic infections, hemorrhage, severe diabetes, and gastrointestinal and psychiatric complications) was significantly higher and MP was definitely better tolerated (6). Another randomized study compared MP with thalidomide and dexamethasone (TD): despite a higher response rate and longer PFS with TD, patients receiving MP presented a significantly longer survival. Patients treated with TD reported more extra-hematological toxicities, mainly related to the HD, and a higher treatment-discontinuation rate. Furthermore, during the first 12 months of therapy, nonmyeloma-related deaths were twice as high in the TD group as compared with those in the MP group, with infections being the primary cause. The difference was even more pronounced in patients older than 72 years with poor performance status (7). These results provided the basis to combine the standard MP with novel agents.

The "New" Standards of Care: Novel Agent-Based Therapies

Thalidomide-Based Therapies

Thalidomide Plus Melphalan and Prednisone. The combination melphalan-prednisone-thalidomide (MPT) has been compared with MP in five randomized studies. In all of them, MPT resulted in higher PR (42–76% vs. 28–48%), higher at least very good partial response (VGPR) or near-complete response (nCR) rate (15–47% vs. 6–8%), and longer PFS (14–27.5 vs. 10–19 months) than did MP (8–13). In the two Intergroupe Francophone du Myelome studies, the PFS advantage observed with MPT translated into a significant overall survival (OS) advantage (45.3–51.6 vs. 27.7–32.2 months) (11,12). These data were not confirmed in the other three trials (8–10,13). In the Nordic study (Nordic Myeloma Study Group), these results were hampered by use of higher doses of melphalan and thalidomide, in a population of patients with a high proportion of subjects older than 75 years and approximately one third with poor performance status (World Health Organization performance status of three or four

in 30% of patients) (13). These data strongly support the use of MPT as the standard of care for elderly patients.

A systematic review using a meta-analytic approach has been recently performed to integrate the existing outcome data related to the efficacy of MP versus MPT. The pooled odds ratio of responding to treatment with MP versus MPT was 0.307 ($P < 0.001$), indicating that MP was worse than MPT in achieving at least a PR. The pooled hazard ratios for PFS and OS were 1.59 ($P < 0.001$) and 1.34 ($P = 0.006$), respectively, in favor of MPT. Although the results from a comprehensive individual patient data pooled analysis would give a more precise estimate, this meta-analysis further confirms that in previously untreated, transplant-ineligible elderly patients with MM, the addition of thalidomide to MP improves PR rate, PFS, and OS compared with the use of MP alone (14).

The main adverse event (AE) associated with this regimen was grade 3 to 4 neutropenia, with an incidence rate ranging from 16% to 48% in newly diagnosed patients. Peripheral neuropathy was reported in 6% to 20% of patients treated with MPT, whereas the incidence of venous thromboembolism (VTE) varies from 3% to 12% (8–12).

Thalidomide Plus Cyclophosphamide and Dexamethasone. Cyclophosphamide, another alkylating agent, has been assessed in combination with thalidomide. In the medical Research Council Myeloma IX trial, the combination of cyclophosphamide plus TD (CTD) was compared with standard MP in 900 patients. Patients given CTD showed higher rates of at least PR (83% vs. 46%) and complete response (CR) (21% vs. 4%) than did those given MP, but this did not translate in improved survival (15).

Bortezomib-Based Therapies

Bortezomib Plus Melphalan and Prednisone. The international VISTA (Velcade as Initial Standard Therapy) trial, which is the largest MP-based phase III study so far (16), explored the combination bortezomib-melphalan-prednisone (VMP) in comparison with standard MP. VMP was significantly superior to MP for all efficacy endpoints: CR rate (30% vs. 4%; $P < 0.001$), median time to progression (TTP) (24 months vs. 16.6 months, $P < 0.001$), and OS at 3 years (72% vs. 59%, $P = 0.0032$). This superiority was confirmed in patients younger and older than 75 years. Overall, these results clearly established VMP as a new standard of care for MM not eligible for ASCT. A subsequent planned updated survival analysis of VISTA trial confirmed the previously demonstrated OS benefit of VMP versus MP, and it examined the efficacy of different rescue therapies. After a median follow-up of more than 3 years, 3-year OS from diagnosis was 68.5% versus 54.0% with VMP and MP, respectively; median survival from start of second-line therapy was 30.2 versus 21.9 months (hazard ratio [HR] = 0.815, $P = 0.21$) in the VMP and MP groups, respectively. This updated analysis of VISTA confirms that VMP results in significantly longer OS compared with MP, despite 50% of MP patients being rescued with bortezomib-based therapy (17).

Bortezomib Plus Thalidomide and Prednisone. A randomized study compared the new standard VMP with a regimen consisting of bortezomib plus thalidomide and prednisone (VTP) as induction therapy. In both arms, bortezomib was administrated, with one 6-week cycle of a twice weekly infusion (days 1, 4, 8, 11, 22, 25, 29, and 32) and five 5-week cycles of a weekly infusion (days 1, 8, 15, and 22). Response rates were similar in both arms: at least PR in 79% of patients treated with VMP and VTP, respectively, with a CR rate of 22% versus 27% (P = nonsignificant [NS]). After a median follow-up of 22 months, there were no significant differences in terms of 2-year TTP (VMP 75% vs. VTP 70%), PFS (VMP 71% vs. VTP 61%), and OS (VMP 81% vs. VTP 84%) between the two treatment groups. Treatment with VTP was correlated with a higher rate of grade 3 to 4 nonhematological AEs, in particular cardiac toxicity (8.5% vs. 0%, $P < 0.001$), thromboembolic events (4% vs. <1%, P = NS), and peripheral neuropathy (9% vs. 5%, P = NS), resulting in a significantly higher rate of

treatment discontinuation (17% vs. 8%, $P = 0.03$). Patients given VMP instead had a higher rate of neutropenia (37% vs. 21%, $P = 0.003$), thrombocytopenia (22% vs. 12%, $P = 0.03$), and infections (7% vs. <1%, $P = 0.01$). Although equally effective, VMP was clearly better tolerated than VTP, thus confirming as standard of care. The subsequent maintenance with bortezomib (bortezomib plus prednisone [VP] in patients treated with VMP, and bortezomib plus thalidomide [VT] in patients treated with VTP induction) contributed to increase the CR rate from 25% (mean obtained after induction therapy) up to 42%, and no significant differences between VT and VP arms were reported (46% and 38%). After a median duration of maintenance of 13 months, a trend in favor of VT in terms of 1-year TTP (84% vs. 71%; $P = 0.05$) was noted, with no differences in 1-year OS (92% for VT vs. 89% for VP) (18).

In another recent U.S. community-based, randomized, phase III b study, the safety and efficacy of three highly active bortezomib-based regimens (bortezomib-thalidomide-dexamethasone [VTD], bortezomib-dexamethasone [VD], and VMP) have been compared in patients with previously untreated MM ineligible for high-dose therapy and ASCT. At least PR rate was 60%, 70%, and 52% in the VD, VTD, and VMP arms, respectively; at least VGPR was 15%, 23%, and 24%, respectively, with CR/near CR rates of 13%, 18%, and 15%. The VD arm had the lowest rate of grade 3 to 4 AEs (58% vs. 71% each in the VTD and VMP arms, respectively), as well as the lowest rate of discontinuations due to AEs (10% vs. 18% and 16% in the VTD and VMP arms, respectively). The VTD arm had the highest rate of serious AEs (50% vs. 39% and 36% in the VD and VMP arms, respectively), as well as peripheral neuropathy of any grade (48% vs. 29% and 30% in the VD and VMP arms, respectively), and rates of serious embolism/thrombosis (8% vs. 6% and 3% in the VD and VMP arms, respectively) (19).

Bortezomib Plus Thalidomide, Melphalan, and Prednisone. A recent phase III trial compared a four-drug combination including MP plus bortezomib and thalidomide (VMPT), followed by maintenance with bortezomib and thalidomide, with VMP not followed by maintenance. The response rates were superior in the VMPT group: at least PR rate (89% vs. 81%, $P = 0.01$), at least VGPR rate (59% vs. 50%, $P = 0.03$), and CR rate (38% vs. 24%, $P = 0.0008$), respectively. After a median follow-up of 17.8 months, the 2-year PFS was significantly longer in the VMPT group (70.0% vs. 58.2%, HR = 0.62, 95% confidence interval = 0.44–0.88, $P = 0.008$). The achievement of CR significantly prolonged PFS in both VMPT ($P < 0.0001$) and VMP ($P = 0.003$) patients. The incidence of grade 3 to 4 neutropenia (37% vs. 28%, $P = 0.02$) and cardiac complications (10% vs. 5%, $P = 0.04$) was higher in the VMPT group, whereas the incidence of other grade 3 to 4 AEs was similar in the two groups: thrombocytopenia (21% vs. 19%), peripheral neuropathy (5% vs. 8%), infections (12% vs. 9%), and gastrointestinal complications (6% vs. 8%) (20). When the standard biweekly schedule of bortezomib (1.3 mg/m^2 on days 1, 4, 8, and 11) was reduced to a weekly infusion (1.3 mg/m^2 on days 1, 8, 15, and 22) (21), the incidence of grade 3 to 4 peripheral neuropathy was considerably reduced in both the VMPT and VMP groups (from 18% to 4%, $P = 0.0002$, and from 13% to 2%, $P = 0.0003$, respectively), without any significant change in PFS (21). This is the first report showing the superiority of a four-drug combination, followed by maintenance in comparison with the most recent standard therapy VMP, and the efficacy and good tolerability of the weekly schedule of bortezomib.

Lenalidomide-Based Therapies

Lenalidomide and Dexamethasone. The thalidomide-analogue lenalidomide has been tested in association with HD (RD) in a phase III randomized trial, in comparison with HD alone: despite higher CR rate (22.1% vs. 3.8%) and 1-year PFS (77% vs. 55%, $P = 0.002$) with RD, no OS advantage was reported. Most important grade 3 to 4 toxicities with RD versus dexamethasone alone were neutropenia (14% vs. 3%) and non neutropenic infections (19% vs. 10%) (22,23).

Another open-label randomized trial evaluated the association of lenalidomide plus low-dose dexamethasone (Rd) versus RD as initial therapy for newly diagnosed MM: despite higher PR rates with RD, the use of HD did not result in superior TTP, PFS, and OS compared with low-dose dexamethasone. OS at 1 year (96% vs. 87%, $P < 0.001$) and at 2 years (87% vs. 75%, $P < 0.001$) were significantly better with low-dose dexamethasone than with HD. HD in a community settings seems more toxic than low-dose dexamethasone, with more early deaths in the first 4 months, increased risk of thromboembolic complications, and higher risk of serious AEs, particularly in patients older than 65 years. Given the better toxicity profile associated with low-dose dexamethasone, all patients enrolled in this trial crossed over from the RD to the Rd cohort, leading to the premature interruption of the protocol. Hence, OS rates at 3 years reported in both groups were similar.

The landmark analysis at 4 months showed the impact of different treatment approaches. Three-year OS for patients who continued on primary therapy beyond 4 months was 79%, whereas in patients who stopped treatment after 4 months, it was 55% (24).

In the light of this, Rd, continued until progression or until tolerated, can be regarded as a reasonable option in patients older than 65 years, although a formal comparison with MP has still not been done.

Lenalidomide Plus Melphalan and Prednisone. Results of the phase I/II dose-escalating study exploring the combination of MP plus lenalidomide showed that at the maximum tolerated dose (lenalidomide 10 mg/daily for 21 days and melphalan 0.18 mg/kg for 4 days every 4–6 weeks, plus prednisone 2 mg/kg days 1–4) PR or better were 81%, including 48% of patients with at least VGPR and 24% of patients with immunofixation-negative CR (25). The 2-year event-free survival (EFS) and OS rates for all patients were 80% and 91%, respectively (26). These results provided the basis for the European Myeloma Network phase III study comparing MP with melphalan-prednisone-lenalidomide (MPR), with or without lenalidomide maintenance. In this study, patients were randomly assigned to receive MPR, followed by lenalidomide maintenance therapy (MPR-R) or MPR followed by placebo maintenance therapy or MP followed by placebo maintenance therapy. At least PR rate was 77% in the MPR-R arm, with at least VGPR in 32% of patients and CR in 18%, significantly higher than in the MP group (at least PR in 49% of patients, at least VGPR in 11%, and CR in 5%) ($P < 0.001$). PFS was significantly improved in patients who received MPR-R compared with those who received MP followed by placebo maintenance (22.5 months vs. 15 months).

No differences were noted in the 1-year OS (92% in both arms). Most important grade 3 to 4 hematological AEs with MPR-R and MP, respectively, were neutropenia (70% vs. 30%) and thrombocytopenia (38% vs. 13%); grade 3 to 4 nonhematological AEs were infections (9% vs. 6%) and fatigue (6% vs. 3%). No grade 3 to 4 peripheral neuropathy was noted (27).

MPR followed by lenalidomide maintenance can be therefore considered a new standard for patients older than 65 years or younger patients not eligible for ASCT.

Table 1 summarizes the efficacy of the main treatment regimens, and Table 2 summarizes the most frequent grade 3 to 4 AEs.

TABLE 1

Efficacy of regimens used as a front-line treatment in elderly patients with MM

		N	CR	≥PR	PFS/EFS/ TTP	OS	Ref.
MP	M: 0.25 mg/kg days 1–7 P: 2 mg/kg days 1–4 for twelve 6-week cycles	112	1%	41%	45% at 24 months	63% at 24 months	Facon et al. (6)
MP	M: 0.25 mg/kg days 1–4 P: 2 mg/kg days 1–4 28–42-day cycle for 9 cycles	144	2%	50%	48% at 24 months	70% at 24 months	Ludwig et al. (7)
TD	T: 200 mg D: 40 mg days 1–4, 15–18 for a 28-day cycle for 9 cycles	145	2%	68%	41% at 24 months	61% at 24 months	Ludwig et al. (7)
MPT	M: 4 mg/m² days 1–7 P: 40 mg/m² days 1–7 for six 4-week cycles T: 100 mg/day until PD	129	16%	76%	50% at 22 months	50% at 45 months	Palumbo et al. (9,10)
MPT	M: 0.25 mg/kg days 1–4 P: 2 mg/kg days 1–4 T: 400 mg/day for twelve 6-week cycles	125	13%	76%	50% at 28 months	50% at 52 months	Facon et al. (11)

Continued

TABLE 1

Efficacy of regimens used as a front-line treatment in elderly patients with MM (*Continued*)

		N	CR	≥PR	PFS/EFS/ TTP	OS	Ref.
MPT	M: 0.25 mg/kg days 1–4 P: 2 mg/kg days 1–4 T: 100 mg/day for twelve 6-week cycles	113	7%	62%	50% at 24 months	50% at 45 months	Hulin et al. (12)
MPT	M: 0.25 mg/kg days 1–4 P: 100 mg days 1–4 T: 200–400 mg/day in a 6-week cycle until plateau T: 200 mg/day until disease progression	182	6%	42%	50% at 20 months	50% at 29 months	Guldbrandsen et al. (8)[a]
MPT	M: 0.25 mg/kg P: 1 mg/days 1–5 T: 200 mg/day for eight 4-week cycles, followed by T: 50 mg/day until disease progression	165	2%	66%	50% at 14 months	50% at 37 months	Wijermans et al. (13)[a]
VMP	M: 9 mg/m^2 days 1–4 P: 60 mg/m^2 days 1–4 V: 1.3 mg/m^2 days 1, 4, 8, 11, 22, 25, 29, 32 for the first four 6-week cycles; days 1, 8, 15, 22 for the subsequent five 6-week cycles	344	30%	71%	50% at 24 months	72% at 36 months	San Miguel et al. (16)
VMP	M: 9 mg/m^2 days 1–4 P: 60 mg/m^2 days 1–4 V: 1.3 mg/m^2 days 1, 8, 15, 22	257	21%	79%	58% at 24 months	89% at 24 months	Palumbo et al. (20)
VMP	M: 9 mg/m^2 days 1–4 P: 60 mg/m^2 days 1–4 V: 1.3 mg/m^2 twice weekly (days 1, 4, 8, 11; 22, 25, 29, and 32) for one 6-week cycle, followed by once weekly (days 1, 8, 15, and 22) for five 5-week cycles	130	22%	79%	72% at 24 months	81% at 24 months	Mateos et al. (18)

Continued

TABLE 1

Efficacy of regimens used as a front-line treatment in elderly patients with MM   (*Continued*)

		N	CR	≥PR	PFS/EFS/ TTP	OS	Ref.
VTP	T: 100 mg/day P: 60 mg/m² days 1–4 V: 1.3 mg/m² twice weekly (days 1, 4, 8, 11; 22, 25, 29, and 32) for one 6-week cycle, followed by once weekly (days 1, 8, 15, and 22) for five 5-week cycles	130	27%	79%	61% at 24 months	84% at 24 months	Mateos et al. (18)
CTD	C: 500 mg days 1, 8, 15 T: 100–200 mg/day D: 40 mg days 1–4, 12–15 in a 3-week cycle	450	23%	82%	ND	ND	Morgan et al. (15)
VMPT	M: 9 mg/m² days 1–4 P: 60 mg/m² days 1–4 V: 1.3 mg/m² days 1, 8, 15, 22 T: 50 mg days 1–42 for nine 5-week cycles followed by Bor: 1.3 mg/m² every 15 days and T: 50 mg/day as maintenance	254	34%	86%	70% at 24 months	90% at 24 months	Palumbo et al. (20)
MPR	M:0.18–0.25 mg/kg days 1–4 P: 2 mg/kg days 1–4 for nine 4-week cycles R: 5–10 mg days 1–21 until relapse or progressive disease	152	18%	45%	55% at 24 months	92% at 12 months	Palumbo et al. (27)
Rd	R: 25 mg days 1–21 d: 40 mg days 1, 8, 15, 22 in a 4-week cycle	222	4%	70%	50% at 25 months	87% at 24 months	Rajkumar et al. (24)

C, cyclophosphamide; CR, complete remission; CTD, cyclophosphamide-thalidomide-dexamethasone; D, high-dose dexamethasone; d, low-dose dexamethasone; EFS, event-free survival; M, melphalan; MM, multiple myeloma; MPR, melphalan-prednisone-lenalidomide; MPT, melphalan-prednisone-thalidomide; N indicates number of patients; NA, not available; OS, overall survival; P, prednisone; PFS, progression-free survival; PR partial response; R, lenalidomide; T, thalidomide; TD, thalidomide and dexamethasone; TTP, time to progression; V, bortezomib; VMP, bortezomib-melphalan-prednisone; VMPT, bortezomib-melphalan-prednisone-thalidomide; VTP, bortezomib-thalidomide-prednisone;

[a] Updated information was presented at the meeting (American Society of Clinical Oncology, European Haematology Association and American Society of Hematology congress).

TABLE 2

Safety (grade 3–4 AE) of regimens used as front-line treatment in elderly patients with MM

Regimen	N	Neutropenia (%)	Thrombocytopenia (%)	Infection (%)	Peripheral Neuropathy (%)	VTE (%)	Ref.
MP	112	15	15	NA	NA	4	Facon et al. (6)
MP	144	15	12	8	NA	4	Ludwig et al. (7)
TD	145	3	1	13	NA	10	Ludwig et al. (7)
MPT	129	16	3	10	8	9	Palumbo et al. (9,10)
MPT	125	48	14	13	6	12	Facon et al. (11)
MPT	113	23	NA	NA	20*	6	Hulin et al. (12)
MPT	165	NA	NA	14	9	3	Wijermans et al. (13)[a]
VMP	344	40	38	11	13	1	S Miguel et al. (16)
VMP	257	28	19	9	5	2	Palumbo et al. (20)
VMP	130	37	22	7	5	<1	Mateos et al. (18)
VTP	130	21	12	<1	9	4	Mateos et al. (18)
VMPT	254	37	21	12	8	5	Palumbo et al. (20)
MPR	152	70	38	9	0	5	Palumbo et al. (27)

AE, adverse events; CTD, cyclophosphamide-thalidomide-dexamethasone; MM, multiple myeloma; MPR, melphalan-prednisone-lenalidomide; MPT, melphalan-prednisone-thalidomide; N indicates number of patients; NA, not available; TD, thalidomide and dexamethasone; VMP, bortezomib-melphalan-prednisone; VMPT, bortezomib-melphalan-prednisone-thalidomide; VTE, venous thromboembolism; VTP, bortezomib-thalidomide-prednisone.

*Grade 2–4.

[a]Updated information was presented at the meeting of the American Society of Clinical Oncology, European Haematology Association and American Society of Hematology Congress.

■ REDUCED-INTENSITY TRANSPLANT

Elderly patients or those with significant comorbidities are generally considered not eligible for standard melphalan 200 mg/m^2 followed by ASCT. A randomized trial exploring the efficacy of high-dose chemotherapy and transplant in patients with newly diagnosed MM actually showed a significant benefit of ASCT in terms of OS in patients younger than 65 years (5-year survival rate of 68% vs. 50%; P = 0.008) (28). Two randomized studies compared intermediate-dose melphalan (Melphalan 100 mg/m^2—Mel 100) and reduced-intensity ASCT with standard MP. In the first study including patients aged 65 to 70 years, ASCT leads to better EFS and OS as compared with MP (29). However, in the second study, including patients aged 65 to 75 years, reduced-intensity ASCT was compared not only with MP but also with MPT: this study showed that PFS and OS were higher with MPT as compared with MP and to Mel100 (11). A recent phase II trial evaluated the efficacy of novel agents incorporated in both pretransplant induction and posttransplant consolidation and maintenance strategy, in patients aged 65 to 75 years, who received reduced-intensity ASCT (Mel100): PR rate was 94% after induction with PAD and 100% following consolidation with LP; the CR rate was 13% after bortezomib induction, 43% after Mel100, and 73% after consolidation-maintenance with lenalidomide. These data indicate that bortezomib as induction and lenalidomide as consolidation-maintenance treatment improve response rates by taking advantage of a sequential exposure to different drugs. During bortezomib induction, grade 3 to 4 toxicities included thrombocytopenia (17%), neutropenia (10%), peripheral neuropathy (16%), and pneumonia (10%). Lenalidomide consolidation-maintenance was well tolerated, with no cumulative or persistent neutropenia (grade 3–4 reported in 16%) and/or thrombocytopenia (reported in 6%); more frequent extra-hematological toxicities were pneumonia (5%) and cutaneous rash (4%) (30). This approach can be used in elderly patients as well as in younger patients with preexisting comorbidities, for whom full-dose chemotherapy and ASCT appears to be too toxic. However, these data need further validation in randomized trials.

■ TREATMENT STRATEGY FOR RELAPSING PATIENTS

There are some key points that help physicians choose the best treatment to manage patients with relapsed/refractory MM:

1. For patients who relapse following a durable response (that is longer than the median PFS expected with the previous therapy), the same treatment (or a similar treatment, using the same agents [rechallenge]) should be repeated.
2. For patients who relapse following a short response (that is, shorter than the median PFS expected with the previous therapy), the patient should be treated with new regimens.
3. Drugs that had already been used before the rechallenge remain secondary options if there

was no clinical evidence of progression under that drug.
4. The choice of drug should always take into account preexisting comorbidities and tolerability reported with previous therapies.

Primary salvage therapy includes bortezomib and dexamethasone, bortezomib and doxorubicin, or lenalidomide and dexamethasone, based on the results of randomized phase III trials, as reported later. Combinations with chemotherapy, such as doxorubicin or cyclophosphamide, or melphalan, or IMIDs, are alternative, less tested options for these patients.

■ THERAPY AT RELAPSE

Bortezomib-Based Therapies

The international, randomized, phase III Assessment of Proteasome Inhibition for Extending Remission (APEX) trial in 2005 led to the approval of bortezomib for the treatment of MM patients who have received at least one prior therapy. In the initial APEX report, single-agent bortezomib demonstrated superior efficacy in comparison with HD in terms of PR rate (38% vs. 18%, $P < 0.001$), TTP (median: 6.2 vs. 3.5 months $P < 0.001$), and OS (1-year OS rate: 80% vs. 66%, $P = 0.003$) (31). In an updated subsequent analysis, median OS was 29.8 months in the bortezomib arm versus 23.7 months in the dexamethasone arm, despite more than 62% of dexamethasone-treated patients crossing over to receive bortezomib (32). These results confirm that, with longer follow-up and despite substantial crossover from HD arm, bortezomib treatment is associated with a significant improvement in survival as compared with dexamethasone.

A phase III international study compared the efficacy and safety of the combination pegylated liposomal doxorubicin (PLD) plus bortezomib with bortezomib monotherapy in patients with relapsed or refractory MM: at least PR rate was 41% for bortezomib and 44% for PLD plus bortezomib, a difference that was not statistically significant, but patients treated with PLD plus bortezomib had a considerably prolonged TTP (9.3 vs. 6.5 months, $P = 0.000004$) and PFS (9.0 vs. 6.5 months, $P = 0.000026$) and a longer duration of response (10.2 vs. 7.0 months, $P = 0.0008$). Furthermore, the 15-month survival rate for PLD plus bortezomib was 76% compared with 65% for bortezomib alone ($P = 0.03$). Therefore, PLD and bortezomib represent an additional new standard of care for this patient population (33).

In relapsed setting, the most common bortezomib-related AEs were neutropenia reported in 14% of patients, and thrombocytopenia, with an incidence ranging from 15% to 30%. Grade 3 to 4 neuropathy was reported in 9% of patients treated with bortezomib and in 4% treated with PLD plus bortezomib (32,33).

Lenalidomide-Based Regimens

Two phase III, placebo-controlled trials investigated the efficacy of lenalidomide plus dexamethasone in relapsed patients in comparison with dexamethasone alone. Response rate (PR + CR) (60–61% vs. 24–19.9%, $P < 0.001$), TTP (median 11.3–11.1 months vs. 4.7 months; $P < 0.001$), and OS (median: 29.6 months vs. 20.2 months, $P < 0.001$) were significantly longer in patients who received lenalidomide plus dexamethasone than in those who received dexamethasone alone. In the two trials, grade 3 to 4 AEs occurred more in the lenalidomide group than in the placebo group, and the most common events were neutropenia (29.5–41.2% vs. 2.3–4.6%, respectively) and VTE (11.4–14.7% vs. 3.4–4.6%, respectively) (34,35).

Because lenalidomide treatment proved to be more efficacious than dexamethasone alone, it can be considered a new standard of care for relapse patients.

Thalidomide-Based Therapies

TD has been compared with HD alone in a single-phase III trial: preliminary results showed higher response rate (PR rate 65% vs. 28%, $P < 0.001$) and longer 1-year PFS (46.5% vs. 31%, $P < 0.001$) in patients treated with TD as compared with patients treated with thalidomide alone. Arterial thrombosis was recorded in 22% of patients in the TD arm, as compared with 7% in the dexamethasone arm ($P = 0.02$). Other frequent side effects were somnolence/mood changes (58% vs. 21%), constipation/nausea (43% vs. 11%), skin/mucosal dryness (26% vs. 9%), and tremor (19% vs. 4%). A symptomatic peripheral neuropathy was observed in 28% and 7% of patients, respectively. Despite toxicity being the main cause of treatment discontinuation (55% vs. 6%, respectively), adding thalidomide to dexamethasone results in higher response rates, and it is a valuable treatment option for patients with relapsed MM (36).

Efficacy and safety of phase III studies in relapsed or refractory MM are summarized in Table 3 and Table 4, respectively.

■ MANAGEMENT OF AES

The efficacy of the treatments described earlier should be balanced against the toxicity profile of the agents used. Toxicity should be graded according to the National Cancer Institute–Common Terminology Criteria (37). Prompt recognition and management of treatment-related AEs can significantly increase treatment efficacy. Furthermore, therapy should be adjusted by reducing drug doses to tailor the treatment approach according to patient age: the higher the age of a patient, the gentler should be the treatment. Therefore, dose reductions are suggested according to the patient's age (Table 5).

Hematological Toxicities

Neutropenia

Neutropenia is quite frequent in patients with MM treated with new drugs in combination with alkylating agents but less frequent when they are used with dexamethasone alone.

TABLE 3
Efficacy of regimens used as treatment in elderly patients with refractory/relapse MM

		N	CR (%)	≥PR (%)	PFS/EFS/ TTP	OS	References
V	V: 1.3 mg/m² days 1, 4, 8, 11 for eight 3-week cycles then days 1, 8, 15, 22 for three 5-week maintenance cycles	333	9	43	50% at 6.2 months	62% at 24 months	Richardson et al. (31)
D	D: 40 mg days 1–4, 9–12, 17–20 for four 5-week cycles then 1–4 for 4-week cycles	336	<1	18	50% at 3.5 months	35% at 24 months	Richardson et al. (31)
V	V: 1.3 mg/m² days 1,4,8,11 for every 21-days cycle	322	2	41	50% at 6.5 months	65% at 15 months	Orlowski et al. (33)
V + PLD	V: 1.3 mg/m² days 1, 4, 8, 11 for every 21-days cycle PLD: 30 mg/m² IV on day 4 of each cycle	324	4	44	50% at 9 months	76% at 15 months	Orlowski et al. (33)
RD	R: 25 mg days 1–21 of a 28 day cycle D: 40 mg days 1–4, 9–12, 17–20 for 4 cycles, after only days 1–4	176	16	60	50% at 11 months	NR	Dimopoulos et al. (35)
D	D: 40 mg days 1–4, 9–12, 17–20 for 4 cycles, after only days 1–4	175	3	24	50% at 4 months	50% at 20 months	Dimopoulos et al. (35)
RD	R: 25 mg days 1–21 of a 28 day cycle D: 40 mg days 1–4, 9–12, 17–20 for 4 cycles, after only days 1–4	177	14	61	50% at 11 months	50% at 30 months	Weber et al. (34)
D	D: 40 mg days 1–4, 9–12, 17–20 for 4 cycles, after only days 1–4	176	0.6	20	50% at 4 months	50% at 20 months	Weber et al. (34)

CR, complete remission; D, dexamethasone; EFS, event-free survival; MM, multiple myeloma; N, number of patients; OS, overall survival; PFS, progression-free survival; PLD, pegylated liposomal doxorubicin; PR partial response; RD, lenalidomide and dexamethasone; TTP, time to progression; V, bortezomib.

TABLE 4
Safety (grade 3–4 AE) of regimens used as treatment in elderly refractory/relapsed patients with MM

Regimen	N	Neutropenia (%)	Thrombocytopenia (%)	Infection (%)	Peripheral Neuropathy (%)	VTE (%)	Study
V	333	14	30	NA	8	NA	Richardson et al. (31)
D	336	1	6	NA	<1	NA	Richardson et al. (31)
V	322	14	15	NA	5	1	Orlowski et al. (33)
V+PLD	324	30	22	NA	3	1	Orlowski et al. (33)
RD	176	29	11	9	NA	11	Dimopoulos et al. (35)
D	175	2	6	6	NA	4	Dimopoulos et al. (35)
RD	177	41	15	21	2	12	Weber et al. (34)
D	176	4	7	12	1	4	Weber et al. (34)

AE, adverse events; D, dexamethasone; MM, multiple myeloma; N, number of patients; NA, not available; PLD, pegylated liposomal doxorubicin; RD, lenalidomide and dexamethasone; V, velcade; VTE, venous thromboembolism.

TABLE 5
Age-adjusted dose reduction

	65–75 years	>75 years	Further Dose Reduction
Dexamethasone weekly	40 mg	20 mg	10 mg
Melphalan days 1–4	0.25 mg/kg	0.18 mg/kg	0.13 mg/kg
Thalidomide per day	200 mg	100 mg	50 mg
Lenalidomide (in combination with dexamethasone) days 1–21	25 mg	15 mg	10 mg
Lenalidomide (in combination with melphalan plus prednisone) days 1–21	10 mg	5 mg	5 mg every other day
Bortezomib	1.3 mg/m^2 twice weekly	1.3 mg/m^2 weekly	1.0 mg/m^2 weekly

The use of granulocyte colony-stimulating factor (G-CSF) is an efficacious and well-tolerated way to decrease/prevent neutropenia. Treatment should be withheld in case of grade 4 neutropenia (neutrophilic count < 500/mm^3) despite G-CSF administration. When the AE resolves to grade 2 (neutrophilic count ≥ 1,000/mm^3), treatment can be restarted with appropriate dose reduction at the beginning of the next cycle. The biggest concern linked to neutropenia is the occurrence of infections. Therefore, prophylaxis with G-CSF is recommended to prevent febrile neutropenia in patients at high risk on the basis of their age, medical history, disease characteristics, and the expected myelotoxicity of the chemotherapy regimen.

Thrombocytopenia

Bortezomib, lenalidomide, alkylating agents, and their combinations may be responsible for the occurrence of thrombocytopenia, whereas it is rare in patients treated with thalidomide alone or plus steroids.

In case thrombocytopenia reaches grade 4 (platelet count < 25,000/mm^3), treatment suspension is needed. Treatment can be restored when thrombocytopenia resolves to grade 2 (platelet count < 50,000/mm^3), but dose reduction of the myelotoxic drug is still necessary.

Anemia

Anemia is generally related to MM and tends to improve with disease response to therapy, but it becomes even more common in patients with recurrent or refractory disease. The use of bortezomib, lenalidomide, and their combinations may rarely cause anemia.

Iron status should be monitored during treatment to prevent functional iron deficiency and support increased erythropoiesis, both for patients receiving erythropoiesis-stimulating agents (ESAs; epoetin and darbepoetin) or not. ESAs can be used to treat treatment-related anemia. ESA treatment is generally recommended when the hemoglobin concentration is less than 9 g/dL; however, treatment can begin earlier at physicians' discretion (hemoglobin 10–12 g/dL) for patients with heart disease or those who have difficulties undertaking regular daily activities. The ESA dose should be adjusted to maintain a hemoglobin concentration around 11 to 12 g/dL, to avoid blood transfusion and anemia-related symptoms. However, with hemoglobin concentration greater than 12 g/dL, serious heart problems may occur and the risk of thrombosis may increase. For patients at high risk for developing blood clots, the risks associated with these drugs need to be balanced against their benefits.

Extra-Hematological Toxicities

Infections

Both the disease (that can cause impairment in immune function) and its treatment (in particular use of HD and therapy-related neutropenia) increase the risk of infections. The risk is higher in case of active disease but decreases with response to therapy. Despite the concomitant use of chemotherapy, and the higher rate of neutropenia, in newly diagnosed patients treated with MPR, severe infections were reported in only 9% of cases. In this trial, ciprofloxacin was administered as antibiotic prophylaxis (25). Herpes zoster infections have been reported as a possible AE associated with bortezomib. In the VMP versus MP trial, patients treated with VMP had a higher incidence of herpes zoster than did patients treated with MP alone (14% vs. 4%), but with acyclovir prophylaxis, incidence decreased to 3% (16).

Trimethoprim-sulphamethoxazole is the most indicated prophylaxis at least during the first 2 to 3 months of chemotherapy or during steroid administration. Acyclovir prophylaxis is recommended for all patients receiving bortezomib-based therapy. Routine antibiotic prophylaxis could be considered for the first 3 months of therapy, where the risk of infection is higher; it is particularly recommended in patients receiving HD, in elderly patients, in patients with comorbidities that increase the risk of infections (i.e., chronic obstructive pulmonary disease, diabetes, renal function impairment), and in patients with an increased infection rate. Treatment can start with oral antibiotics, but in case of severe systemic infections, intravenous administration is more appropriate.

Peripheral Neuropathy

Peripheral neuropathy is a common AE linked to bortezomib- and thalidomide-based therapies. Incidence of grade 3 to 4 neuropathy is similar in thalidomide- or bortezomib-based regimen, in both relapsed and newly diagnosed settings (9–12,16–18,31,33). Both thalidomide and bortezomib-related neuropathies are cumulative and linked to the administration dose. However, bortezomib-related neuropathy may improve after discontinuation, in contrast to thalidomide-related neuropathy (38,39).

By contrast, grade 3 to 4 peripheral neuropathy is very rare in patients treated with lenalidomide, and lenalidomide has been administered to patients who have received prior thalidomide treatment without further deterioration of preexisting thalidomide-related neuropathy (34,35).

There are no pharmacological drugs available so far to effectively relieve neuropathic symptoms. Therefore, immediate dose reduction and modifications of the treatment schedule are the most effective means to treat this condition. In case of grade 1 with pain or grade 2 peripheral neuropathy, a dose reduction of bortezomib to 1.0 mg/m² is recommended; for grade 2 with pain or grade 3 peripheral neuropathy, interruption of bortezomib is recommended until peripheral neuropathy resolves, and then it can be restarted at 0.7 mg/m²; treatment should be discontinued in case of grade 4 peripheral neuropathy (38). Results of the VMP versus VMPT study suggest that a good alternative can be to reduce the biweekly infusion (starting dose 1.3 mg/m² twice a week for a total of four doses every treatment cycle) to a weekly infusion (same dose 1.3 mg/m² once weekly for a total of four doses every treatment cycle) in case of grade 1 painful neuropathy or grade 2 sensory peripheral neuropathy. Treatment interruption is needed if grade 2 painful neuropathy or grade 3 neuropathy occurs. It can then be restarted on a weekly basis (1.0 mg/m² once weekly for a total of four doses every treatment cycle) when neuropathy improves to at least grade 1. If further dose reductions are needed, 0.7 mg/m² per week can be considered; in case of grade 4 peripheral neuropathy, patients should stop treatment (21).

Patients treated with thalidomide should be instructed on how to recognize peripheral neuropathy, decrease the dose, or discontinue the drug when sensory paresthesia is complicated by pain, motor deficiency, or an interference with daily function. With grade 1 neuropathy, the assigned dose should still be maintained; with grade 2 neuropathy, thalidomide dose should be reduced by 50%; in case of grade 3 neuropathy, thalidomide discontinuation is necessary, and it can be resumed at a decreased dose when neuropathy improves to grade 1 (39).

Thrombosis

In patients with MM, incidence of VTE varies from 3% to 10%. The type of drug used to treat the disease is an important factor determining the risk of VTE. It has been observed that bortezomib-based therapies do not contribute to increase the risk of VTE, nor do thalidomide and lenalidomide alone. On the other hand, the risk of VTE substantially increases when dexamethasone or chemotherapy is added to IMIDs, in particular in newly diagnosed patients, whereas the risk of VTE at relapse is lower, especially in thalidomide-treated patients (40). It should be noticed that in the Italian study, VTE incidence significantly decreased (from 20% to 3%) after the introduction of prophylactic enoxaparin (9). In newly diagnosed patients treated with RD, VTE has been observed in 26% of patients; incidence significantly decreased with the use of low-dose dexamethasone (12% with the Rd combination) (24); in patients treated with MPR, VTEs are reported in about 5% of cases (25). In both studies, aspirin was recommended as antithrombotic prophylaxis.

At present, there are no data on which is the best thromboprophylaxis to use in patients with MM treated with IMIDs. To address this issue, the Italian Myeloma Network GIMEMA designed a phase III study to compare the efficacy and safety of low-molecular-weight heparin (LMWH), low-fixed-dose warfarin (1.25 mg/day), or low-dose aspirin as VTE prophylaxis in newly diagnosed patients, who received primary induction with thalidomide-based regimens: preliminary results showed that grade 3 to 4 VTE incidence was not significantly different in patients treated with ASA compared with LMWH (3.6% of patients vs. 2.7% of patients, respectively, $P = 0.17$), but significantly higher in warfarin patients compared with LMWH patients (6.4% of patients vs. 2.7% of patients, respectively, P = 0.02) (41). Similarly, no differences were reported in another phase III trial comparing ASA with LMWH in newly diagnosed patients treated with Rd induction (VTE rate 2% vs. 1%, respectively, P = NS) (42).

In asymptomatic patients, baseline coagulation tests and screening for VTE are not required. Presence of risk factors for thrombosis in patients with MM treated with IMIDs should be evaluated. In patients with MM, thromboprophylaxis should be carefully chosen on the basis of the presence of risk factors (classified as individual risk factors [history of VTE, inherited thrombophilia age, obesity, comorbidities such as cardiac disease, chronic renal disease, diabetes, infections, immobilization, presence of central venous catheter, and surgical procedures]; myeloma-related risk factors [diagnosis and hyperviscosity]; therapy-related risk factors [HD, doxorubicin, or multi-agent chemotherapies, or immunomodulatory compounds]). Therapy-related risk factors should be considered per se as high-risk risk factors. If none or one individual or one myeloma-related risk factor is present, aspirin (81–325 mg/day) is considered the most appropriate prophylaxis. If two or more individual or myeloma-related risk factors are observed, LMWH (equivalent of enoxaparin 40 mg/day) or full-dose warfarin (international normalized ratio target 2–3) is preferred. Overall, LMWH or full-dose warfarin is recommended for patients with therapy-related risk factor. Prophylaxis is generally recommended for at least the first 4 to 6 months. Patients who experienced VTE during treatment can either continue the treatment or they can suspend it and then be retreated after stabilization. Patients who experienced VTE despite being given aspirin should receive LMWH; patients treated with prophylactic LMWH should be switched to therapeutic doses (40).

Renal Toxicity

Factors involved in the pathogenesis of renal failure include the capacity of the light-chain component of the immunoglobulin to cause proximal tubular damage, dehydration, hypercalcemia, hyperuricemia, infections, and use of nephrotoxic drugs. If patients experience renal failure, no dose modification of agents such as thalidomide and bortezomib should be made. Lenalidomide can be used, but hematological function should be constantly monitored, especially in the early cycles. Lenalidomide dose reductions are compulsory on the basis of creatinine clearance values: between 30 and 60 mL/min, the recommended dose of lenalidomide is 10 mg/day; with a value lower than 30 mL/min, the recommended dose is 15 mg every other day, if the patient does not require dialysis; if creatinine clearance is inferior to 30 mL/min and the patient requires dialysis, lenalidomide dose is 5 mg/day after dialysis and only on dialysis days.

Bone Disease

Skeletal complications (43,44), such as vertebral compression or collapse from osteoporosis, and pain arising from these complications are common in patients with MM. Systemic analgesia, local measures, and chemotherapy can be used to relieve the pain. Local radiotherapy is effective for pain relief of bone disease (45,46).

Vertebroplasty too (47) leads to local pain relief and bone strengthening, but it does not restore vertebral height. However, a recent randomized phase III study of balloon kyphoplasty showed marked reduction in back disability and pain at 1 month after procedure (48). Long-term bisphosphonate is increasingly being used to try to prevent these problems. Osteonecrosis of the jaw is an uncommon but potentially serious complication of intravenous bisphosphonate.

Gastrointestinal AEs

Gastrointestinal events are common side effects of myeloma therapy. Rarely are they related to myeloma, the only exception is constipation related to severe hypercalcemia. Constipation is the most common gastrointestinal AE related to thalidomide treatment. The main frequent gastrointestinal event in lenalidomide-treated patients is diarrhea. Both constipation and diarrhea have been reported with bortezomib-based regimens.

Patients suffering from diarrhea should maintain a high fluid intake; antidiarrheal drugs can be used in case of diarrhea, after exclusion of active infections. In case of severe (grade 3–4) toxicity, a 50% dose reduction of the drug is recommended. Also in case of constipation, patients should maintain a high fluid intake, and a high fiber diet, if medically appropriate, can be of help. If necessary, stool softeners and osmotic laxatives can be administered.

Dermatological AEs

Both thalidomide and lenalidomide can cause dermatological toxicity, most frequently rash, dry skin, and mouth and atrophic lesions. These events are generally mild to moderate and easily manageable. Toxic epidermic necrolysis and Stevens-Johnson syndrome (SJS) are serious AEs, but they are quite rare (39). Dermatological toxicity is rare with bortezomib-based regimens (the higher rate reported with the association of bortezomib and PLD in relapsed patients, where the main AE was hand-foot syndrome related to PLD) (31,33).

A particular attention should be paid when coadministering thalidomide or lenalidomide and agents with known dermatological toxicity (e.g., sulfonamides, allopurinol, cotrimoxazole). In these cases, a close monitoring is needed. When mild toxicities occur, temporary discontinuation is generally the best method to solve the rash. If necessary, treatment should begin with antihistamines; if rash persists, low-dose prednisone (10–20 mg/day for up to 14 days) should be added. In case of grade 3 to 4 AEs, treatment can be resumed after complete resolution and with 50% dose reductions. After toxic epidemic necrolysis or the SJS, readministration of the responsible drug is contraindicated.

CONCLUSION

The combination of conventional chemotherapy or low-dose dexamethasone with new drugs has substantially changed the treatment paradigm for patients with MM, increasing therapeutic options available for this disease. Randomized phase III studies have shown that MPT, MP plus bortezomib, and MPR are all better than MP; hence, they can now be regarded as new standards of care for patients ineligible for ASCT, according to age or comorbidities. Preliminary results suggest that Rd could be a valid alternative option as well.

Physicians can now tailor specific therapies according to the patient characteristics and comorbidities, by balancing efficacy and toxicity of the treatment regimens. Patients with renal impairment can be treated with both thalidomide- and bortezomib-based regimens, without any dose modification, whereas lenalidomide may be taken into account as a valid option after appropriate dose reduction. Lenalidomide-based regimens should be preferred for patients with preexisting neuropathy. Patients with risk factors for VTE can be safely treated with bortezomib-based regimens, without increasing their risk of thrombosis; IMIDs can be administered with appropriate antithrombotic prophylaxis.

Having a wider variety of treatment options available enables physicians to choose the best and more personalized option for the patient, leading to both improved quality of life and outcome.

ACKNOWLEDGMENTS

Our thanks to Giorgio Schirripa for help in writing the manuscript.

REFERENCES

1. Jemal A, Murray T, Ward E, et al. Cancer statistics, 2005. *CA Cancer J Clin* 2005;55(1):10–30.
2. Kyle RA, Rajkumar SV. Multiple myeloma. *N Engl J Med* 2004;351(18):1860–1873.
3. Kyle RA, Rajkumar SV. Criteria for diagnosis, staging, risk stratification and response assessment of multiple myeloma. *Leukemia* 2009;23(1):3–9.
4. Myeloma trialists' Collaborative Group. Combination chemotherapy versus melphalan plus prednisone as

treatment for multiple myeloma: an overview of 6,633 patients from 27 randomized trials. *J Clin Oncol* 1998;16:3832–3842.

5. Rajkumar SV, Kyle RA. Treatment of newly diagnosed multiple myeloma. In: Rajkumar SV, Kyle RA, eds. *Treatment of Multiple Myeloma and Related Disorders.* Minnesota, MN: Mayo Clinic, 2009:26–35

6. Facon T, Mary JY, Pégourie B, et al.; Intergroupe Francophone du Myélome (IFM) group. Dexamethasone-based regimens versus melphalan-prednisone for elderly multiple myeloma patients ineligible for high-dose therapy. *Blood* 2006; 107(4):1292–1298.

7. Ludwig H, Hajek R, Tóthová E, et al. Thalidomide-dexamethasone compared with melphalan-prednisolone in elderly patients with multiple myeloma. *Blood* 2009;113(15):3435–3442.

8. Guldbrandsen N, Waage A, Gimsin P, et al. A randomised placebo controlled study with melphalan/prednisone vs melphalan/prednisone/thalidomide: quality of life and toxicity [abstract 0209]. *Haematologica* 2008;93:84.

9. Palumbo A, Bringhen S, Caravita T, et al.; Italian Multiple Myeloma Network, GIMEMA. Oral melphalan and prednisone chemotherapy plus thalidomide compared with melphalan and prednisone alone in elderly patients with multiple myeloma: randomised controlled trial. *Lancet* 2006;367(9513):825–831.

10. Palumbo A, Bringhen S, Liberati AM, et al. Oral melphalan, prednisone, and thalidomide in elderly patients with multiple myeloma: updated results of a randomized controlled trial. *Blood* 2008;112(8):3107–3114.

11. Facon T, Mary JY, Hulin C, et al.; Intergroupe Francophone du Myélome. Melphalan and prednisone plus thalidomide versus melphalan and prednisone alone or reduced-intensity autologous stem cell transplantation in elderly patients with multiple myeloma (IFM 99–06): a randomised trial. *Lancet* 2007;370(9594):1209–1218.

12. Hulin C, Facon T, Rodon P, et al. Efficacy of melphalan and prednisone plus thalidomide in patients older than 75 years with newly diagnosed multiple myeloma: IFM 01/01 trial. *J Clin Oncol* 2009;27(22):3664–3670.

13. Wijermans P, Schaafsma M, van Norden Y, et al. Melphalan + prednisone versus melphalan + prednisone + thalidomide in induction therapy for multiple myeloma in elderly patients: final analysis of the Dutch cooperative group HOVON 49 study [Abstract]. *Blood* 2008;112:649.

14. Kapoor P, Rajkumar V, Dispenzieri A, et al. Melphalan and prednisone (MP) versus melphalan, prednisone and thalidomide (MPT) as initial therapy for previously untreated elderly and/or transplant ineligible patients with multiple myeloma: a meta-analysis of randomized controlled trials [Abstract 615]. *Blood* 2009.

15. Morgan GJ, Faith ED, Walter MG, et al. The addition of thalidomide to the induction treatment of newly presenting myeloma patients increases the CR rate which is likely to translate into improved PFS and OS [Abstract 352]. *Blood* 2009;114.

16. San Miguel JF, Schlag R, Khuageva NK, et al.; VISTA Trial Investigators. Bortezomib plus melphalan and prednisone for initial treatment of multiple myeloma. *N Engl J Med* 2008;359(9):906–917.

17. Mateos MV, Richardson PG, Schlag R, et al. Bortezomib plus melphalan–prednisone continues to demonstrate a survival benefit vs melphalan–prednisone in the phase III VISTA trial in previously untreated multiple myeloma after 3 years' follow-up and extensive subsequent therapy use [Abstract 3859]. Poster presented at: 51st Annual Meeting and Exposition of the American Society of Hematology; December 5–8, 2009; New Orleans, LA.

18. Mateos MV, Oriol A, Martinez J, et al. A prospective, multicenter, randomized, trial of bortezomib/melphalan/prednisone (VMP) versus bortezomib/thalidomide/prednisone (VTP) as induction therapy followed by maintenance treatment with bortezomib/thalidomide (VT) versus bortezomib/prednisone (VP) in elderly untreated patients with multiple myeloma older than 65 years [Abstract 3]. *Blood* 2009;114:3.

19. Niesvizky R, Reeves J, Flinn IW, et al. Phase 3b UPFRONT study: interim results from a community practice-based prospective randomized trial evaluating three bortezomib-based regimens in elderly, newly diagnosed myeloma patients [Abstract 129]. *Blood* 2009.

20. Palumbo A, Bringhen S, Rossi D, et al. Bortezomib, melphalan, prednisone and thalidomide (VMPT) followed by maintenance with bortezomib and thalidomide for initial treatment of elderly multiple myeloma patients [Abstract 128]. *Blood* 2009;114(22).

21. Gay F, Bringhen S, Genuardi M, et al. The weekly infusion of bortezomib reduces peripheral neuropathy [Abstract 3887]. *Blood* 2009.

22. Zonder JA, Crowley J, Hussein MA, et al. Superiority of lenalidomide (len) plus high-dose dexamethasone (HD) compared to HD alone as treatment of newly-diagnosed multiple myeloma (NDMM):

results of the randomized, double-blinded, placebo-controlled SWOG trial S0232 [Abstract 77]. *Blood* 2007;110(11):77.

23. Zonder JA, Crowley J, Bolejack V, et al. A randomized Southwest Oncology Group study comparing dexamethasone (D) to lenalidomide + dexamethasone (LD) as treatment of newly-diagnosed multiple myeloma (NDMM): impact of cytogenetic abnormalities on efficacy of LD, and updated overall study results [Abstract 8521]. *J Clin Oncol* 2008;26.

24. Rajkumar SV, Jacobus S, Callander NS, et al.; Eastern Cooperative Oncology Group. Lenalidomide plus high-dose dexamethasone versus lenalidomide plus low-dose dexamethasone as initial therapy for newly diagnosed multiple myeloma: an open-label randomised controlled trial. *Lancet Oncol* 2010;11(1):29–37.

25. Palumbo A, Falco P, Corradini P, et al.; GIMEMA–Italian Multiple Myeloma Network. Melphalan, prednisone, and lenalidomide treatment for newly diagnosed myeloma: a report from the GIMEMA–Italian Multiple Myeloma Network. *J Clin Oncol* 2007;25(28):4459–4465.

26. Palumbo A, Falco P, Falcone A, et al. Melphalan, prednisone, and lenalidomide for newly diagnosed myeloma: kinetics of neutropenia and thrombocytopenia and time-to-event results. *Clin Lymphoma Myeloma* 2009;9(2):145–150.

27. Palumbo A, Meletios A, Dimopoulos MA, et al. A phase III study to determine the efficacy and safety of lenalidomide in combination with melphalan and prednisone (MPR) in elderly patients with newly diagnosed multiple myeloma [Abstract 613]. *Blood* 2009;114:253.

28. Barlogie B, Tricot G, Anaissie E, et al. Thalidomide and hematopoietic-cell transplantation for multiple myeloma. *N Engl J Med* 2006;354(10):1021–1030.

29. Palumbo A, Bringhen S, Petrucci MT, et al. Intermediate-dose melphalan improves survival of myeloma patients aged 50 to 70: results of a randomized controlled trial. *Blood* 2004;104(10):3052–3057.

30. Palumbo A, Gay F, Falco P, et al. Bortezomib as induction before autologous transplantation, followed by lenalidomide as consolidation-maintenance in untreated multiple myeloma patients. *J Clin Oncol* 2010;28(5):800–807.

31. Richardson PG, Sonneveld P, Schuster MW, et al.; Assessment of Proteasome Inhibition for Extending Remissions (APEX) Investigators. Bortezomib or high-dose dexamethasone for relapsed multiple myeloma. *N Engl J Med* 2005;352(24):2487–2498.

32. Richardson PG, Sonneveld P, Schuster M, et al. Extended follow-up of a phase 3 trial in relapsed multiple myeloma: final time-to-event results of the APEX trial. *Blood* 2007;110(10):3557–3560.

33. Orlowski RZ, Nagler A, Sonneveld P, et al. Randomized phase III study of pegylated liposomal doxorubicin plus bortezomib compared with bortezomib alone in relapsed or refractory multiple myeloma: combination therapy improves time to progression. *J Clin Oncol* 2007;25(25):3892–3901.

34. Weber DM, Chen C, Niesvizky R, et al.; Multiple Myeloma (009) Study Investigators. Lenalidomide plus dexamethasone for relapsed multiple myeloma in North America. *N Engl J Med* 2007;357(21):2133–2142.

35. Dimopoulos M, Spencer A, Attal M, et al.; Multiple Myeloma (010) Study Investigators. Lenalidomide plus dexamethasone for relapsed or refractory multiple myeloma. *N Engl J Med* 2007;357(21):2123–2132.

36. Fermand J-P, Jaccard A, Macro M, et al. A randomized comparison of dexamethasone + thalidomide (dex/thal) vs dex + placebo (dex/p) in patients (pts) with relapsing multiple myeloma (MM) [Abstract 3563]. *Blood* 2006;108.

37. National Cancer Institute. Common Terminology Criteria for Adverse Events, v3.0, (CTCAE) http://ctep.cancer.gov/protocolDevelopment/electronic_applications/ctc.htm#ctc_v30. Accessed December 1, 2009.

38. Argyriou AA, Iconomou G, Kalofonos HP. Bortezomib-induced peripheral neuropathy in multiple myeloma: a comprehensive review of the literature. *Blood* 2008;112(5):1593–1599.

39. Palumbo A, Facon T, Sonneveld P, et al. Thalidomide for treatment of multiple myeloma: 10 years later. *Blood* 2008;111(8):3968–3977.

40. Palumbo A, Rajkumar SV, Dimopoulos MA, et al., International Myeloma Working Group. Prevention of thalidomide- and lenalidomide-associated thrombosis in myeloma. *Leukemia* 2008;22(2):414–423.

41. Palumbo A, Cavo M, Bringhen S, et al. A phase III study of enoxaparin vs aspirin vs low-dose warfarin as thromboprophylaxis for newly diagnosed myeloma patients treated with thalidomide based-regimens [Abstract 492]. *Blood* 2009;114.

42. Palumbo A, Cavallo F, Yehuda, et al. A prospective, randomized study of melphalan, prednisone, lenalidomide (MPR) versus melphalan (200 mg/m^2) and autologous transplantation (Mel200) in newly diagnosed myeloma patients: an interim analysis [Abstract 350]. *Blood* 2009;114.

43. Smith A, Wisloff F, Samson D. Guidelines on the diagnosis and management of multiple myeloma. *Br J Hematol* 2005;132:410–451.

44. Sezer O. Myeloma bone disease: recent advances in biology, diagnosis, and treatment. *Oncologist* 2009; 14(3):276–283.

45. Mill WB, Griffith R. The role of radiation therapy in the management of plasma cell tumors. *Cancer* 1980;45(4):647–652.

46. Leigh BR, Kurtts TA, Mack CF, Matzner MB, Shimm DS. Radiation therapy for the palliation of multiple myeloma. *Int J Radiat Oncol Biol Phys* 1993;25(5):801–804.

47. Hussein MA, Vrionis FD, Allison R, et al.; International Myeloma Working Group. The role of vertebral augmentation in multiple myeloma: International Myeloma Working Group Consensus Statement. *Leukemia* 2008;22(8):1479–1484.

48. Berenson JR, Tillman JB, Hussein MA, et al. A phase III trial of kyphoplasty versus nonsurgical care for cancer patients with vertebral fractures [Abstract 204]. *Clin Lymphoma Myeloma* 2009;28.

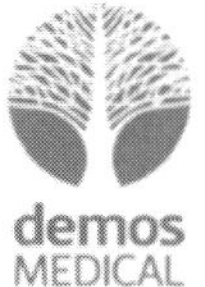

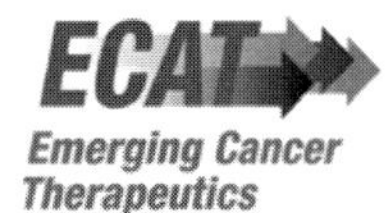

Relapsed and Refractory Multiple Myeloma

Taiga Nishihori* and Melissa Alsina

*H. Lee Moffitt Cancer Center and Research Institute,
University of South Florida, Tampa, FL*

■ ABSTRACT

Relapsed refractory multiple myeloma remains incurable and poses significant clinical challenges. Conventional chemotherapy and high-dose therapy followed by hematopoietic cell transplantation have been historically the mainstay of therapy. However, recent advancement and insights into the biology of myeloma and availability of novel therapeutic agents have changed the landscape of myeloma treatment. This chapter reviews the recent literatures for the treatment of relapsed and refractory myeloma including established regimens and newer regimens incorporating thalidomide, bortezomib and lenalidomide, with additional discussion on emerging therapeutics including carfilzomib and pomalidomide which may prove beneficial to patients with relapsed myeloma.

■ INTRODUCTION

Recent significant advances in the treatment of myeloma with the emergence of novel drugs and combination induce response rates in more than 90% of patients upfront. However, in most cases the disease eventually progresses, requiring subsequent therapeutic interventions. Despite the increased number of treatment options for these patients, relapsed and refractory multiple myeloma (MM) remains a significant clinical challenge, and there is an unmet medical need to improve the current status of its treatment outcomes. Median survival of patients with relapsed and refractory myeloma before the introduction of novel agents had been traditionally shorter and lasted approximately 10 months (1,2). Responses to chemotherapy in this setting are usually short.

---

*Corresponding author, H. Lee Moffitt Cancer Center and Research Institute, University of South Florida, Tampa, FL
E-mail addresses: taiga.nishihori@moffitt.org

Emerging Cancer Therapeutics 1:2 (2010) 383–402.
© 2010 Demos Medical Publishing LLC. All rights reserved.
DOI: 10.5003/2151–4194.1.2.383

demosmedpub.com/ecat

The traditional definitions of relapse and refractory MM are as follows. Relapse from a complete response (CR) is defined as reappearance of the serum or urinary paraprotein, ≥5% bone marrow plasma cells, new lytic bone lesions or soft-tissue plasmacytomas, an increase in the size of residual bone lesions, and/or development of hypercalcemia (corrected serum calcium > 11.5 mg/dL) not attributable to another cause (3). Criteria for progressive disease when a CR has not been achieved include new or expanding bone lesions, hypercalcemia and a > 25% increase in serum monoclonal paraprotein concentration, 24-hour urinary light chain excretion, or plasma cells within a bone marrow. Relapsed MM refers to a clinical scenario where a patient treated to the point of maximal response suffers from progressive disease, whereas refractory MM refers to one in which a patient is either unresponsive to the therapy or progresses within 60 days of last treatment. The International Myeloma Working Group has published criteria for relapsed and refractory MM, which is defined as those patients who have achieved minimal response (MR), relapse, and then progress while on salvage therapy (i.e., unresponsive to the therapy), or those who experience progression within 60 days of last therapy (4).

In the era prior to the development of novel biologics-based therapy for myeloma, including immunomodulatory drugs as well as proteasome inhibitors, relapse from successive treatment regimens resulted in progressively shorter response durations, which typically reflected emerging drug resistance, as well as changes in disease biology within each patient, with tumor cells expressing a more aggressive phenotype, higher proliferative fraction, and lower apoptotic rates. The ability of the immunomodulatory agents and proteasome inhibitors to overcome drug resistance was shown in preclinical models and confirmed in the context of clinical trials, leading to the US Food and Drug Administration approval of thalidomide, lenalidomide, and bortezomib in the treatment armamentarium for relapse and refractory MM.

Several prognostic factors have been identified for newly diagnosed MM; however, prognostic factors in relapsed and refractory myeloma have not been comprehensively defined. Nonetheless, within the overall adverse prognosis of relapsed and refractory myeloma, patients with poorer risk include those with t(4;14) or t(14;16) translocations, deletion of chromosome 17 or 13, hypodiploidy, high β2-microglobulin, and low serum albumin. Other clinical features including light chain myeloma, IgA isotype, renal failure, extramedullary disease, oligosecretory myeloma, and advanced bone disease may pose additional clinical challenges.

The advent of novel therapies targeting disease biology and tumor microenvironment has significantly improved the outlook and changed the landscape for patients with relapsed and refractory myeloma. Bortezomib, a first-in-class proteasome inhibitor, and the immunomodulatory agents, including thalidomide and lenalidomide, now constitute the backbone of contemporary myeloma regimens. We will focus on available treatment options and emerging agents for patients with relapsed and refractory MM.

■ THALIDOMIDE

The recognition of antiangiogenic properties of thalidomide led to its use in MM based on elevated levels of circulating angiogenic cytokines such as vascular endothelial growth factor and increased bone marrow vascularization (5–7). Further delineation of relationships between myeloma cells and the bone marrow microenvironment has shed light onto other more active and, perhaps, important biological properties of thalidomide that may contribute to antimyeloma activity (8). Thalidomide could also augment T-cell– and natural killer cell–mediated immunological responses, induce caspase-8–mediated apoptosis, block IL-6 production within the bone marrow microenvironment, and sensitize myeloma cells to other agents (9–12).

In the initial phase II study of thalidomide, of 84 patients with relapsed and refractory myeloma, most had relapsed after autologous transplant; 32% responded to single-agent thalidomide (13). In an update where 169 patients received thalidomide 200 to 800 mg per day, the initial results were confirmed with responses (≥50% reduction in M-protein) in 30% of patients with a 2% CR rate; 2-year event-free survival (EFS) and overall survival (OS) in this study were 26% and 48%, respectively. Toxicities of grade 3 or higher included the central nervous system and gastrointestinal and peripheral neuropathy (14). Nine years after the initiation of the trial, 10 patients remained event free and 17 alive, whereas 25% of patients had remained event free 2 years after discontinuing thalidomide. The presence of karyotypic abnormalities and λ light chain isotype were the major adverse prognostic factors affecting both EFS and OS (15). A systematic review of 42 studies with target dose of single-agent thalidomide ranging from 50 mg per day to 800 mg per day that included 1,629 patients has been reported (16). At least a partial response (PR) was noted in 29.4% (95% confidence interval [CI], 27–32%) with an additional 25% of patients achieving minor responses or disease stabilization and a median OS in all trials of approximately 14 months. Across studies, grade 3/4 adverse events included constipation, somnolence, neutropenia, and neuropathy. Toxicities appeared both cumulative and dose dependent. The incidences of somnolence, peripheral neurotoxicity, and thromboembolism were all higher at doses higher than 200 mg per day and worsened over time (16).

The optimal dose of thalidomide has not been adequately defined due to various doses used in many trials. Only a few patients could tolerate doses greater than 400 mg per day (13,15), and dose escalation beyond 400 mg per day seemed to increase toxicity rather than responses. The Intergroupe Francophone du Myeloma conducted a randomized trial in patients with relapsed or refractory myeloma to receive either 100 mg per day or 400 mg per day of thalidomide; dexamethasone was added for patients who did not respond after 3 months of therapy with single-agent thalidomide (17). Response rates in the 100 mg per day arm were lower (15% vs. 28%), but OS at 1 year was similar; toxicity was significantly higher in the 400-mg group. There was no difference in the rate of deep venous thrombosis (DVT) between the two groups. After the addition of dexamethasone, response rates were similar between 100-mg and 400-mg groups indicating that the addition of dexamethasone might increase thalidomide activity and permit lower thalidomide dose. Lower doses of thalidomide are preferred, particularly in individuals who may not tolerate thalidomide-related side effects.

Preclinical data indicate that thalidomide enhances antimyeloma activity of dexamethasone on myeloma cells (10). This observation was confirmed in several phase II studies showing the clinical activity of this combination (18–20). In a retrospective study, Thal/dex was as effective as a second autologous transplant in terms of response rate and progression-free survival (PFS), but it was associated with improved OS after first relapse compared with a second autologous transplant (21). In a systematic review, thal/dex was found to be superior (overall response rate [ORR], 51%; 95% CI, 45–57%) to single-agent thalidomide (ORR, 29%; 95% CI, 27–32%) (22). Responses with thal/dex are rapid with median time to response of approximately 1 month. When lower doses of thalidomide are used, there are fewer side effects including less neurotoxicity, sedation, somnolence, and constipation. However, the risk of DVT increases substantially, approaching 10% of patients treated with thal/dex for relapsed and refractory multiple myeloma developing DVT. Therefore, prophylaxis for DVT is required in this setting (23). Thal/dex remains a convenient oral regimen for patients with relapsed and refractory myeloma; however, the risk of neurotoxicity should be considered. The decision to use thal/dex at relapse may depend on the duration of response to prior thalidomide therapy, the time from prior thalidomide exposure, and the presence of neuropathy.

TABLE 1

Selected thalidomide + chemotherapy regimens for relapsed and refractory multiple myeloma

Reference	Regimen	N	ORR	PFS/EFS/TTP	Survival
Lee et al. (24)	[DTPACE] Dex 40 mg/day, days 1–4 Thal 400 mg/day Cisplatin 10 mg/m^2/day, CI days 1–4 Doxorubicin 10 mg/m^2/day, CI days 1–4 Cyclophosphamide 400 mg/m^2/day, CI days 1–4 Etoposide 40 mg/m^2/day, CI days 1–4 4-week cycles	236	32% (CR/nCR: 15%)	NR	NR
Moehler et al. (25)	[TCED] Thal 400 mg/day Dex 40 mg/day orally days 1–4 Cyclophosphamide 400 mg/m^2 CI days 1–4 Etoposide 40 mg/m^2 CI days 1–4 4-week cycle, up to 6 cycles	50	72% (CR 4%)	PFS: 16 months	Not reached
Offidani et al. (27)	Thal 400 mg/day Dex 40 mg/day, days 1–4, 9–12 Liposomal doxorubicin 40 mg/m^2 on day 1 4-week cycles	50	76% (CR/nCR 32%, VGPR 6%)	EFS: 17 months	Not reached
Kropff et al. (26)	[Hyper CDT] Cyclophosphamide 300 mg/m^2 IV over 3 hours every 12 hours days 1–3 Dex 20 mg/m2/day orally days 1–4, 9–12, 17–20 Thalidomide 100–400mg/day	60	72%	EFS: 11 months	19 months
Garcia-Sanz et al. (29)	[ThaCyDex] Thal 200–800 mg/day Dex 40 mg/day × 4days Cyclophosphamide orally 50 mg/day 3-week cycles	71	55% (CR 10%)	2-year PFS:57%	2-year OS: 66%

Continued

TABLE 1

Selected thalidomide + chemotherapy regimens for relapsed and refractory multiple myeloma   (*Continued*)

Reference	Regimen	N	ORR	PFS/EFS/TTP	Survival
Kyriakou et al. (30)	[Weekly CDT] Thal 100–300 mg/day Dex 40 mg/day; days 1–4 monthly Cyclophosphamide 300 mg/m^2 orally weekly	52	79% (CR 17%)	2-year EFS: 34%	2-year OS: 73%
Dimopoulos et al. (31)	[Pulsed CDT] Thal 400 mg/day; days 1–5 and 14–18 Dex 20 mg/m^2 orally days 1–5 and 14–18 Cyclophosphamide M150 mg/m^2 orally every 12 hours on days 1–5 4-week cycles for 3 cycles	53	≥ 60% PR	TTP: 12 months	17.5 months
Hussein et al. (108)	[DVd-T] Pegylated liposomal doxorubicin 40 mg/m^2 IV day 1 Vincristine 2 mg IV day 1 Dexamethasone 40 mg/m^2 orally days 1–4 Thalidomide 150–400 mg orally daily 4-week cycles, minimum of 6 cycles	49	75%	PFS: 15.5 months	OS: 39.9 months

CDT, cyclophosphamide, dexamethasone, thalidomide; CI, continuous infusion; CR, complete response; Dex, dexamethasone; DTPACE, dexamethasone, thalidomide, infusional cisplatin, doxorubicin, cyclophosphamide, and etoposide; DVd-T, pegylated liposomoal doxorubicin, vincristine, dexamethasone, thalidomide; EFS, event-free survival; IV, intravenously; nCR, near complete response; NR, not reported; ORR, overall response rate; OS, overall survival; PFS, progression-free survival; PR, partial response; TCED, thalidomide, cyclophosphamide, etoposide, dexamethasone; ThaCyDex, thalidomide, cyclophosphamide, dexamethasone; Thal, thalidomide; TTP, time to progression; VGPR, very good partial response.

Thalidomide has also been used in combination with other chemotherapeutic agents in the management of relapsed and refractory MM (Table 1). Response rates ranging from 32% to 76% have been reported but with increased toxicity and higher risk of DVT (24–28). The oral combination of cyclophosphamide, thalidomide, and dexamethasone has been used frequently especially in the elderly and in patients who are not heavily pretreated (29–31). Thalidomide, cyclophosphamide, and dexamethasone resulted in an ORR of 60% with 5% CR/near CR (nCR) rate (31). Time to progression (TTP) was 8.2 months, and OS was 17.5 months. Grade 3/4 neutropenia was reported in 26% of patients. Thalidomide and dexamethasone have been combined with cyclophosphamide and pegylated liposomal doxorubicin (PLD) (27). ORR for the combination of thalidomide, PLD, and dexamethasone was 76%, with 26% CR rate. EFS and PFS were 17 and 22 months, respectively. OS was not reached. Significant toxicities included neutropenia, DVT (12%), and severe infection (15%) (27). The access to thalidomide is currently restricted to individuals who participate in the System for Thalidomide Education and Prescription Safety (STEPS) program, implemented by the drug's manufacturer, due in part to the association between thalidomide and severe birth defects in the 1960s. An important safety consideration with thalidomide is the risk of DVT, which increases substantially when thalidomide is combined with corticosteroids and some chemotherapeutic agents, but not bortezomib (23,32). Other notable side effects associated with thalidomide include bradycardia, hypothyroidism, liver toxicity, and skin rash with a severe form being Stevens Johnson syndrome.

■ LENALIDOMIDE

In an effort to reduce the toxicity and enhance the activity of thalidomide, thalidomide analogues have been synthesized. Lenalidomide is an immunomodulatory derivative of thalidomide that demonstrates higher in vitro potency and greater activity than thalidomide in MM cell lines, suggesting that it may be effective in thalidomide-resistant patients (33). Following considerable promise and excellent tolerability of lenalidomide in relapsed myeloma in a series of phase I and II trials (33,34), two large, randomized, multicenter, double-blind, placebo-controlled phase III clinical trials comparing lenalidomide plus high-dose dexamethasone to high-dose dexamethasone alone have been reported

(35,36). In both studies, patients were randomly assigned to receive 25 mg of oral lenalidomide or placebo on days 1 to 21 of a 28-day cycle. All patients received dexamethasone on days 1 to 4, 9 to 12, and 17 to 20 for the first four cycles and subsequently, after the fourth cycle, only on days 1 to 4. In the North American study (MM-009), 171 patients were treated with lenalidomide plus dexamethasone; the ORR of 61% with 13% CR rate was encouraging. Furthermore, TTP was 11.1 months and median OS was 29.6 months. Of note, grade 3 or higher toxicities were neutropenia, DVT (including pulmonary embolism), thrombocytopenia, anemia, pneumonia, atrial fibrillation, fatigue, and diarrhea (35). In the European/Israeli/Australian study (MM-010), 176 patients were treated with lenalidomide plus high-dose dexamethasone. ORR was remarkable at 60.2% with 15.9% CR rate. TTP in this study was similar at 11.3 months and OS has not been reached. Reported grade 3 or higher toxicities also included neutropenia, thrombocytopenia, anemia, and DVT (36).

Lenalidomide has also been used in combination with both alkylating agents and anthracyclines in the treatment of relapsed and refractory MM (Table 2). In a phase II study involving 21 patients with relapsed and refractory disease, lenalidomide (25 mg on days 1–21), cyclophosphamide (500 mg on days 1, 8, 15, and 21), and dexamethasone (40 mg on days 1–4 and 12–15) produced an odds ratio rate of 65%, including 5% CR and 15% very good partial response (VGPR) (37). The combination of lenalidomide, doxorubicin, and dexamethasone was evaluated involving 69 patients with relapsed and refractory MM (38). This regimen produced an ORR of 73% in heavily treated patients. Deletion 17p and an elevated β2-microglobulin were associated with inferior outcomes. Single-agent lenalidomide has not been associated with an increased risk of thromboembolism (33). The combination of lenalidomide with higher-dose dexamethasone is associated with a higher risk of DVT, particularly with concomitant use of erythropoietin (39). Moreover, this

TABLE 2

Selected lenalidomide-based regimens for relapsed and refractory multiple myeloma

Reference	Regimen	N	ORR	PFS/EFS/TTP	Survival
Richardson et al. (34)	Len 30 mg/day or 15 mg twice a day, days 1–21 Dex 40 mg × 4 days, every 14 days for suboptimal response 4-week cycles	67 (QD) 35 (twice a day)	24% 29%	TTP: 7.7 months TTP: 3.9 moths	OS: 27 months OS: 27 months
Weber et al. [MM-009] (35)	Len 25 mg/day; days 1–21 Dex 40 mg/day; days 1–4, 9–12, 17–20 Dex 40 mg/day; days 1–4 only from cycle 5	170	61% (CR/ nCR 13%)	TTP: 11.1 months	OS: 29.6 months
Dimopoulos et al. [MM-010] (36)	Len 25 mg/day; days 1–21 Dex 40 mg/day; days 1–4, 9–12, 17–20 Dex 40 mg/day; days 1–4 only from cycle 5	176	60.2% (CR/ nCR 15%)	TTP: 11.3 months	Not reached
Morgan et al. (37)	Len 25 mg/day; days 1–21 Dex 40 mg/day; days 1–4 and 12–15 Cyclophosphamide 500 mg orally days 1, 8, 15, 21 4-week cycles for 9 cycles	21	65% (CR 5%; VGPR 15%)	NR	NR
Baz et al. (109)	Len 5–25 mg/day; orally days 1–21 Pegylated liposomal doxorubicin 40 mg/m^2 IV day 1 Vincristine 2mg IV day 1 Dex 40 mg/day; days 1–4 4-week cycle	52	75% (CR/ nCR 29%)	PFS: 12 months	Not reached

CR, complete response; Dex, dexamethasone; EFS, event-free survival; IV, intravenously; nCR, near complete response; Len, lenalidomide; NR, not reported; ORR, overall response rate; PFS, progression-free survival; PR, partial response; TTP, time to progression; QD, daily; VGPR, very good partial response.

risk appears to be elevated in patients who have had prior therapy with thalidomide and effective thromboprophylaxis would be a vital intervention (40). Lenalidomide is rarely associated with peripheral neuropathy. Myelosuppression, especially neutropenia, was the most common toxicity in the phase III trials of lenalidomide (35,36). Skin rash may occur in approximately a third of patients who receive lenalidomide (41). The teratogenic potential of lenalidomide in humans is unknown, but the access to lenalidomide is restricted to individuals who participate in the RevAssist program, administered by the drug's manufacturer. Other side effects of lenalidomide include fatigue, myalgia, and diarrhea. Patients with renal impairment (defined as a creatinine clearance less than 50 mL/min) could receive lenalidomide at the cost of higher rates of thrombocytopenia. Based on a pharmacokinetic study, specific dose adjustments have been proposed for various degrees of renal function as follows: no dose reduction for creatinine clearance ≥ 50 mL/min; 10 mg/day for creatinine clearance 30 to 50 mL/min; 15 mg every other day for patients with creatinine clearance < 30 mL/min but not on dialysis; and 15 mg three times per week after each dialysis on patient requiring dialysis (42).

■ BORTEZOMIB

Bortezomib is the first proteasome inhibitor to be used in humans with significant antiproliferative, proapoptotic, antiangiogenic, and antitumor activity through inhibition of proteasomal degradation of regulatory protein. It was granted accelerated approval for patients with relapsed and refractory myeloma in 2003.

Two phase II studies (SUMMIT and CREST) demonstrated activity of bortezomib in patients with relapsed and refractory myeloma (43,44). An international, randomized phase III (Assessment of Proteasome Inhibition for Extending Remissions [APEX]) trial compared bortezomib with high-dose dexamethasone in 669 patients with relapsed and refractory MM (45). The trial was stopped when the interim analysis demonstrated the superiority of single-agent bortezomib in terms of response rates, median TTP, and survival compared with high-dose dexamethasone. Final results of this trial confirmed these findings, as well as superior ORR of 43%, including a 15% CR/nCR with bortezomib monotherapy. Updated analysis with extended follow-up again confirmed that use of bortezomib resulted in a 6-month survival advantage (29.8 months vs. 23.7 months), despite more than 62%

rate of crossover to bortezomib from the high-dose dexamethasone arm (46).

Prolonged administration of bortezomib beyond 6 months or retreatment with bortezomib may be safe (47). Retrospective analyses have also shown that retreatment with bortezomib in patients who had an initial response to bortezomib is feasible and can result in objective responses without excess peripheral neuropathy (48,49). The most frequently reported grade 3/4 side effects leading to bortezomib discontinuation is peripheral neuropathy. The other side effects include fatigue and gastrointestinal symptoms. Careful assessment of neuropathy is the prerequisite especially in patients with pre-existing peripheral neuropathy from thalidomide, disease, or diabetes. Dose adjustment of bortezomib must be made before severe neuropathy develops. Bortezomib-induced peripheral neuropathy is generally reversible in the majority of patients. Bortezomib-related cytopenias (i.e., thrombocytopenia and neutropenia) are transient and cyclical. Patients with pre-existing mild thrombocytopenia may be at increased risk of grade 3/4 thrombocytopenia (50). Bortezomib has been demonstrated to be safe and active in patients with impaired renal function, even those patients requiring hemodialysis (51,52). Bortezomib-based combination regimens may improve renal function in patients with myeloma-related renal failure (53,54). There was a higher incidence of herpes zoster reactivation in APEX trial among patients who received bortezomib with dexamethasone (45). Viral prophylaxis is strongly recommended for patients receiving bortezomib-based therapy. Rare lung complications of bortezomib, including bronchiolitis obliterans with organizing pneumonia, diffuse alveolar hemorrhage, and pulmonary fibrosis have been reported (55–57).

Combination chemotherapy has been an area of active investigation (Table 3). Bortezomib has been shown to have significant activity in thalidomide-refractory patients (44,45), and may act synergistically with thalidomide (12). The combination of thalidomide and bortezomib may be a concern due to potential cumulative neurotoxicity

TABLE 3
Selected bortezomib-based regimens for relapsed and refractory multiple myeloma

Reference	Regimen	N	ORR	PFS/EFS/TTP	Survival
Orlowski et al. [MMY-3001] (64)	Bortezomib 1.3 mg/m^2 days 1, 4, 8, 11 Liposomal doxorubicin 30 mg/m^2 on day4 3-week cycles	324	44% (CR/nCR 13%)	TTP: 9.3 months	145 months OS: 76%
Palumbo et al. (110)	Bortezomib 1.3 mg/m^2 days 1, 4, 8, 11 Dex 40 mg/day; days 1–4 Doxorubicin 20 mg/m^2 days 1, 4 (34 patients) orLiposomal doxorubicin 30 mg/m^2 day 1 4-week cycle	64	67% (VGPR 25%)	1-year EFS: 34%	1-year OS: 66%
Berenson et al. (68)	Bortezomib 0.7–1.0 mg/m^2 IV days 1, 4, 8, 11 Melphalan 0.025–0.25 mg orally days 1–4 4-week cycle	46	50% (CR 4%)	PFS: 9 months	OS: 32 months
Kropff et al. (66)	Bortezomib 1.3 mg/m^2 IV days 1, 4, 8, 11 every 3 weeks ×8, then on days 1, 8, 15, 22 every 5 weeks ×3 Cyclophosphamide 50 mg orally daily Dexamethasone 20 mg/day; orally on the day of bortezomib	50	66% (CR 16%)	EFS: 12 months	OS: 20 months
Palumbo et al. (59)	Bortezomib 1.0–1.6mg/m2 IV days 1, 4, 15, 22 Melphalan 6 mg/m2/day; orally for 5 days Dexamethasone 60 mg/m2/day; for 5 days Thalidomide 50 mg/day; for 35 days Every 35 days for 6 cycles	30	67% (CR 17%)	1-year PFS: 61%	1-year OS: 84%

CR, complete response; Dex, dexamethasone; EFS, event-free survival; IV, intravenously; nCR, near complete response; NR, not reported; ORR, overall response rate; OS, overall survival; PFS, progression-free survival; PR, partial response; TTP, time to progression; VGPR, very good partial response.

from both agents; however, clinical trials have suggested that it is manageable. Bortezomib, thalidomide, and dexamethasone in heavily pretreated refractory patients with abnormal cytogenetics resulted in 63% PR rate and 22% nCR rate (58). Four-drug combinations of bortezomib, melphalan, prednisone/dexamethasone, and thalidomide either daily (VMPT) or intermittently (VMDT) showed significant ≥ 63% to 67% PR rate and ≥ 40% to 43% VGPR rate (59,60). Addition of other agents including doxorubicin or liposomal doxorubicin to the bortezomib/thalidomide combination also demonstrated significant responses (61–63). The result of a large phase III study comparing bortezomib and PLD with bortezomib alone in 636 relapsed patients was reported (64). TTP was significantly longer with the combination than with bortezomib alone (9.3 months vs. 6.5 months, respectively). Toxicities were somewhat higher with the combination, including higher rates of grade 3 or higher thrombocytopenia and neutropenia; rates of peripheral neuropathy were similar in the two treatment arms.

Lenalidomide is less neurotoxic compared with thalidomide; hence, combinations with bortezomib may have more favorable toxicity profile although increased myelosuppression may ensue. Preclinical data indicated sensitization of myeloma cells to bortezomib and dexamethasone by addition of lenalidomide (10). In a phase I multicenter dose-escalation study, the combination of lenalidomide and bortezomib was given to patients with relapse and refractory MM, including patients who had prior lenalidomide, bortezomib, thalidomide, or high-dose melphalan therapy (65). The maximum tolerated dose for lenalidomide was determined at 15 mg per day for 14 days and for bortezomib at 1.0 mg/m² on days 1, 4, 8, and 11 of a 21-day cycle. Toxicity was manageable; no significant peripheral neuropathy was reported and no anticoagulant prophylaxis was given. Among 36 evaluable patients, 39% achieved ≥ PR including 6% with CR/nCR. Responses were durable (median, 6 months). Bortezomib and dexamethasone have also been combined with cyclophosphamide (66).

In 50 patients, ORR was 82% with 12% CR/nCR; EFS was 12 months and OS was not reached at the time of presentation. Dose-limiting grade 3/4 toxicities with this combination included thrombocytopenia, infection, peripheral neuropathy, herpes zoster infection, fatigue, cardiovascular complications, diarrhea, and orthostatic hypotension (66). In a smaller study including prednisone in place of dexamethasone, the ORR was 45% with CR/nCR rate of 15% (67). Bortezomib has also been combined with low-dose melphalan. In 21 evaluable patients, the ORR was 47%, with 15% CR/nCR rate; PFS was 8 months. Grade 3/4 toxicities included neutropenia, thrombocytopenia, anemia, and hypocalcemia (68).

Bortezomib has, in addition, been combined with a new emerging agent. Histone acetylation modulates gene expression, cellular differentiation, and survival; it is regulated by the opposing activity of histone acetyltransferases and histone deacetylases (HDACs). HDAC inhibition induces differentiation and/or apoptosis in transformed cells, and it has been hypothesized that HDAC inhibition could act as a "master switch" that may simultaneously affect multiple cellular pathways critical for survival in MM cells. Based on preclinical data (69,70), a phase I dose escalation of oral vorinostat, a histone deacetylase inhibitor (at 200, 250, and 300 mg orally twice a day for 5 consecutive days followed by 2 days of rest), was administered every month in patients with relapsed and refractory MM (71). In combination with bortezomib, 2 pilot studies have been conducted using vorinostat (72,73). Eight patients (50%) achieved PR or nCR.

■ EMERGING THERAPEUTICS

Carfilzomib

Second-generation proteasome inhibitors and the new immunomodulatory compounds are undergoing active evaluation in clinical trials in patients with relapsed and refractory MM. Two second-generation proteasome inhibitors—carfilzomib (PR-171) and salinosporamide (NPI-0052)—have shown significant antimyeloma activity in preclinical models and are being investigated in clinical trials (74,75). Both agents irreversibly inhibit the proteasome in contrast to the reversible nature of bortezomib-induced proteasome inhibition and have the potential for oral administration. Unlike bortezomib, carfilzomib has activity only against the chymotryptic-like activity of the 20S proteasome (75), whereas salinosporamide inhibits the tryptic-like and caspase-like activity of the 20S proteasome as well as chymotryptic-like activity (74). In vitro studies have suggested that both agents possess activity against bortezomib-refractory disease (74,75). In two phase II clinical trials of carfilzomib, patients were treated with 20 mg/m² of carfilzomib intravenously on days 1, 2, 8, 9, 15, and 16 every 28 days, for up to 12 cycles (76–79). In the updated 51 patients, ORR was 45% with 1 CR and 4 VGPR (78). An additional 18% of patients had MR and 20% experienced stable disease (SD). The most common adverse events were fatigue (59%), nausea (41%), dyspnea (36%), and anemia (29%). Dose modifications were rarely required. Peripheral neuropathy of any grade was infrequent (12%). Of 12 patients with impaired renal function at baseline, none required dose modifications due to renal adverse events. The study is ongoing and subjects are now permitted to be on dose level of 27 mg/m². In the bortezomib-treated cohort (33 patients), ORR was 18% with 1 CR and 5 PRs. An additional 12% of patients had MR and 39% had SD (79). In a phase Ib dose-escalating trial, carfilzomib was combined with lenalidomide and low-dose dexamethasone (CRd) (80). An active dose of carfilzomib at 20 mg/m² in combination with full-dose lenalidomide (25 mg) and low-dose dexamethasone has been established as a tolerated dose. A phase III trial of CRd versus lenalidomide plus low-dose dexamethasone is planned.

Pomalidomide

Pomalidomide (CC4047), an analog of the immunomodulatory drugs thalidomide and lenalidomide, exerts antimyeloma activity through various mechanisms (10–12). At least when measured in in vitro studies, pomalidomide is a more potent immunomodulatory agent (81–83). Previously reported two phase I clinical trials in patients with relapsed and refractory MM showed that pomalidomide was well tolerated in doses ranging from 1 to 5 mg per day and produced a PR rate of at least 50% (84,85). The first phase II trial of pomalidomide combined with low-dose dexamethasone in patients with relapsed or refractory MM was reported (86). Sixty patients were enrolled. Pomalidomide was given orally at a dose of 2 mg daily on days 1 through 28 of a 28-day cycle. Dexamethasone was given orally at a dose of 40 mg daily on days 1, 8, 15, and 22 of each cycle. Aspirin 325 mg orally daily was given as prophylaxis for thromboembolic disease. ORR was 63% with 5% of CR and 28% VGPR. Responses were seen in 40% of lenalidomide-refractory, 37% of thalidomide-refractory, and 60% of bortezomib-refractory patients. Toxicity consisted primarily of myelosuppression. Neutropenia was seen in 35% of patients. One patient had a thromboembolic event. In truly lenalidomide-refractory (relapsing on or within 60 days of stopping lenalidomide) heavily pretreated additional 34 patients, pomalidomide and dexamethasone were administered with the same schedule (87). Nine (26%) demonstrated PR and 53% had SD suggesting non–cross-resistant nature of pomalidomide with lenalidomide.

Other Investigational Agents

There are a number of new investigational compounds targeting novel pathways that have entered early phases of clinical trials. Those compounds would include but are not limited to perifosine (an AKT inhibitor, KRX-0401), panobinostat (a second HDAC inhibitor, LBH589), and CNTO 328 (IL-6 monoclonal antibody). Selected results of these new compounds are summarized in Table 4.

TABLE 4
Selected investigational agents for relapsed and refractory multiple myeloma

Reference	Regimen	N	PR/CR
Richardson et al. (111)	Perifosine 50–100 mg/day; orally, days 1–21 Bortezomib 1–1.3 mg/m²/day; IV days 1, 4, 8, 11 Dex 20 mg/day; orally days 1, 2, 4, 5, 8.9, 11, 12	57	PR 16%; CR 4%
Rossi et al. (112)	CNTO 328 6 mg/kg/day; IV, every 2 weeks Bortezomib 1.3 mg/m²/day; IV days 1, 4, 8, 11	21	PR 57%; CR 14%
Voorhees et al. (113)	CNTO 328 6 mg/kg IV every 2 weeks Dexamethasone 40 mg orally days 1–4, 9–12, 17–20	36	PR 19%; CR 0%
Siegel et al. (114)	Panobinostat 10–20 mg/day orally three times per week Bortezomib 1 mg/m²/day IV days 1, 4, 8, 11 Dexamethasone after cycle 1 for progression	14	PR 29%; CR 7%
Hofmeister et al. (115)	NPI-0052 0.025–0.6 mg/m² IV days 1, 8, 15	17	PR 0%; CR 0%
Harrison et al. (116)	Bortezomib 1.3 mg/m²/day; IV days 1, 4, 8, 11 Dexamethasone 20 mg/day orally days 1, 2, 4, 5, 8, 9, 11, 12 Romidepsin 8–10 mg/m²/day IV days 1, 8, 18	18	PR 67%; CR/nCR 22%
Jakubowiak et al. (117)	Pomalidomide 50–100 mg/day orally days 1–28 Lenalidomide 15–25 mg/day orally days 1–21 Dexamethasone 20 mg/day orally days 1–4, 9–12, 17–20 for 4 cycles, then 20 mg/day days 1–4	32	PR 6%; CR 0%

CR, complete response; Dex, dexamethasone; IV, intravenously; nCR, near complete response; NR, not reported; PR partial response.

■ TRANSPLANT APPROACH

Autologous

Preclinical data have shown that increased doses of alkylating agents may overcome resistance to conventional chemotherapy leading to the introduction of high-dose melphalan for patients with refractory myeloma. Barlogie et al (88) pioneered the use of high-dose melphalan with or without autologous bone marrow infusion in patients with refractory myeloma in the 1980s. Although most patients responded, remission duration was short-lived and significant treatment-related mortality was observed in those who did not receive autologous marrow infusion. The same group studied a more intensive regimen including high-dose melphalan and total body irradiation (TBI) with autologous bone marrow support, which was found to have both significant activity and toxicity (89). A retrospective analysis of refractory myeloma patients who underwent various high-dose therapy regimens demonstrated significant mortality in patients receiving TBI. Melphalan at a dose of 200 mg/m² with stem cell support and low β2-microglobulin levels was associated with improved outcomes (90). Myeloablative conditioning in refractory myeloma may be more efficacious when administered early in the course of the disease. Retrospective comparisons have suggested that patient with primary resistant disease could benefit from early myeloablative therapy, but this was not the case in patients with long-standing resistant disease (91,92). It has been shown that some patients who relapse after one or two autologous transplant(s) could still be salvaged from high-dose melphalan (93,94). A randomized trial exploring the optimal timing for autologous transplantation has demonstrated similar survival in patients who received high-dose melphalan upfront compared with those who received salvage transplants (95). Among patients who received salvage high-dose melphalan, 2-year survival was 59% for those with relapsing disease and 57% for those with primary refractory disease. The current role of high-dose melphalan followed by autologous hematopoietic cell transplantation in the management of relapsed and refractory MM may be limited due to the availability and ease of novel agents. However, for those patients who achieve long-term treatment-free interval after the first transplantation, a second high-dose chemotherapy with autologous hematopoietic cell transplantation may be offered with a significant probability of long-term remission. Unfortunately, those patients who did not demonstrate reasonable response after a first autologous transplant will not be likely to benefit from a second course of transplant at relapse.

Allogeneic

Allogeneic hematopoietic cell transplantation could be an option for selected patients with an HLA-matched donor. Allogeneic transplant could induce molecular remissions in certain refractory myeloma cases. However, allogeneic hematopoietic cell transplantation is associated with significant toxicity and mortality, largely due to graft-versus-host disease and infectious complications. In a retrospective comparison, allogeneic transplantation may offer superior PFS and OS than

autologous transplant, at the expense of significantly higher transplant-related complications and toxic deaths (94). Reduced-intensity conditioning regimens have been introduced in order to minimize transplant-related toxicity while exploiting potential benefit of graft-versus-myeloma effect. However, the graft-versus-tumor effect may be less potent in myeloma compared to those in leukemia or lymphoma. Initial reports with reduced-intensity conditioning regimens demonstrated that prior cytoreduction was essential to produce good responses after allogeneic transplant which was later confirmed by an analysis of transplant registry dataset (96). Donor lymphocyte infusion at the time of relapse after allogeneic transplant may remain a viable option inducing remissions in some cases. In the context of exploiting graft-versus-myeloma effect, high-dose melphalan and autologous hematopoietic cell transplantation followed by reduced-intensity conditioning and allogeneic transplantation was given in 54 patients, of whom 26 (48%) had refractory or relapsed disease. Transplant-related mortality was 22%, but 57% of patients achieved CR (97). The Arkansas group reported similar results using melphalan 100 mg/m^2 followed by reduced-intensity conditioning of TBI and fludarabine at the expense of higher transplant mortality (98). Others have also identified that relapse after prior high-dose melphalan and autologous transplant is associated with poor outcome after reduced-intensity allogeneic transplant (99,100), while a study comparing autologous to reduced-intensity allogeneic transplant following relapse from autologous transplant found no significant difference in PFS or OS (101). Prior high-dose melphalan may also be a poor prognostic factor for treatment-related mortality in patients receiving allogeneic transplant (102). The role of allogeneic hematopoietic cell transplant for the treatment strategy for patients with relapsed and refractory MM remains controversial. This option is usually limited to selected young patients with an HLA-matched donor, and should be further explored in the context of well-designed clinical trials.

■ CHOICE OF TREATMENT STRATEGY

A number of factors will be considered when determining appropriate therapy for a patient with relapsed and refractory MM. These would include comorbidities, previous therapy, time from previous treatment, mode of drug administration, potential role of autologous or allogeneic hematopoietic cell transplantation, and patient preference. The disease risk level could also be obtained using the International Staging System at the time of initial treatment, the plasma cell labeling index, and conventional as well as florescence in situ hybridization (FISH)-based cytogenetic analysis, which may influence treatment decision. Those patients who have responded to a first or subsequent line of treatment and maintained long-lasting response (i.e., 1 or 2 years), a reintroduction of the same agent or regimen could be considered and may be beneficial. Patients who had prior autologous hematopoietic cell transplantation and relapse within 1 year after high-dose chemotherapy have a poor prognosis (103). These patients should be encouraged to participate in clinical trials of novel agents when available. Otherwise, these patients are candidates for lenalidomide plus dexamethasone or bortezomib plus dexamethasone or other combinations. Retrospective analysis of phase III study have suggested that when these agents are given at first relapse, they are associated with a more superior outcome than when given at a later stage of the disease (45). Patients who relapse after thalidomide-based treatment may respond to lenalidomide- or bortezomib-based treatments (40,45).

Certain clinical scenarios may favor one treatment strategy over another. Thalidomide may be appropriate for patients with clinically significant cytopenias due to its less myelosuppressive potential. Lenalidomide is the preferred agent for patients with pre-existing peripheral neuropathy and for those who prefer oral formulation of the therapy and could not accommodate frequent clinical visits. Lenalidomide requires careful dose adjustment and close follow-up of the renal function. Bortezomib may be strongly considered in patients with high-risk disease based on cytogenetic information, those with significant underlying renal impairment, especially those with myeloma-related renal failure, as well as those with advanced bone disease due to its ability to both inhibit osteoclastogenesis and promote osteoblast differentiation and proliferation (104,105). Bortezomib-based combinations are associated with a significant probability of renal function improvement. Bortezomib-induced neuropathy in most cases improves within 6 months after discontinuing bortezomib therapy, and in many patients who achieve reasonable response to bortezomib, this agent could be reintroduced perhaps at a lower dose (47–49). Both bortezomib and lenalidomide have been shown to overcome the poor prognosis conferred by the deletion of chromosome 13 (106). Bortezomib has also been shown to overcome the poor prognostic factors of elevated β2-microglobulin and low serum albumin, as well as being active in patients with advanced bone disease, plasmacytoma, and extramedullary involvement (107). As noted throughout this chapter, combination regimens of these agents are appropriate for certain patients with relapsed and refractory MM. Chemotherapy may also be an option for the treatment. Anthracyclines, either doxorubicin or liposomal formulations, and cyclophosphamide have shown significant activity when they are combined with novel agents and may even be given to patients with moderate renal impairment. Low-dose chemotherapy with cyclophosphamide, with alternate-date low-dose corticosteroids, may also be an option for those patients with limited performance status.

■ CONCLUSIONS

Until recently, management strategies for patients with relapsed and refractory MM have been limited to conventional chemotherapy and occasionally autologous stem cell transplantation. Given that patients with recurring disease typically are more symptomatic, with potential comorbidities, may be older, and are characteristically resistant to treatment, relapsed and refractory disease remains especially challenging for clinicians to treat. Although development of the novel agents thalidomide, lenalidomide, and bortezomib as well as the combinations of these agents and other chemotherapy agents have improved outcomes for patients with relapsed and refractory MM, the disease unfortunately remains incurable. Relapsed and refractory MM constitutes an important area of ongoing research efforts. Characterization of disease at molccular level and bone marrow microenvironment has provided the platform for the development of the novel agents as well as emerging new compounds. Newer drugs are showing promise in clinical trials, specifically carfilzomib and pomalidomide. The drug combinations that target different oncogenic pathways may express greater antimyeloma activity and are expected to make progress in the treatment of patients with relapsed and refractory disease. Treatment-associated toxicities and effects on quality of life should also be considered to inform decisions in terms of the treatment choice for an individual patient.

■ REFERENCES

1. Dalton WS, Crowley JJ, Salmon SS, et al. A phase III randomized study of oral verapamil as a chemosensitizer to reverse drug resistance in patients with refractory myeloma. A Southwest Oncology Group study. *Cancer* 1995;75(3):815–820.
2. Kyle RA, Gailani S, Seligman BR, et al. Multiple myeloma resistant to melphalan: treatment with cyclophosphamide, prednisone, and BCNU. *Cancer Treat Rep* 1979;63(8):1265–1269.
3. Bladé J, Samson D, Reece D, et al. Criteria for evaluating disease response and progression in patients with multiple myeloma treated by high-dose therapy and haemopoietic stem cell transplantation. Myeloma Subcommittee of the EBMT. European Group for Blood and Marrow Transplant. *Br J Haematol* 1998;102(5):1115–1123.
4. Durie BG, Harousseau JL, Miguel JS, et al.; International Myeloma Working Group. International uniform response criteria for multiple myeloma. *Leukemia* 2006;20(9):1467–1473.
5. D'Amato RJ, Loughnan MS, Flynn E, Folkman J. Thalidomide is an inhibitor of angiogenesis. *Proc Natl Acad Sci USA* 1994;91(9):4082–4085.
6. Vacca A, Ribatti D, Roncali L, et al. Bone marrow angiogenesis and progression in multiple myeloma. *Br J Haematol* 1994;87(3):503–508.
7. Vacca A, Di Loreto M, Ribatti D, et al. Bone marrow of patients with active multiple myeloma: angiogenesis and plasma cell adhesion molecules LFA-1, VLA-4, LAM-1, and CD44. *Am J Hematol* 1995; 50(1):9–14.
8. Mitsiades CS, Mitsiades NS, Munshi NC, Richardson PG, Anderson KC. The role of the bone microenvironment in the pathophysiology and therapeutic management of multiple myeloma: interplay of growth factors, their receptors and stromal interactions. *Eur J Cancer* 2006;42(11):1564–1573.
9. Anderson KC. Lenalidomide and thalidomide: mechanisms of action–similarities and differences. *Semin Hematol* 2005;42(4 suppl 4):S3–S8.
10. Hideshima T, Chauhan D, Shima Y, et al. Thalidomide and its analogs overcome drug resistance of human multiple myeloma cells to conventional therapy. *Blood* 2000;96(9):2943–2950.
11. Davies FE, Raje N, Hideshima T, et al. Thalidomide and immunomodulatory derivatives augment natural killer cell cytotoxicity in multiple myeloma. *Blood* 2001;98(1):210–216.
12. Mitsiades N, Mitsiades CS, Poulaki V, et al. Apoptotic signaling induced by immunomodulatory thalidomide analogs in human multiple myeloma cells: therapeutic implications. *Blood* 2002;99(12):4525–4530.
13. Singhal S, Mehta J, Desikan R, et al. Antitumor activity of thalidomide in refractory multiple myeloma. *N Engl J Med* 1999;341(21):1565–1571.
14. Barlogie B, Desikan R, Eddlemon P, et al. Extended survival in advanced and refractory multiple myeloma after single-agent thalidomide: identification of prognostic factors in a phase 2 study of 169 patients. *Blood* 2001;98(2):492–494.
15. van Rhee F, Dhodapkar M, Shaughnessy JD Jr, et al. First thalidomide clinical trial in multiple myeloma: a decade. *Blood* 2008;112(4):1035–1038.
16. Glasmacher A, Hahn C, Hoffmann F, et al. A systematic review of phase-II trials of thalidomide monotherapy in patients with relapsed or refractory multiple myeloma. *Br J Haematol* 2006;132(5):584–593.

17. Yakoub-Agha I, Attal M, Dumontet C, et al. Thalidomide in patients with advanced multiple myeloma: a study of 83 patients report of the Intergroupe Francophone du Myélome (IFM). *Hematol J* 2002;3(4):185–192.

18. Dimopoulos MA, Zervas K, Kouvatseas G, et al. Thalidomide and dexamethasone combination for refractory multiple myeloma. *Ann Oncol* 2001;12(7):991–995.

19. Anagnostopoulos A, Weber D, Rankin K, Delasalle K, Alexanian R. Thalidomide and dexamethasone for resistant multiple myeloma. *Br J Haematol* 2003; 121(5):768–771.

20. Palumbo A, Giaccone L, Bertola A, et al. Low-dose thalidomide plus dexamethasone is an effective salvage therapy for advanced myeloma. *Haematologica* 2001;86(4):399–403.

21. Palumbo A, Falco P, Ambrosini MT, et al. Thalidomide plus dexamethasone is an effective salvage regimen for myeloma patients relapsing after autologous transplant. *Eur J Haematol* 2005;75(5):391–395.

22. von Lilienfeld-Toal M, Hahn-Ast C, Furkert K, et al. A systematic review of phase II trials of thalidomide/dexamethasone combination therapy in patients with relapsed or refractory multiple myeloma. *Eur J Haematol* 2008;81(4):247–252.

23. Palumbo A, Rajkumar SV, Dimopoulos MA, et al.; International Myeloma Working Group. Prevention of thalidomide- and lenalidomide-associated thrombosis in myeloma. *Leukemia* 2008;22(2):414–423.

24. Lee CK, Barlogie B, Munshi N, et al. DTPACE: an effective, novel combination chemotherapy with thalidomide for previously treated patients with myeloma. *J Clin Oncol* 2003;21(14):2732–2739.

25. Moehler TM, Neben K, Benner A, et al. Salvage therapy for multiple myeloma with thalidomide and CED chemotherapy. *Blood* 2001;98(13):3846–3848.

26. Kropff MH, Lang N, Bisping G, et al. Hyperfractionated cyclophosphamide in combination with pulsed dexamethasone and thalidomide (HyperCDT) in primary refractory or relapsed multiple myeloma. *Br J Haematol* 2003;122(4):607–616.

27. Offidani M, Corvatta L, Marconi M, et al. Low-dose thalidomide with pegylated liposomal doxorubicin and high-dose dexamethasone for relapsed/refractory multiple myeloma: a prospective, multicenter, phase II study. *Haematologica* 2006;91(1):133–136.

28. Zangari M, Barlogie B, Thertulien R, et al. Thalidomide and deep vein thrombosis in multiple myeloma: risk factors and effect on survival. *Clin Lymphoma* 2003;4(1):32–35.

29. García-Sanz R, González-Porras JR, Hernández JM, et al. The oral combination of thalidomide, cyclophosphamide and dexamethasone (ThaCyDex) is effective in relapsed/refractory multiple myeloma. *Leukemia* 2004;18(4):856–863.

30. Kyriakou C, Thomson K, D'Sa S, et al. Low-dose thalidomide in combination with oral weekly cyclophosphamide and pulsed dexamethasone is a well tolerated and effective regimen in patients with relapsed and refractory multiple myeloma. *Br J Haematol* 2005;129(6):763–770.

31. Dimopoulos MA, Hamilos G, Zomas A, et al. Pulsed cyclophosphamide, thalidomide and dexamethasone: an oral regimen for previously treated patients with multiple myeloma. *Hematol J* 2004;5(2):112–117.

32. Hussein MA. Thromboembolism risk reduction in multiple myeloma patients treated with immunomodulatory drug combinations. *Thromb Haemost* 2006;95(6):924–930.

33. Richardson PG, Schlossman RL, Weller E, et al. Immunomodulatory drug CC-5013 overcomes drug resistance and is well tolerated in patients with relapsed multiple myeloma. *Blood* 2002;100(9):3063–3067.

34. Richardson PG, Blood E, Mitsiades CS, et al. A randomized phase 2 study of lenalidomide therapy for patients with relapsed or relapsed and refractory multiple myeloma. *Blood* 2006;108(10):3458–3464.

35. Weber DM, Chen C, Niesvizky R, et al.; Multiple Myeloma (009) Study Investigators. Lenalidomide plus dexamethasone for relapsed multiple myeloma in North America. *N Engl J Med* 2007;357(21):2133–2142.

36. Dimopoulos M, Spencer A, Attal M, et al.; Multiple Myeloma (010) Study Investigators. Lenalidomide plus dexamethasone for relapsed or refractory multiple myeloma. *N Engl J Med* 2007;357(21):2123–2132.

37. Morgan GJ, Schey SA, Wu P, et al. Lenalidomide (Revlimid), in combination with cyclophosphamide and dexamethasone (RCD), is an effective and tolerated regimen for myeloma patients. *Br J Haematol* 2007;137(3):268–269.

38. Knop S, Gerecke C, Liebisch P, et al. Lenalidomide, adriamycin, and dexamethasone (RAD) in patients with relapsed and refractory multiple myeloma: a report from the German Myeloma Study Group DSMM (Deutsche Studiengruppe Multiples Myelom). *Blood* 2009;113(18):4137–4143.

39. Knight R, DeLap RJ, Zeldis JB. Lenalidomide and venous thrombosis in multiple myeloma. *N Engl J Med* 2006;354(19):2079–2080.

40. Wang M, Dimopoulos MA, Chen C, et al. Lenalidomide plus dexamethasone is more effective than dexamethasone alone in patients with relapsed or refractory multiple myeloma regardless of prior thalidomide exposure. *Blood* 2008;112(12):4445–4451.

41. Sviggum HP, Davis MD, Rajkumar SV, Dispenzieri A. Dermatologic adverse effects of lenalidomide therapy for amyloidosis and multiple myeloma. *Arch Dermatol* 2006;142(10):1298–1302.

42. Chen N, Lau H, Kong L, et al. Pharmacokinetics of lenalidomide in subjects with various degrees of renal impairment and in subjects on hemodialysis. *J Clin Pharmacol* 2007;47(12):1466–1475.

43. Jagannath S, Barlogie B, Berenson J, et al. A phase 2 study of two doses of bortezomib in relapsed or refractory myeloma. *Br J Haematol* 2004;127(2): 165–172.

44. Richardson PG, Barlogie B, Berenson J, et al. A phase 2 study of bortezomib in relapsed, refractory myeloma. *N Engl J Med* 2003;348(26):2609–2617.

45. Richardson PG, Sonneveld P, Schuster MW, et al.; Assessment of Proteasome Inhibition for Extending Remissions (APEX) Investigators. Bortezomib or high-dose dexamethasone for relapsed multiple myeloma. *N Engl J Med* 2005;352(24):2487–2498.

46. Richardson PG, Sonneveld P, Schuster M, et al. Extended follow-up of a phase 3 trial in relapsed multiple myeloma: final time-to-event results of the APEX trial. *Blood* 2007;110(10):3557–3560.

47. Berenson JR, Jagannath S, Barlogie B, et al. Safety of prolonged therapy with bortezomib in relapsed or refractory multiple myeloma. *Cancer* 2005;104(10):2141–2148.

48. Wolf J, Richardson PG, Schuster M, LeBlanc A, Walters IB, Battleman DS. Utility of bortezomib retreatment in relapsed or refractory multiple myeloma patients: a multicenter case series. *Clin Adv Hematol Oncol* 2008;6(10):755–760.

49. Conner TM, Doan QD, Walters IB, LeBlanc AL, Beveridge RA. An observational, retrospective analysis of retreatment with bortezomib for multiple myeloma. *Clin Lymphoma Myeloma* 2008;8(3):140–145.

50. Lonial S, Waller EK, Richardson PG, et al.; SUMMIT/CREST Investigators. Risk factors and kinetics of thrombocytopenia associated with bortezomib for relapsed, refractory multiple myeloma. *Blood* 2005;106(12):3777–3784.

51. Chanan-Khan AA, Kaufman JL, Mehta J, et al. Activity and safety of bortezomib in multiple myeloma patients with advanced renal failure: a multicenter retrospective study. *Blood* 2007;109(6):2604–2606.

52. San-Miguel JF, Richardson PG, Sonneveld P, et al. Efficacy and safety of bortezomib in patients with renal impairment: results from the APEX phase 3 study. *Leukemia* 2008;22(4):842–849.

53. Dimopoulos MA, Roussou M, Gavriatopoulou M, et al. Reversibility of renal impairment in patients with multiple myeloma treated with bortezomib-based regimens: identification of predictive factors. *Clin Lymphoma Myeloma* 2009;9(4):302–306.

54. Roussou M, Kastritis E, Migkou M, et al. Treatment of patients with multiple myeloma complicated by renal failure with bortezomib-based regimens. *Leuk Lymphoma* 2008;49(5):890–895.

55. Zappasodi P, Dore R, Castagnola C, et al. Rapid response to high-dose steroids of severe bortezomib-related pulmonary complication in multiple myeloma. *J Clin Oncol* 2007;25(22):3380–3381.

56. Miyakoshi S, Kami M, Yuji K, et al. Severe pulmonary complications in Japanese patients after bortezomib treatment for refractory multiple myeloma. *Blood* 2006;107(9):3492–3494.

57. Duek A, Feldberg E, Haran M, Berrebi A. Pulmonary fibrosis in a myeloma patient on bortezomib treatment. A new severe adverse effect of a new drug. *Am J Hematol* 2007;82(6):502–503.

58. Pineda-Roman M, Zangari M, van Rhee F, et al. VTD combination therapy with bortezomib-thalidomide-dexamethasone is highly effective in advanced and refractory multiple myeloma. *Leukemia* 2008;22(7):1419–1427.

59. Palumbo A, Ambrosini MT, Benevolo G, et al.; Italian Multiple Myeloma Network; Gruppo Italiano Malattie Ematologicche dell'Adulto. Bortezomib, melphalan, prednisone, and thalidomide for relapsed multiple myeloma. *Blood* 2007;109(7):2767–2772.

60. Terpos E, Kastritis E, Roussou M, et al. The combination of bortezomib, melphalan, dexamethasone and intermittent thalidomide is an effective regimen for relapsed/refractory myeloma and is associated with improvement of abnormal bone metabolism and angiogenesis. *Leukemia* 2008;22(12): 2247–2256.

61. Chanan-Khan A, Miller KC. Velcade, Doxil and Thalidomide (VDT) is an effective salvage regimen for patients with relapsed and refractory multiple myeloma. *Leuk Lymphoma* 2005;46(7):1103–1104.

62. Ciolli S, Leoni F, Casini C, Breschi C, Santini V, Bosi A. The addition of liposomal doxorubicin to bortezomib, thalidomide and dexamethasone significantly improves clinical outcome of advanced multiple myeloma. *Br J Haematol* 2008;141(6):814–819.

63. Chanan-Khan A, Miller KC, Musial L, et al. Bortezomib in combination with pegylated liposomal doxorubicin and thalidomide is an effective steroid independent salvage regimen for patients with relapsed or refractory multiple myeloma: results of a phase II clinical trial. *Leuk Lymphoma* 2009;50(7):1096–1101.

64. Orlowski RZ, Nagler A, Sonneveld P, et al. Randomized phase III study of pegylated liposomal doxorubicin plus bortezomib compared with bortezomib alone in relapsed or refractory multiple myeloma: combination therapy improves time to progression. *J Clin Oncol* 2007;25(25):3892–3901.

65. Richardson PG, Weller E, Jagannath S, et al. Multicenter, phase I, dose-escalation trial of lenalidomide plus bortezomib for relapsed and relapsed/refractory multiple myeloma. *J Clin Oncol* 2009;27(34): 5713–5719.

66. Kropff M, Bisping G, Schuck E, et al.; Deutsche Studiengruppe Multiples Myelom,. Bortezomib in combination with intermediate-dose dexamethasone and continuous low-dose oral cyclophosphamide for relapsed multiple myeloma. *Br J Haematol* 2007;138(3):330–337.

67. Reece DE, Rodriguez GP, Chen C, et al. Phase I-II trial of bortezomib plus oral cyclophosphamide and prednisone in relapsed and refractory multiple myeloma. *J Clin Oncol* 2008;26(29):4777–4783.

68. Berenson JR, Yang HH, Sadler K, et al. Phase I/II trial assessing bortezomib and melphalan combination therapy for the treatment of patients with relapsed or refractory multiple myeloma. *J Clin Oncol* 2006;24(6):937–944.

69. Richardson P, Mitsiades C, Colson K, et al. Phase I trial of oral vorinostat (suberoylanilide hydroxamic acid, SAHA) in patients with advanced multiple myeloma. *Leuk Lymphoma* 2008;49(3):502–507.

70. Mitsiades N, Mitsiades CS, Richardson PG, et al. Molecular sequelae of histone deacetylase inhibition in human malignant B cells. *Blood* 2003;101(10):4055–4062.

71. Richardson PG, Mitsiades CS, Colson K, et al. Final results of a phase I trial of oral vorinostat (suberoylanilide hydroxamic acid, SAHA) in patients with advanced multiple myeloma. ASH Annual Meeting Abstracts [Abstract 1179]. *Blood* 2007;110(11).

72. Weber DM, Jagannath S, Sobecks R, et al. Combination of vorinostat plus bortezomib for the treatment of patients with multiple myeloma who have previously received bortezomib. ASH Annual Meeting Abstracts [Abstract 3711]. *Blood* 2008;112(11).

73. Weber DM, Jagannath S, Mazumder A, et al. Phase I trial of oral vorinostat (suberoylanilide hydroxamic acid, SAHA) in combination with bortezomib in patients with advanced multiple myeloma. ASH Annual Meeting Abstracts [Abstract 1172]. *Blood* 2007;110(11).

74. Chauhan D, Catley L, Li G, et al. A novel orally active proteasome inhibitor induces apoptosis in multiple myeloma cells with mechanisms distinct from Bortezomib. *Cancer Cell* 2005;8(5):407–419.

75. Kuhn DJ, Chen Q, Voorhees PM, et al. Potent activity of carfilzomib, a novel, irreversible inhibitor of the ubiquitin-proteasome pathway, against preclinical models of multiple myeloma. *Blood* 2007;110(9):3281–3290.

76. Jagannath S, Vij R, Stewart AK, et al. Initial Results of PX-171–003, An open-label, single-arm, phase II study of carfilzomib (CFZ) in patients with relapsed and refractory multiple myeloma (MM). ASH Annual Meeting Abstracts [Abstract 864]. *Blood* 2008;112(11).

77. Vij R, Wang M, Orlowski R, et al. Initial results of PX-171–004, an open-label, single-arm, phase II study of carfilzomib (CFZ) in patients with relapsed myeloma (MM). ASH Annual Meeting Abstracts [Abstract 865]. *Blood* 2008;112(11).

78. Wang L, Siegel D, Kaufman JL, et al. Updated results of bortezomib-naive patients in PX-171–004, an ongoing open-label, phase II study of single-agent carfilzomib (CFZ) in patients with relapsed or refractory myeloma (MM). ASH Annual Meeting Abstracts [Abstract 302]. *Blood* 2009;114(22).

79. Siegel D, Wang L, Orlowski RZ, et al. PX-171–004, An ongoing open-label, phase II study of single-agent carfilzomib (CFZ) in patients with relapsed or refractory myeloma (MM): updated results from the bortezomib-treated cohort. ASH Annual Meeting Abstracts [Abstract 303]. *Blood* 2009; 114(22).

80. Niesvizky R, Wang L, Orlowski RZ, et al. Phase Ib multicenter dose escalation study of carfilzomib plus lenalidomide and low dose dexamethasone (CRd) in relapsed and refractory multiple myeloma (MM). In: 51st American Society of Hematology Annual Meeting and Exposition; December 5–8, 2009; New Orleans, LA. Abstract 304.

81. Galustian C, Meyer B, Labarthe MC, et al. The anti-cancer agents lenalidomide and pomalidomide inhibit the proliferation and function of T regulatory cells. *Cancer Immunol Immunother* 2009;58(7):1033–1045.

82. Verhelle D, Corral LG, Wong K, et al. Lenalidomide and CC-4047 inhibit the proliferation of malignant B cells while expanding normal CD34+ progenitor cells. *Cancer Res* 2007;67(2):746–755.

83. Shalapour S, Zelmer A, Pfau M, et al. The thalidomide analogue, CC-4047, induces apoptosis signaling and growth arrest in childhood acute lymphoblastic leukemia cells *in vitro* and in vivo. *Clin Cancer Res* 2006;12(18):5526–5532.

84. Schey SA, Fields P, Bartlett JB, et al. Phase I study of an immunomodulatory thalidomide analog, CC-4047, in relapsed or refractory multiple myeloma. *J Clin Oncol* 2004;22(16):3269–3276.

85. Streetly M, Hunt BJ, Parmar K, Jones R, Zeldis J, Schey S. Markers of endothelial and haemostatic function in the treatment of relapsed myeloma with the immunomodulatory agent Actimid (CC-4047) and their relationship with venous thrombosis. *Eur J Haematol* 2005;74(4):293–296.

86. Lacy MQ, Hayman SR, Gertz MA, et al. Pomalidomide (CC4047) plus low-dose dexamethasone (Pom/dex) is highly effective therapy in relapsed multiple myeloma. ASH Annual Meeting Abstracts [Abstract 866]. *Blood* 2008;112(11).

87. Lacy MQ, Gertz MA, Hayman SR, et al. Pomalidomide (CC4047) plus low dose dexamethasone (Pom/dex) is active and well tolerated in lenalidomide refractory multiple myeloma (MM). ASH Annual Meeting Abstracts [Abstract 429]. *Blood* 2009;114(22).

88. Barlogie B, Hall R, Zander A, Dicke K, Alexanian R. High-dose melphalan with autologous bone marrow transplantation for multiple myeloma. *Blood* 1986;67(5):1298–1301.

89. Barlogie B, Alexanian R, Dicke KA, et al. High-dose chemoradiotherapy and autologous bone marrow transplantation for resistant multiple myeloma. *Blood* 1987;70(3):869–872.

90. Vesole DH, Barlogie B, Jagannath S, et al. High-dose therapy for refractory multiple myeloma: improved prognosis with better supportive care and double transplants. *Blood* 1994;84(3):950–956.

91. Alexanian R, Dimopoulos MA, Hester J, Delasalle K, Champlin R. Early myeloablative therapy for multiple myeloma. *Blood* 1994;84(12):4278–4282.

92. Alexanian R, Dimopoulos M, Smith T, Delasalle K, Barlogie B, Champlin R. Limited value of myeloablative therapy for late multiple myeloma. *Blood* 1994;83(2):512–516.

93. Fassas AB, Barlogie B, Ward S, et al. Survival after relapse following tandem autotransplants in multiple myeloma patients: the University of Arkansas total therapy I experience. *Br J Haematol* 2003;123(3):484–489.

94. Lee CK, Barlogie B, Zangari M, et al. Transplantation as salvage therapy for high-risk patients with myeloma in relapse. *Bone Marrow Transplant* 2002;30(12):873–878.

95. Fermand JP, Ravaud P, Chevret S, et al. High-dose therapy and autologous peripheral blood stem cell transplantation in multiple myeloma: up-front or rescue treatment? Results of a multicenter sequential randomized clinical trial. *Blood* 1998;92(9): 3131–3136.

96. Crawley C, Iacobelli S, Björkstrand B, Apperley JF, Niederwieser D, Gahrton G. Reduced-intensity conditioning for myeloma: lower nonrelapse mortality but higher relapse rates compared with myeloablative conditioning. *Blood* 2007;109(8):3588–3594.

97. Maloney DG, Molina AJ, Sahebi F, et al. Allografting with nonmyeloablative conditioning following cytoreductive autografts for the treatment of patients with multiple myeloma. *Blood* 2003;102(9):3447–3454.

98. Lee CK, Badros A, Barlogie B, et al. Prognostic factors in allogeneic transplantation for patients with high-risk multiple myeloma after reduced intensity conditioning. *Exp Hematol* 2003;31(1):73–80.

99. Giralt S, Aleman A, Anagnostopoulos A, et al. Fludarabine/melphalan conditioning for allogeneic transplantation in patients with multiple myeloma. *Bone Marrow Transplant* 2002;30(6):367–373.

100. Einsele H, Schäfer HJ, Hebart H, et al. Follow-up of patients with progressive multiple myeloma undergoing allografts after reduced-intensity conditioning. *Br J Haematol* 2003;121(3):411–418.

101. Qazilbash MH, Saliba R, De Lima M, et al. Second autologous or allogeneic transplantation after the failure of first autograft in patients with multiple myeloma. *Cancer* 2006;106(5):1084–1089.

102. Kröger N, Perez-Simon JA, Myint H, et al. Relapse to prior autograft and chronic graft-versus-host disease are the strongest prognostic factors for outcome of melphalan/fludarabine-based dose-reduced allogeneic stem cell transplantation in patients with multiple myeloma. *Biol Blood Marrow Transplant* 2004;10(10):698–708.

103. Kumar S, Mahmood ST, Lacy MQ, et al. Impact of early relapse after auto-SCT for multiple myeloma. *Bone Marrow Transplant* 2008;42(6):413–420.

104. Dawson MA, Opat SS, Taouk Y, et al. Clinical and immunohistochemical features associated with a

response to bortezomib in patients with multiple myeloma. *Clin Cancer Res* 2009;15(2):714–722.

105. von Metzler I, Krebbel H, Hecht M, et al. Bortezomib inhibits human osteoclastogenesis. *Leukemia* 2007;21(9):2025–2034.

106. Jagannath S, Richardson PG, Sonneveld P, et al. Bortezomib appears to overcome the poor prognosis conferred by chromosome 13 deletion in phase 2 and 3 trials. *Leukemia* 2007;21(1):151–157.

107. Richardson PG, Sonneveld P, Schuster MW, et al. Safety and efficacy of bortezomib in high-risk and elderly patients with relapsed multiple myeloma. *Br J Haematol* 2007;137(5):429–435.

108. Hussein MA, Baz R, Srkalovic G, et al. Phase 2 study of pegylated liposomal doxorubicin, vincristine, decreased-frequency dexamethasone, and thalidomide in newly diagnosed and relapsed-refractory multiple myeloma. *Mayo Clin Proc* 2006;81(7):889–895.

109. Baz R, Walker E, Karam MA, et al. Lenalidomide and pegylated liposomal doxorubicin-based chemotherapy for relapsed or refractory multiple myeloma: safety and efficacy. *Ann Oncol* 2006;17(12):1766–1771.

110. Palumbo A, Gay F, Bringhen S, et al. Bortezomib, doxorubicin and dexamethasone in advanced multiple myeloma. *Ann Oncol* 2008;19(6):1160–1165.

111. Richardson P, Wolf J, Jakubowiak A, et al. Phase I/II Results of a Multicenter Trial of Perifosine (KRX-0401) + Bortezomib in Patients with Relapsed or Relapsed/Refractory Multiple Myeloma Who Were Previously Relapsed from or Refractory to Bortezomib. ASH Annual Meeting Abstracts [Abstract 870]. *Blood* 2008;112(11).

112. Rossi J-F, Manges RF, Sutherland HJ, et al. Preliminary Results of CNTO 328, An Anti-Interleukin-6 Monoclonal Antibody, in Combination with Bortezomib in the Treatment of Relapsed or Refractory Multiple Myeloma. ASH Annual Meeting Abstracts [Abstract 867]. *Blood* 2008;112(11).

113. Voorhees PM, Manges RF, Somlo G, et al. A phase II multicenter study of CNTO 328, an anti-IL-6 monoclonal antibody, in patients (pts) with relapsed or refractory multiple myeloma (MM) [Abstract 8527]. *J Clin Oncol* 2009;27:15S.

114. Siegel Dd, Sezer O, San Miguel JF, et al. A phase IB, multicenter, open-label, dose-escalation study of oral panobinostat (LBH589) and I.V. bortezomib in patients with relapsed multiple myeloma. ASH Annual Meeting Abstracts [Abstract 2781]. *Blood* 2008;112(11).

115. Hofmeister CC, Richardson P, Zimmerman T, et al. Clinical trial of the novel structure proteasome inhibitor NPI-0052 in patients with relapsed and relapsed/refractory multiple myeloma (r/r MM) [Abstract 8505]. *J Clin Oncol* 2009;27:15S.

116. Harrison SJ, Quach H, Yuen K, et al. High response rates with the combination of bortezomib, dexamethasone and the pan-histone deacetylase inhibitor romidepsin in patients with relapsed or refractory multiple myeloma in a phase I/II clinical trial. *ASH Annual Meeting Abstracts*. 2008;112(11):3698.

117. Jakubowiak A, Richardson P, Zimmerman TM, et al. Phase I results of perifosine (KRX-0401) in combination with lenalidomide and dexamethasone in patients with relapsed or refractory multiple myeloma (MM). In: American Society of Hematology Annual Meeting; 2008. Abstract 3691.

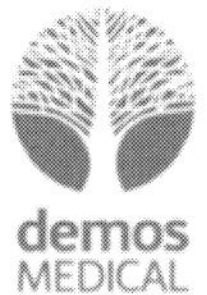

demos
MEDICAL

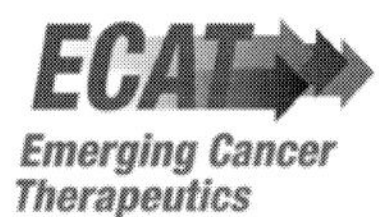

ECAT
Emerging Cancer
Therapeutics

Management of Treatment Complications and Supportive Care

Francis Buadi*

Mayo Clinic, Rochester, MN

■ ABSTRACT

Multiple myeloma is a malignancy involving plasma cells. This typically results in hypercalcemia (C), renal insufficiency (R), anemia (A), and lytic bone lesions or osteoporosis (B), referred to as CRAB and defined by the myeloma working group. The management of these complications is vital in the management of multiple myeloma. Approximately 20,000 cases of myeloma are diagnosed each year, with about 10,000 deaths occurring each year in the United States. The major cause of death in patients with multiple myeloma is infection and renal failure. The current armamentarium of drugs for the management of multiple myeloma is extensive, and these have changed significantly over the last decade. The traditional agents such as alkylators, anthracyclines, and platinum have given way to immunomodulatory drugs (thalidomide and lenalidomide) and the proteosome inhibitor bortezomib. In addition to the primary complications of multiple myeloma, all these drugs also do come with their own peculiar side effects, which will have to be effectively monitored and managed during their use.

Multiple myeloma is a malignancy involving plasma cells. However, in contrast to other malignancies, the mere presence of a clonal plasma cell disorder is not sufficient to assign the diagnosis of multiple myeloma (1). One is only classified as having active multiple myeloma when one has a clonal plasma cell disorder in association with organ damage and complications attributed to the proliferation of the clonal plasma cells (2,3). These primarily include hypercalcemia (C), renal insufficiency (R), anemia (A), and lytic bone lesions or osteoporosis (B), referred to as CRAB and defined by the myeloma working group (4). The management of these complications is vital in the management of multiple myeloma. In a study at the Mayo Clinic, anemia was the presenting sign in 73% of

*Corresponding author, Division of Hematology, Mayo Clinic, 200 First St, SW, Rochester, MN 55905
   E-mail addresses: Buadi.francis@mayo.edu

Emerging Cancer Therapeutics 1:2 (2010) 403–422.
© 2010 Demos Medical Publishing LLC. All rights reserved.
DOI: 10.5003/2151–4194.1.2.403

demosmedpub.com/ecat

the patients, lytic bone lesions in 66%, hypercalcemia in 13%, and renal insufficiency in 19% (5). Approximately 20,000 cases of myeloma are diagnosed each year, with about 10,000 deaths occurring each year in the United States of America. The major cause of death in patients with multiple myeloma is infection and renal failure, and the management of these is of vital importance in the long-term survival of these patients (6). The current armamentarium of drugs for the management of multiple myeloma is extensive, and these have changed significantly over the last decade. The traditional agents such as alkylators, anthracyclines, and platinum (7–10) have given way to immuno-modulatory drugs (thalidomide and lenalidomide) and the proteosome inhibitor bortezomib (11–14). In addition to the primary complications of multiple myeloma, all these drugs also do come with their own peculiar side effects, which will have to be effectively monitored and managed during their use. In this chapter, we will review the management of some of these complications.

■ ANEMIA

Anemia is the most common presentation of multiple myeloma. Published case series form the Mayo Clinic and other institutions have showed that about 50% to 80% of patients with multiple myeloma have anemia at the time of diagnosis (3,5,15). In the British and Chilean series, at least 50% had hemoglobulin less the 10 g/dL. Severe anemia requiring transfusion support was seen in 8% of patients in the study of 1,027 newly diagnosed patients published by Kyle et al. (5). The anemia is typically normocytic normochromic, and the usual symptom is fatigue. Almost all patients with progressive disease do develop anemia. Bone marrow failure as a result of replacement by plasma cells is the usual cause of the anemia, although decreased erythropoiesis mediated by cytokines such as tumor necrosis factor-alpha (TNFα), interleukin-1 (IL-1), and IL-6 may also occur (16,17). Anemia of chronic disease with its various mechanisms

such as ineffective erythropoiesis, decreased red cell survival, dysfunctional iron metabolism, and impaired erythropoietin response is well known. Other factors such as vitamin deficiency, chronic renal failure, and iron deficiency may play a role. Case reports of hemolytic anemia in patients with multiple myeloma have been reported (18–20).

The anemia usually should improve or resolve with treatment. Persistent anemia during therapy may be related to the effects of chemotherapy or disease progression. Lack of improvement in anemia should prompt evaluation for other causes of anemia such as vitamin and erythropoietin deficiency. Figure 1 shows an algorithm that can be used in the evaluation and management of anemia in patients with multiple myeloma. Certain chemotherapy regimen may worsen the anemia, but in these situations, baseline hemoglobulin should improve with subsequent therapy in responding patients.

Those presenting with severe symptomatic anemia should receive red cell transfusion. The benefit of packed red blood cell transfusion in this situation far outweighs the risk of transfusion-associated complications. This usually results in improvement of symptoms such as fatigue and general weakness. The need for transfusion support should decrease with disease response to therapy. Most patients will have had basic evaluation of their anemia as part of the initial diagnostic evaluation of their multiple myeloma. If anemia, however, persists, despite adequate response to therapy, other causes such as nutritional deficiencies should be considered. Vitamin B12 deficiency has been reported in patients with multiple myeloma (21–24). With the median age of multiple myeloma of 65 years, it is certainly not unusual to encounter vitamin deficiencies. Appropriate vitamin B12 replacement therapy should be instituted and is usually associated with improvement in hemoglobulin. Folate levels must also be assessed, because a small percentage of patients with multiple myeloma may have simultaneous amyloidosis with malabsorption syndrome leading to folate deficiency. Iron deficiency anemia must

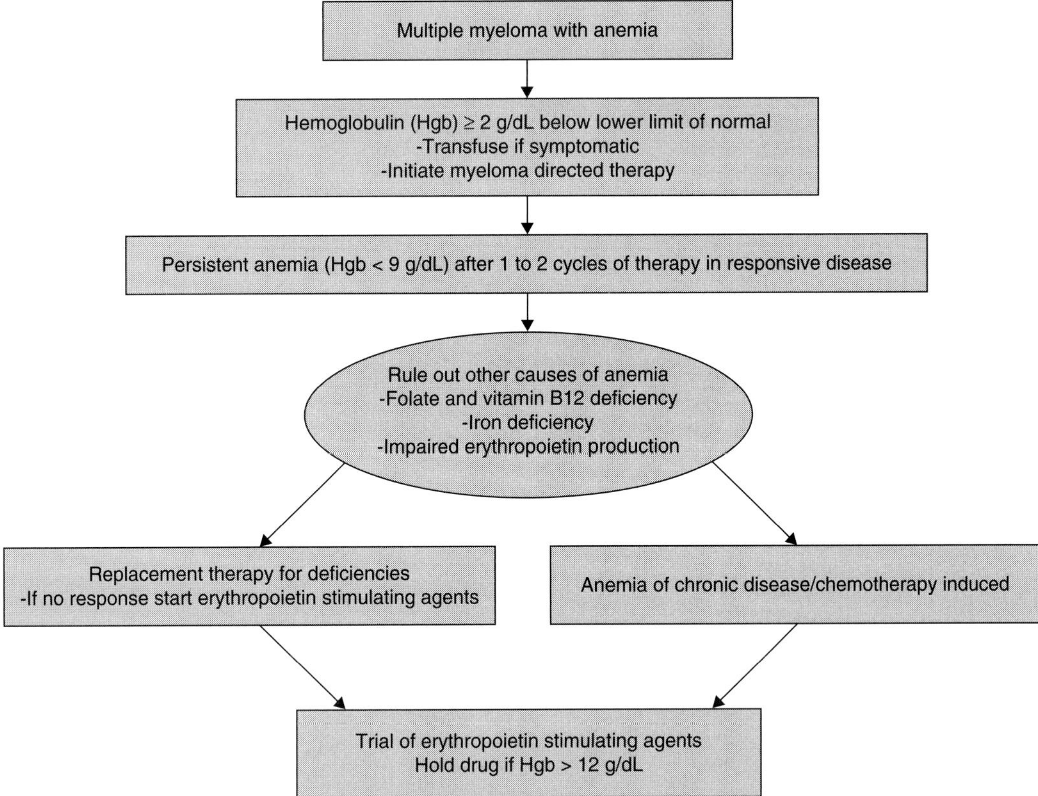

FIGURE 1

Algorithm for the management of anemia in multiple myeloma.

also be ruled out especially in patients who need erythropoietin stimulating agents (ESA) for the management of their anemia.

Renal failure is seen in about 19% of patients with multiple myeloma at presentation (5). Renal insufficiency with relative erythropoietin deficiency is common in this population. In these patients, anemia may be related to relative erythropoietin deficiency, and such patients may benefit from replacement therapy. The use of ESA in multiple myeloma, however, should not be routine. In particular, most patients will maintain a reasonable hemoglobulin on initiation of therapy for their multiple myeloma and will not require ESA. It should, however, be considered for those with persistent symptomatic multiple myeloma-associated anemia, renal insufficiency, and chemotherapy-induced anemia. The goal of therapy should be to improve quality of life and reduce or eliminate the need for red cell transfusion. The role and benefit of appropriate use of ESA have been shown in multiple studies (16,25–29). The use of ESA has been associated with improvement in hemoglobulin in about 60% to 75% of patients and also a better quality of life. Although the use of ESA is accepted by all societies (National Comprehensive Cancer Network, European Organisation for Research and Treatment of Cancer, The American Society of Clinical Oncology and The American Society of Hematology) involved in the use of these agents, the threshold for initiation varies (30–33). Most recommend starting ESA for hemoglobulin of less than 10 g/dL with a target hemoglobulin of 11 to 12 g/dL. The ESA available include erythropoietin alpha, beta, and darbepoetin, and they are of equivalent efficacy. The recommended starting dose of erythropoietin alpha or beta is 150 units/kg three times a week or 40,000 units weekly given subcutaneously. Darbepoetin is given at a dose of 2.25 mcg/kg weekly or 500 mcg subcutaneously every 3 weeks. In our practice at the Mayo Clinic, we do recommend initiating ESA for hemoglobulin less than 9 gm/dL and prefer darbepoetin 200 mcg every 2 weeks. Responses are usually seen in about 6 to 8 weeks, and dose adjustments, typically doubling of the dose, should be made at this time if no improvement in anemia is observed. Adequate iron stores are required for effective response to erythropoietin. A ferritin and iron saturation level should be checked and should be greater than 100 ng/dL and 20%, respectively. Iron replacement should be given if levels are inadequate. Treatment should be discontinued if there is no improvement in red cell transfusion requirement or improvement in hemoglobulin. If desired hemoglobulin is achieved, adjusting dose down by 25% to 40% may be required to maintain acceptable hemoglobulin level. Treatment should be discontinued if hemoglobulin exceeds 12 g/dL. The use of ESA is associated with complications such as thromboembolism 3% to 7%, hypertension 4% to 30%, and renal failure 12% (34–37). These complications are also common in multiple myeloma, especially thromboembolism (38), which may be exacerbated in the setting of immunomodulatory drugs such as thalidomide and lenalidomide (39). These patients should be monitored closely and full-dose anticoagulation with low-molecular-weight heparin (LMWH) or warfarin should be considered.

■ INFECTION

Infections are one of the major causes of mortality and morbidity in multiple myeloma (6,40–42). The reported incidence of infection in commonly used chemotherapy regimen for multiple myeloma is shown in Table 1 (11,43–47). The increased risk of infection is due to multiple factors, including

TABLE 1

Infection risk with commonly used multiple myeloma induction chemotherapy regimen[a]

Study	Regimen	No. of Patients	Neutropenia (%)	Infection Rate (%)	Death Due to Infection
Weber et al. (43)	Thal/Dex	68	0	14	1
Cavo et al. (44)	Thal/Dex	100	0	4	2
	VAD	100	12	5	0
Rajkumar et al. (11)	Thal/Dex	102	9	10	3
	Dex	102	6	7	1
Rajkumar et al. (45)	Len/Dex	34	44	3	1
Palumbo et al. (46)	MPT	129	16	10	5
	MP	126	17	2	2
Richardson et al. (47)	Bort/Dex	331	19	35	0

Bort, bortezomib; Dex, dexamethasone; Len/Dex, lenalidomide + dexamethasone; MP, melphalan, prednisone; MPT, melphalan, prednisone, thalidomide; Thal/Dex, thalidomide+dexamethasone; VAD, vincristine, adriamycin, dexamethasone.

[a]No reported antibiotic prophylaxis.

immunodeficiency (polyclonal hypogammaglobulinemia) and neutropenia as a result of disease and chemotherapy (48–51) and also the use of intravenous catheters. Poor ventilation and impaired control of respiratory secretions as a result of pain also increases the risk of pulmonary infections (52). In a study of 3,107 newly diagnosed cases of multiple myeloma by the Medical Research Council of United Kingdom, 299 died within the first 60 days of diagnosis, and out of this 135 (45%) were attributed to infections (6). Specifically, pneumonia occurred in 89 (66%) of 135 bacterial infections. Thoracic pain was identified in 22 (25%) of 89 patients with pneumonia. Suggesting that, better pain control may reduce this risk. Most of the patients did not have severe neutropenia, and at the time of diagnosis, only 11 of the 135 deaths from infection were classified as having neutropenia. The most common organisms cultured were *Pneumococcus pneumoniae, Staphylococcus aureus,* and *Escherichia coli.* The risk and type of infection vary depending on whether the individual is newly diagnosed, receiving induction chemotherapy, in plateau phase, or at relapse (52–56). Hargreaves et al. followed 102 patients in plateau phase and found that the risk of infection was four times at the time of active disease (53). In Perri's study, the incidence of infection per patient years in the first 2 months was 4.68 compared with 1.04 for subsequent months (54). The pattern of infection has changed over the years, especially in the era of early diagnosis, more use of effective novel therapy rather than cytotoxic chemotherapy, and the decrease use of corticosteroids (42,57). Although there is less neutropenia with these new agents, the risk of bacterial infections ranges between 10% and 40%. Rajkumar reported 10% incidence of infection in patients treated with thalidomide and dexamethasone, similar to an infection rate of 14% reported by Weber et al. (11,43). These novel therapies do also bring their own peculiar increased risk of certain infection, for example, high risk of herpes zoster with bortezomib (58–60). The reported incidence is about 13% in this population (61). In our quest to increase complete response rates because this has

been associated with better survival, more combination chemotherapy regimens and prolonged treatments are being used that are associated with cytopenias and more immunosuppression.

The use of prophylaxis has therefore become an integral part of the management of multiple myeloma. Although there are no large randomized studies available, the few published literature suggest a benefit. This is even more important during periods of neutropenia and the first few months of therapy (62). In a study conducted by Oken and colleagues, 54 patients with newly diagnosed multiple myeloma were randomized to receive prophylaxis with trimethoprim–sulfamethoxazole (TMP-SMX) 160/800 mg twice a day (n = 28) versus placebo (n = 26) for 2 months and followed for 3 months (63). The incidence of bacterial infection was significantly lower in the prophylaxis group (n = 2) compared with placebo (n = 11). Most clinical trials using combination chemotherapy associated with increased risk of neutropenia recommend antibiotic prophylaxis (64,65). Bacterial prophylaxis using TMP-SMX 80/400 daily is therefore recommended. Quinolones have also been shown to be effective (62); a quinolone or penicillin can be substituted for patients allergic to sulfa and also those receiving an immunomodulatory drug-based induction treatment because of the increased risk of rash associated with these drugs. The need for long-term bacterial prophylaxis should be reassessed after completion of induction therapy. Although uncommon, *Pneumocystis jiroveci* (PCP), formerly referred to as *Pneumocystis carinii*, is associated with a high mortality (66–69). This is even more important in those receiving consolidation and maintenance chemotherapy containing corticosteroids after stem cell transplantation. If patients are to remain on long-term corticosteroid therapy, TMP-SMX for PCP prophylaxis is recommended, especially those on high doses of corticosteroids (68,70,71). Antiviral prophylaxis for *Varicella zoster* is recommended for all patients receiving bortezomib-based chemotherapy because of the high incidence of herpes zoster. Acyclovir at 400 mg twice a day or valacyclovir 500 mg daily is typically used (72,73).

The value of vaccination against pneumococcus and influenza in patients with multiple myeloma is not clearly defined, and some studies suggest no benefit (74). The median age of patients with myeloma puts them at high risk for pneumococcal infection, and efficacy of Pneumovax has been documented in this population (75). Most studies, however, have shown some immune response even in patients with myeloma compared with baseline (56,76–78). In view of the low risk associated with this vaccination, Pneumovax and influenza vaccination should be offered to all newly diagnosed patients.

Intravenous immunoglobulin (IVIG) has been available for several decades and has been frequently used in patients with multiple myeloma. However, randomized studies on the use of IVIG in multiple myeloma are limited (79–81). In a randomized, double-blind, placebo-controlled, multicentre trial, 82 patients with stable multiple myeloma received monthly infusions of IVIG at 0.4 g/kg body weight or an equivalent volume of placebo (0.4% albumin) intravenously for 1 year (82). There were no episodes of septicemia or pneumonia in patients receiving IVIG compared with 10 in placebo patients ($P = 0.002$). IVIG also protected against recurrent infections in 60 patients who completed a year of treatment ($P = 0.021$). Before treatment, 54 of the patients who were immunized with Pneumovax had specific IgG responses measured. A poor pneumococcal IgG antibody response (less than twofold increase) identified patients who had maximum benefit from IVIG. No clear survival benefit, however, has been shown with the prophylactic use of IVIG. Although its use is not routinely recommended, it may be beneficial in reducing recurrent infection in a limited population.

■ ACUTE RENAL FAILURE

Impaired renal function may be present at initial presentation of multiple myeloma or can occur during the course of the disease. Approximately 20% of patients will present with some degree of renal insufficiency and up to 50% during the course of the disease (5,83). In a review of 423 multiple myeloma cases by Blade, 94 (22.2%) had renal impairment similar to the Mayo Clinic series of 19% (5,84). This is usually due to light chain cast nephropathy, hypercalcemia, dehydration, renal tubular dysfunction, nephrotoxic medications, and intravenous contrast dye. In a small percentage, this may be related to the simultaneous presence of renal diseases associated with monoclonal gammopathy such as light chain deposition disease, membranoproliferative glomerulonephritis, and amyloidosis (85).

Effective management of acute renal failure and rapid reversal of renal damage are not only essential for the ability to allow adequate dosing and to use all known effective medications, but data suggest that lack of improvement in renal function has a significant effect on long-term survival (86). Approximately 20% to 70% of patients will recover their renal function with aggressive management of the renal failure and effective multiple myeloma therapy (87).

In the blade series, the median survival of the 94 patients with renal failure was 8.6 months, whereas that of the 329 patients with normal renal function was 34.5 months ($P < 0.001$). The median survival was 28.3 months in those who recovered their renal function, not significantly different from those with normal renal function at presentation ($P = 0.97$). The Greek myeloma study group evaluation of 756 newly diagnosed patients also showed that the presence of renal failure at diagnosis was associated with inferior survival of 19.5 months versus 40.4 months for patients without renal failure ($P < 0.001$) (83). The frequency and reversibility of renal failure in 775 patients with multiple myeloma were studied by the Nordic myeloma group (86). Renal failure was observed in 29% of the cases at the time of diagnosis. Normalization of renal function was seen in 58% by the end of the first year of diagnosis, with most occurring within the first 3 months. Reversibility of renal failure was more frequently observed in patients with moderate renal failure, hypercalcemia, and low Bence-Jones protein excretion. Patients who needed dialysis had a poor prognosis, with a median survival of 3.5 months. A 12-month landmark analysis showed that reversibility of renal failure was an important prognostic factor and that reversibility of renal failure improves long-term survival similar to the finding by Blade. Renal failure with need for dialysis is generally irreversible; however, some patients may benefit from intensive management and survive for a longer period with good quality of life.

Hypercalcemia is seen in about 13% of multiple myeloma cases and does contribute to acute renal failure in these patients. It should be treated aggressively with hydration and forced diuresis (88,89). Bisphosphonate therapy should be an integral part of the management. Both pamidronate and zolendronic acid are effective; however, dose adjustment is needed for zolendronic acid in the setting of acute renal failure (90–94). Calcitonin alone or in combination with glucocorticoids is also effective and may be beneficial especially in cases refractory to bisphosphonates (95–97).

The role of plasma exchange in the management of acute renal failure in patients with multiple myeloma remains controversial. This is probably because not all renal failures in patients with multiple myeloma are related to light chain cast nephropathy. The largest randomized study to date from the Canadian apheresis group looked at 104 patients randomized to conventional chemotherapy therapy in addition to plasma exchange (n = 61) or conventional chemotherapy alone (n = 43) (98). The primary outcome was a composite measure of death, dialysis dependence, or glomerular filtration rate less than 30 mL/min per 1.73 m^2. This occurred in 33 of 57 (57.9%) patients in the plasma exchange group and in 27 of 39 (69.2%) patients in the control group (difference between groups, 11.3% [95% confidence interval, CI, −8.3–29.1]; P = 0.36). Concluding that, there was no benefit in the use of plasma exchange. One of the criticisms of this study was that kidney biopsies were not performed, and therefore there is the possibility of other causes of renal failure which are not responsive to plasma exchange.

Two other small randomized studies have also looked at the role of plasma exchange in multiple myeloma-associated acute renal failure. In 1990, Johnson and colleagues published a study of 21 patients who were randomly assigned either to plasma exchange and chemotherapy or to chemotherapy alone (99). There was no significant difference in renal recovery or patient survival; however, in the plasma exchange group, three out of dialysis-dependent patients were able to come of dialysis, compared with none in the control group (43% vs. 0%). This difference was not statistically significant, probably because of the small sample size.

The second study by Zucchelli and colleagues, however, reported a positive outcome with the use of plasma exchange in addition to chemotherapy (100). This study randomized 29 patients to plasma exchange (n = 15) in addition chemotherapy and hemodialysis when needed or to chemotherapy (n = 14) in addition to preemptive intermittent peritoneal dialysis. The outcomes were changes in renal function and patient survival. At 2 months, 11 out of 13 (85%) patients in the plasma exchange group had recovered sufficient renal function to stop dialysis, compared with 2 out of 11 (18%) in the control group (P < 0.01). Patient survival at 1 year was also superior in the plasma exchange group: 66% compared with 28% in the control group. In view of the fact that two of these studies showed the possibility of improvement in renal function, which has been shown to impact survival, plasma exchange should be considered in selected cases of myeloma-related acute renal failure. Patients who most probably will benefit are those with high circulating immunoglobulin light chain and light chain cast nephropathy on a kidney biopsy. Where possible, a kidney biopsy should be considered.

The primary goal in these situations should be rapid reduction of tumor burden using effective chemotherapy. Response rates in the range of 60% to 90% have been seen with the current chemotherapy regimen available for multiple myeloma (12,14,101,102). Most of these drugs have been used in patients with myeloma with acute renal failure (87,103–107). Table 2 (87,105,106,108–110) shows some of the reported outcomes in patients with renal failure treated with combination chemotherapy regimens incorporating newer novel agents. Thalidomide in combination with dexamethasone was given to 20 patients with refractory multiple myeloma and renal insufficiency; 45% achieved a

partial response and 25% minor response (105). Recovery to a normal renal function was observed in 12 of 15 responsive patients. Bortezomib has been well studied in patients with myeloma with renal failure. The safety and efficacy of bortezomib were detailed in a study of 10 patients with creatinine clearance (CrCl) less than 30 mL/min by Jagannath and colleagues (109). Seven patients completed eight cycles of treatment; four patients received the full dose of 1.3 mg/m², and three

TABLE 2
Outcome of multiple myeloma patients with renal failure treated with novel agents

Study	N	Regimen	Median Cr (Range)	HRR (%)	Post-therapy Median Cr	Number on HD	HD Discontinued	RRR (%)
Kastritis 2007 (87)	41	VAD (26) Thal + Dex (15)[a]	3.4 (2–12.8) mg/dL	46 64	83% had Cr < 2 mg/dL	10	8	18 (69) 12 (80)
Tosi 2004 (105)	20	Thal + Dex	All had Cr > 130 umol/L	75	12 had Cr < 130 umol/L	3	0	12 (60)
Ludwig 2007 (108)	8	Bort + Dex (5) VDD (3)	9.05 (5.2– 12.0) mg/dL	75	2.1 (0.8–2.4) mg/dL	5	–	5 (63)
Jagannath 2005 (109)	10	Bort + Dex	247.5 umol/L (124–389)	30	Mean serum Cr improved	0	–	–
Channan-Khan 2007 (110)	24	Bort + Dex (8) VTD (4) BDT (7) Others (5)[b]	6.8 (3.1– 12.8) mg/dL	75	–	23	3	4 (16)
Roussou 2008 (106)	20	Bort + Dex (8) VTD (2) VDD (3) VMTD (7)	3.9 (2–11.9) mg/dL	65	<2 mg/dL	5	1	10 (50)

BDT, bortezomib, doxil, thalidomide; Bort, bortezomib; Cr, creatinine; Dex, dexamethasone; HD, hemodialysis; HRR, hematologic response rate; RRR, renal response; Thal, thalidomide; VAD, vincristine, adriamycin, dexamethasone; VDD, bortezmib, doxil, dexamthasone; VMTD, bortezomib, melphalan, thalidomide, dexamethasone; VTD, bortezomib, thalidomide, dexamethasone.

[a] Two patients in that group received bortezomib.

[b] Various bortezomib containing regimen

patients received 1.0 mg/m^2. Responses were seen in these heavily pretreated patients, with no increased toxicity compared with those with normal renal function. Renal function did not appear to affect the 1-hour postdose proteasome inhibition or its recovery. Ludwig reported eight patients with myeloma-associated renal failure and a median creatine of 9.05 (5.2–12.0) mg/mL treated with bortezomib 1.0 mg/m^2 or 1.3 mg/m^2 on days 1, 4, 8, and 11 on a 3-week cycle (108). Five out of the eight patients experienced reversal of renal failure, with their median creatinine level decreasing from 9.05 mg/dL (5.2–12.0 mg/dL) to 2.1 mg/dL (0.8–2.4 mg/dL). All of the improvements were seen in 2½ months after starting therapy and were associated with disease response to chemotherapy. A multicenter retrospective study of 24 patients with renal failure all requiring dialysis except one, treated with bortezomib-based chemotherapy regimen, showed an overall hematologic response rate of 75%. One patient was spared dialysis, and three others were able to discontinue dialysis (110). In view of all these studies, patients with myeloma with renal insufficiency should be treated with bortezomib-based chemotherapy regimen.

For those patients who are well enough to proceed to an autologous stem cell transplant as part of their myeloma therapy, further recovery in renal function may occur (111,112). The largest study so far showing the benefit of autologous stem cell transplant in patients with myeloma with renal failure was published by Badros and colleagues (112). They reviewed 81 patients with multiple myeloma with renal failure (creatinine > 176.8 micromol/L) at the time of autologous stem cell transplantation (auto-SCT), including 38 patients on dialysis. Conditioning regimen was melphalan 200 mg/m^2 in 60 patients (27 on dialysis). The remaining 21 patients (11 on dialysis) received melphalan 140 mg/m^2 because of excessive toxicity. Thirty-one patients (38%) completed tandem auto-SCT, including 11 on dialysis. Complete hematologic remission was achieved in 21 patients (26%) after first auto-SCT and 31 patients (38%) after tandem auto-SCT. Two patients discontinued

dialysis after auto-SCT. Probabilities of event-free survival and overall survival at 3 years were 48% and 55%, respectively. The same group also looked at 59 patients on dialysis at the time of autologous stem cell transplant (113). A total of 37 patients had been on dialysis for more than 6 months. Of 54 patients evaluable for renal function improvement, 13 (24%) became dialysis independent at a median of 4 months after auto-SCT (range: 1–16). Dialysis duration 6 months or less prior to first auto-SCT and pretransplant CrCl more than 10 mL/min were significant for renal function recovery. This treatment option should be offered to patients with myeloma with renal failure who are otherwise eligible for autologous stem cell transplant and early in the disease course because of the potential benefit.

■ BONE DISEASE

Bone destruction presenting in the form of osteolytic lesion, osteopenia, osteoporosis, and skeletal fractures is common in multiple myeloma and in a significant number of cases is the initial presenting feature (5). The bone destruction is initiated and maintained by increased osteoclastic activity due to the effect of cytokines such as IL-1, IL-6, and TNF secreted by myeloma cells and bone marrow stromal cells (17,114,115). These usually may manifest as bone pain, pathologic fractures, or vertebra compression fracture. These skeletal complications are associated with significant morbidity. Detailed radiologic evaluation of all bones should be performed with metastatic bone survey. Magnetic resonance imaging and whole-body computerized tomography scanning with positron emission tomography may be required for better evaluation of abnormal bony lesions or any areas of concern. Pathologic fractures or areas at risk for pathologic fractures especially weight-bearing bones must be evaluated by an orthopedic surgeon and appropriate intervention instituted.

Intractable bone pain should be treated with analgesics or radiation treatment. Adequate analgesic therapy including nonsteroidal antiinflammatory drugs (NSAIDs) and narcotics may be required to control pain. However, one must be careful with the use of NSAID in the setting of renal insufficiency because 20% of multiple myeloma patients will present with some degree of renal failure. Palliative radiation is associated with rapid pain and disease control (116). When using local radiotherapy, the recommended dose for control of bone pain in myeloma is 10 to 20 Gy given over 5 to 10 fractions (117–119). Radiation therapy should, however, be used with caution so as to limit the extent of bone marrow exposure which may affect hematopoietic reserve.

Vertebral compression fractures may be treated with vertebroplasty, balloon kyphoplasty, or radiation therapy (120–123). The VERTOS study evaluated the short-term clinical outcome of patients with subacute or chronic painful osteoporotic vertebral compression fractures treated with percutaneous vertebroplasty (PV) compared with optimal pain medication (OPM) (124). Thirty-four patients were enrolled in the study. Eighteen patients were randomized to be treated by PV and 16 patients by OPM. Pain relief and improvement of mobility, function, and stature after PV were immediate and significantly better in the short term compared with OPM treatment. A randomized multicenter balloon kyphoplasty trial also looked at 300 patients assigned to kyphoplasty treatment ($n = 149$) or nonsurgical care ($n = 151$) (125). At 1 month, the mean physical component score (36 physical component summary score on a 0–100 scale) improved by 7.2 points (95% CI, 5.7–8.8) in the kyphoplasty group and by 2.0 points (0.4–3.6) in the nonsurgical group ($P < 0.0001$). There, however, have been questions about the real benefit of these vertebral procedures in pain management. One of such studies looked at 78 patients randomized to vertebroplasty ($n = 38$) and placebo ($n = 40$) with a 6-month follow-up (126). Vertebroplasty did not result in a significant advantage in any measured outcome at any time point. At 3 months, the mean (±SD) reductions in the score for pain in the vertebroplasty and control groups were 2.6 ± 2.9

and 1.9 ± 3.3, respectively. Similar improvements were seen in both groups with respect to pain at night and at rest, physical functioning, quality of life, and perceived improvement. A larger study by the Investigational Vertebroplasty Efficacy and Safety Trial, a randomized controlled trial of PV, is currently underway to help resolve the role of these vertebral procedures (127). Until this is resolved, these vertebral procedures should be individualized.

The benefit of bisphosphonate therapy (pamidronate or zoledronic acid) in reducing skeletal events in multiple myeloma has been shown in multiple clinical studies (128–130). However, the enthusiasm for routine and continuous use of bisphosphonates has been influenced by the risk of osteonecrosis of the jaw (131–134). This risk, however, may be reduced by good dental hygiene and referral of patients with chronic periodontal problems to a dentist for treatment and dental extraction prior to starting bisphosphonate therapy (135–137). Antibiotic prophylaxis before dental procedures may be helpful in patients on bisphosphonates (138). Patients should be continuously evaluated for the development of osteonecrosis of the mandible. Although both pamidronate and zoledronic acid do cause osteonecrosis of the jaw, the incidence seems to be slightly higher in zoledronic acid. In our practice, pamidronate is therefore favored over zoledronic acid (139). Pamidronate is given intravenously over 2 hours at a dose of 90 mg every 4 weeks. No dosage adjustment is recommended in renal impairment when given monthly. Zoledronic acid is administered as an intravenous infusion over 15 minutes at a dose of 4 mg every 4 weeks. Dose adjustment is, however, required for patients with renal impairment. Oral calcium and vitamin D supplements should be recommended for all patients on bisphosphonate therapy. The duration of therapy is not clearly defined. Long-term use has been associated with stress fractures (140–142). Treatment is therefore recommended for a total of 2 years, and frequency of administration can be reduced to every 3 months in the second

TABLE 3
Mayo Clinic practice guidelines for bisphosphonate use in multiple myeloma (MM)

Clinical Scenario	Recommendation
MM and lytic disease evident on plain radiographs	Intravenous bisphosphonates should be administered monthly
	Oral calcium and Vitamin D Supplement for all patients on bisphosphonates
MM with osteopenia or osteoporosis but no lytic disease	Reasonable to start if osteopenia or osteoporosis is evident on bone mineral density studies
Duration of therapy	Monthly for first year; every 3 months for second year:
	At 2 years, if in stable plateau phase, discontinue therapy
	If still active treatment, continue every 3 months
Choice of bisphosphonate	Pamidronate
Follow-up of patients taking bisphosphonates	Comprehensive dental evaluation before treatment
	Maximize preventive care
	Withhold bisphosphonate treatment for at least 1 month before dental procedure and do not resume until the patient has fully recovered and healing of the surgery is complete
	Consider prophylactic antibiotics for dental procedures

Adapted from Lacy et al. (139).

year for those who achieve complete response and/or plateau phase (139). For patients whose disease is active, or who have threatening bone disease beyond 2 years, therapy can be decreased to every 3 months. The Mayo Clinic consensus guidelines are shown in Table 3 (139).

■ NEUROPATHY

Monoclonal gammopathies have long been known to be associated with neurologic disorders. Some of the well-described conditions include primary amyloidosis, POEMS syndrome (osteosclerotic myeloma), cryoglobulinemia, and the most common of all monoclonal gammopathy-associated peripheral neuropathy (143–147). Patients with overt myeloma may also have neuropathy as a complication of their disease (148,149). In a small number of patients, this is due to a structural abnormality such as infiltration of tumor into the spinal cord or peripheral nerve. However, in a larger number of cases, the primary mechanism is not well understood (150). These neurologic complications at diagnosis, however, are significantly low compared with the neuropathies that are associated with the therapeutic interventions use to control their multiple myeloma. Although this has always been a major problem even with traditional chemotherapy agents used in the treatment of multiple myeloma such as vincristine and cisplatin (151–153), the incidence has significantly increased in the era of immunomodulatory drugs and proteosome inhibitors. Thalidomide, the first approved immunomodulatory drug for the management of myeloma, is associated with a 25% to 80% incidence of neuropathy (154,155). This is related to dose and duration of therapy as seen in a study by Mileshkin and colleagues, in which neuropathy increased from 38% at 6 months to 73% at 12 months, with 81% of responding patients developing this complication (154). The second-generation immunomodulatory drug lenalidomide, however, has a significantly lower incidence of neuropathy, with most studies reporting about 3% to 23% incidence and only 3% with greater than grade 3 neuropathy (156–160). The first-generation proteosome inhibitor bortezomib is associated with a 35% to 80% incidence of neuropathy (47,102,161).

In a phase II study of bortezomib in 64 patients with newly diagnosed multiple myeloma, sensory polyneuropathy developed during treatment in 64% of patients (grade 3 in 3%), but this resolved in 85% within a median of 98 days (160). Underlying neuropathy, duration, and frequency of therapy, in addition to dose, seem to be the risk factors for the development of neuropathy (149,160).

Bortezomib-associated neuropathy, although a common toxicity, is reversible in most patients, if identified early and appropriate intervention such as discontinuation of drug or dose adjustment is instituted (161,162).

These drugs are highly effective in the management of multiple myeloma, and higher response rates are seen when used in combination. Therefore, preemptive evaluation and early management of neuropathy must be incorporated in the management of all patients with multiple myeloma. Prior to starting therapy, patients should be evaluated for signs and symptoms of peripheral neuropathy and educated about the symptoms and the importance of reporting them. There should be continuing evaluation during treatment so that appropriate interventions can be employed if necessary. This should begin with exclusion of other treatable causes of neuropathy such as vitamin B12 deficiency (22–24). Specific management strategies are based on the severity of the peripheral neuropathy. In mild cases, modification of dose and schedule will prevent progression. In the case of bortezomib, weekly dosing has been associated with less neuropathy (163,164). In severe cases, treatment will initially have to be discontinued and resumed at lower doses after resolution of symptoms.

Therapeutic interventions include analgesic and antiepileptic agents, and these may improve mood, sleep disturbance, and quality of life.

Tricyclic antidepressants (amitriptyline) and anticonvulsants (gabapentin and pregabalin) have become the primary treatment for chemotherapy-induced peripheral neuropathy. The antiepileptic agent gabapentin has shown benefit in managing peripheral neuropathy. The starting dose should be 300 mg daily, and this can be escalated to 2,700 mg depending on response. In diabetic-associated peripheral neuropathy, pregabalin was found to be safe and effective in decreasing pain (165,166). The literature on its use in cancer and chemotherapy-associated neuropathy is limited. In a study of 30 children (median age 13.5 years) with chemotherapy-induced neuropathic pain, pregabalin was given at a daily dose of 150 to 300 mg for 8 weeks (167). A significant and long-lasting pain relief was noted in 86% of these patients. If pharmacologic therapy is required, we do recommend gabapentin 300 to 2,700 mg daily or pregabalin 150 to 300 mg daily. In most cases, patients do require analgesic therapy. In severe cases, narcotic analgesics or the monoaminergic drug tramadol have been shown to be beneficial (168). In our practice, a topical formulation containing ketamine 0.5%, lidocaine 2%, and amitriptyline 2% have been used with good symptomatic pain control. Other measures that may reduce pain and also reduce injury include wearing soft loose fit shoes and minimal bedding over feet at night. Regular screening and monitoring, combined with patient education and effective management strategies, can reduce the risk of these treatment-related complications as well as their consequences.

■ THROMBOSIS

The increased risk of thrombosis in cancer has been well known (169–171). The risk of thrombosis in multiple myeloma is estimated at about 3% (38,172). Prior to the era of immunomodulatory drugs, thrombosis in myeloma was attributed to the disease, immobilization as a result of bone pain, fractures, and dexamethasone therapy. The recent introduction of immunomodulatory drugs as an integral part of myeloma therapy has increase the risk significantly. Thalidomide and lenalidomide in combination with dexamethasone has been associated with about 10% to 30% risk of thrombosis (173–176). Preemptive intervention is therefore recommended in all patients receiving immunomodulatory drugs (177). All patients on immunomodulatory drugs should be monitored closely for the development of thrombosis. Preventive therapies have included aspirin, LMWH, and warfarin (159,178–182). All of these therapies have been shown to reduce the risk of thrombosis, but there are no comparative studies to show which therapy is superior. LMWH and warfarin, however, do come with an increased risk of bleeding, and because they have not been shown to be superior to aspirin, we do recommend aspirin as the initial thrombosis prophylaxis. Patients with prior history of thrombosis or other increase risk of thrombosis should be treated with full anticoagulation with LMWH or warfarin (183). Those on immunomodulatory drugs who develop thrombosis while on aspirin should have their drug held and started on full anticoagulation. This can be resumed after they are well anticoagulated (179).

■ REFERENCES

1. Kyle RA, Remstein ED, Therneau TM, et al. Clinical course and prognosis of smoldering (asymptomatic) multiple myeloma. *N Engl J Med* 2007;356(25): 2582–2590.
2. Bladé J, Rosiñol L. Complications of multiple myeloma. *Hematol Oncol Clin North Am* 2007;21(6):1231–1246, xi.
3. Conte LG, Figueroa MG, Lois VV, et al. Clinical features and survival of Chilean patients with multiple myeloma [in Spanish]. *Rev Med Chil* 2007;135(9):1111–1117.
4. International Myeloma Working Group. Criteria for the classification of monoclonal gammopathies, multiple myeloma and related disorders: a report of the International Myeloma Working Group. *Br J Haematol* 2003;121(5):749–757.
5. Kyle RA, Gertz MA, Witzig TE, et al. Review of 1027 patients with newly diagnosed multiple myeloma. *Mayo Clin Proc* 2003;78(1):21–33.
6. Augustson BM, Begum G, Dunn JA, et al. Early mortality after diagnosis of multiple myeloma: analysis of patients entered onto the United kingdom Medical Research Council trials between 1980 and 2002–Medical Research Council Adult Leukaemia Working Party. *J Clin Oncol* 2005;23(36): 9219–9226.
7. Barlogie B, Smith L, Alexanian R. Effective treatment of advanced multiple myeloma refractory to alkylating agents. *N Engl J Med* 1984;310(21):1353–1356.
8. Alexanian R, Barlogie B, Tucker S. VAD-based regimens as primary treatment for multiple myeloma. *Am J Hematol* 1990;33(2):86–89.
9. Dimopoulos MA, Kastritis E. Is there still place for VAD as primary treatment for patients with multiple myeloma who are candidates for high-dose therapy? *Leuk Lymphoma* 2006;47(11):2271–2272.
10. Kyle RA, Rajkumar SV. Treatment of multiple myeloma: a comprehensive review. *Clin Lymphoma Myeloma* 2009;9(4):278–288.
11. Rajkumar SV, Blood E, Vesole D, Fonseca R, Greipp PR; Eastern Cooperative Oncology Group. Phase III clinical trial of thalidomide plus dexamethasone compared with dexamethasone alone in newly diagnosed multiple myeloma: a clinical trial coordinated by the Eastern Cooperative Oncology Group. *J Clin Oncol* 2006;24(3):431–436.
12. Rajkumar SV, Jacobus S, Callander NS, et al.; Eastern Cooperative Oncology Group. Lenalidomide plus high-dose dexamethasone versus lenalidomide plus low-dose dexamethasone as initial therapy for newly diagnosed multiple myeloma: an open-label randomised controlled trial. *Lancet Oncol* 2010;11(1):29–37.
13. Richardson PG, Sonneveld P, Schuster M, et al. Extended follow-up of a phase 3 trial in relapsed multiple myeloma: final time-to-event results of the APEX trial. *Blood* 2007;110(10):3557–3560.
14. Harousseau JL, Attal M, Leleu X, et al. Bortezomib plus dexamethasone as induction treatment prior to autologous stem cell transplantation in patients with newly diagnosed multiple myeloma: results of an IFM phase II study. *Haematologica* 2006;91(11): 1498–1505.
15. Prognostic features in the third MRC myelomatosis trial. Medical Research Council's Working Party on Leukaemia in Adults. *Br J Cancer* 1980;42(6): 831–840.
16. Musto P, Falcone A, D'Arena G, et al. Clinical results of recombinant erythropoietin in transfusion-dependent patients with refractory multiple myeloma:

role of cytokines and monitoring of erythropoiesis. *Eur J Haematol* 1997;58(5):314–319.

17. Carter A, Merchav S, Silvian-Draxler I, Tatarsky I. The role of interleukin-1 and tumour necrosis factor-alpha in human multiple myeloma. *Br J Haematol* 1990;74(4):424–431.

18. Vaiopoulos G, Kyriakou D, Papadaki H, Fessas P, Eliopoulos GD. Multiple myeloma associated with autoimmune hemolytic anemia. *Haematologica* 1994;79(3):262–264.

19. Friedland M, Schaefer P. Myelomatosis and hemolytic anemia. Hemolytic anemia, a rare complication of multiple myeloma, is successfully managed by splenectomy. *R I Med J* 1979;62(12):469–471.

20. Wada H, Yata K, Mikami M, et al. Multiple myeloma complicated by autoimmune hemolytic anemia. *Intern Med* 2004;43(7):595–598.

21. Vlasveld LT. Low cobalamin (vitamin B12) levels in multiple myeloma: a retrospective study. *Neth J Med* 2003;61(8):249–252.

22. Heyerdahl F, Kildahl-Andersen O. [Myelomatosis and low level of vitamin B12]. *Tidsskr Nor Laegeforen* 1999;119(29):4321–4322.

23. Perillie PE. Myeloma and pernicious anemia. *Am J Med Sci* 1978;275(1):93–98.

24. Hansen OP, Drivsholm A, Hippe E, Quadros E, Linnell JC. Interrelationships between Vitamin B12 and folic acid in myelomatosis: cobalamin coenzyme and tetrahydrofolic acid function. *Scand J Haematol* 1978;20(4):360–370.

25. Ludwig H, Fritz E, Kotzmann H, Höcker P, Gisslinger H, Barnas U. Erythropoietin treatment of anemia associated with multiple myeloma. *N Engl J Med* 1990;322(24):1693–1699.

26. Osterborg A, Brandberg Y, Molostova V, et al.; Epoetin Beta Hematology Study Group. Randomized, double-blind, placebo-controlled trial of recombinant human erythropoietin, epoetin Beta, in hematologic malignancies. *J Clin Oncol* 2002;20(10):2486–2494.

27. Dammacco F, Castoldi G, Rödjer S. Efficacy of epoetin alfa in the treatment of anaemia of multiple myeloma. *Br J Haematol* 2001;113(1):172–179.

28. Garton JP, Gertz MA, Witzig TE, et al. Epoetin alfa for the treatment of the anemia of multiple myeloma. A prospective, randomized, placebo-controlled, double-blind trial. *Arch Intern Med* 1995;155(19):2069–2074.

29. Cazzola M, Messinger D, Battistel V, et al. Recombinant human erythropoietin in the anemia associated with multiple myeloma or non-Hodgkin's lymphoma: dose finding and identification of predictors of response. *Blood* 1995;86(12):4446–4453.

30. Rizzo JD, Somerfield MR, Hagerty KL, et al.; American Society of Clinical Oncology; American Society of Hematology. Use of epoetin and darbepoetin in patients with cancer: 2007 American Society of Clinical Oncology/American Society of Hematology clinical practice guideline update. *J Clin Oncol* 2008;26(1):132–149.

31. Straus DJ, Testa MA, Sarokhan BJ, et al. Quality-of-life and health benefits of early treatment of mild anemia: a randomized trial of epoetin alfa in patients receiving chemotherapy for hematologic malignancies. *Cancer* 2006;107(8):1909–1917.

32. Charu V, Saidman B, Ben-Jacob A, et al. A randomized, open-label, multicenter trial of immediate versus delayed intervention with darbepoetin alfa for chemotherapy-induced anemia. *Oncologist* 2007;12(10):1253–1263.

33. Osterborg A, Boogaerts MA, Cimino R, et al. Recombinant human erythropoietin in transfusion-dependent anemic patients with multiple myeloma and non-Hodgkin's lymphoma—a randomized multicenter study. The European Study Group of Erythropoietin (Epoetin Beta) Treatment in Multiple Myeloma and Non-Hodgkin's Lymphoma. *Blood* 1996;87(7):2675–2682.

34. Bennett CL, Silver SM, Djulbegovic B, et al. Venous thromboembolism and mortality associated with recombinant erythropoietin and darbepoetin administration for the treatment of cancer-associated anemia. *JAMA* 2008;299(8):914–924.

35. Vanrenterghem Y, Bárány P, Mann JF, et al.; European/Australian NESP 970200 Study Group. Randomized trial of darbepoetin alfa for treatment of renal anemia at a reduced dose frequency compared with rHuEPO in dialysis patients. *Kidney Int* 2002;62(6):2167–2175.

36. Steurer M, Sudmeier I, Stauder R, Gastl G. Thromboembolic events in patients with myelodysplastic syndrome receiving thalidomide in combination with darbepoietin-alpha. *Br J Haematol* 2003;121(1):101–103.

37. Singh AK, Szczech L, Tang KL, et al.; CHOIR Investigators. Correction of anemia with epoetin alfa in chronic kidney disease. *N Engl J Med* 2006;355(20):2085–2098.

38. Catovsky D, Ikoku NB, Pitney WR, Galton DA. Thromboembolic complications in myelomatosis. *Br Med J* 1970;3(5720):438–439.

39. Galli M, Elice F, Crippa C, Comotti B, Rodeghiero F, Barbui T. Recombinant human erythropoietin and the risk of thrombosis in patients receiving

thalidomide for multiple myeloma. *Haematologica* 2004;89(9):1141–1142.

40. Doughney KB, Williams DM, Penn RL. Multiple myeloma: infectious complications. *South Med J* 1988;81(7):855–858.

41. Paradisi F, Corti G, Cinelli R. Infections in multiple myeloma. *Infect Dis Clin North Am* 2001;15(2): 373–84, vii.

42. Espersen F, Birgens HS, Hertz JB, Drivsholm A. Current patterns of bacterial infection in myelomatosis. *Scand J Infect Dis* 1984;16(2):169–173.

43. Weber D, Rankin K, Gavino M, Delasalle K, Alexanian R. Thalidomide alone or with dexamethasone for previously untreated multiple myeloma. *J Clin Oncol*. 2003;21(1):16–19.

44. Cavo M, Zamagni E, Tosi P, et al. Superiority of thalidomide and dexamethasone over vincristine-doxorubicin dexamethasone (VAD) as primary therapy in preparation for autologous transplantation for multiple myeloma. *Blood*, 2005;106(1):35–9.

45. Rajkumar SV, Hayman SR, Lacy MQ, et al. Combination therapy with lenalidomide plus dexamethasone (Rev/Dex) for newly diagnosed myeloma. *Blood*, 2005;106(13):4050–3.

46. Palumbo A, Bringhen S, Caravita T, et al. Oral melphalan and prednisone chemotherapy plus thalidomide compared with melphalan and prednisone alone in elderly patients with multiple myeloma: randomised controlled trial. *Lancet*, 2006;367(9513):825–31.

47. Richardson PG, Sonneveld P, Schuster MW, et al.; Assessment of Proteasome Inhibition for Extending Remissions (APEX) Investigators. Bortezomib or high-dose dexamethasone for relapsed multiple myeloma. *N Engl J Med* 2005;352(24):2487–2498.

48. Hopen G, Glette J, Halstensen A, Kalager T, Schreiner A, Solberg CO. Granulocyte function in malignant monoclonal gammopathy. *Scand J Haematol* 1983;31(2):133–143.

49. Jacobson DR, Zolla-Pazner S. Immunosuppression and infection in multiple myeloma. *Semin Oncol* 1986;13(3):282–290.

50. Cesana C, Nosari AM, Klersy C, et al. Risk factors for the development of bacterial infections in multiple myeloma treated with two different vincristine-adriamycin-dexamethasone schedules. *Haematologica* 2003;88(9):1022–1028.

51. Cheson BD, Plass RR, Rothstein G. Defective opsonization in multiple myeloma. *Blood* 1980;55(4):602–606.

52. Goranov S. Clinical problems of infectious complications in patients with multiple myeloma. *Folia Med (Plovdiv)*. 1994;36(1):41–46.

53. Hargreaves RM, Lea JR, Griffiths H, et al. Immunological factors and risk of infection in plateau phase myeloma. *J Clin Pathol*. 1995;48(3):260–266.

54. Perri RT, Hebbel RP, Oken MM. Influence of treatment and response status on infection risk in multiple myeloma. *Am J Med*. 1981;71(6):935–940.

55. Savage DG, Lindenbaum J, Garrett TJ. Biphasic pattern of bacterial infection in multiple myeloma. *Ann Intern Med*. 1982;96(1):47–50.

56. Einarsdóttir HM, Erlendsdóttir H, Kristinsson KG, Gottfredsson M. Nationwide study of recurrent invasive pneumococcal infections in a population with a low prevalence of human immunodeficiency virus infection. *Clin Microbiol Infect*. 2005;11(9): 744–749.

57. Shaikh BS, Lombard RM, Appelbaum PC, Bentz MS. Changing patterns of infections in patients with multiple myeloma. *Oncology*. 1982;39(2):78–82.

58. Kim SJ, Kim K, Kim BS, et al.; Korean Multiple Myeloma Working Party. Bortezomib and the increased incidence of herpes zoster in patients with multiple myeloma. *Clin Lymphoma Myeloma* 2008;8(4):237–240.

59. Hasegawa Y, Kawahara F, Nagai H, et al. [Prophylaxis with acyclovir for herpes zoster infection during bortezomib-dexamethasone combination therapy]. *Rinsho Ketsueki* 2009;50(6):488–494.

60. Basler M, Lauer C, Beck U, Groettrup M. The proteasome inhibitor bortezomib enhances the susceptibility to viral infection. *J Immunol* 2009;183 (10):6145–6150.

61. Chanan-Khan A, Sonneveld P, Schuster MW, et al. Analysis of herpes zoster events among bortezomib-treated patients in the phase III APEX study. *J Clin Oncol* 2008;26(29):4784–4790.

62. Reuter S, Kern WV, Sigge A, et al. Impact of fluoroquinolone prophylaxis on reduced infection-related mortality among patients with neutropenia and hematologic malignancies. *Clin Infect Dis* 2005;40(8):1087–1093.

63. Oken MM, Pomeroy C, Weisdorf D, Bennett JM. Prophylactic antibiotics for the prevention of early infection in multiple myeloma. *Am J Med* 1996; 100(6):624–628.

64. Lee CK, Barlogie B, Munshi N, et al. DTPACE: an effective, novel combination chemotherapy with thalidomide for previously treated patients with myeloma. *J Clin Oncol* 2003;21(14):2732–2739.

65. Reeder CB, Reece DE, Kukreti V, et al. Cyclophosphamide, bortezomib and dexamethasone induction for newly diagnosed multiple myeloma:

high response rates in a phase II clinical trial. *Leukemia* 2009;23(7):1337–1341.

66. van der Lelie J, Venema D, Kuijper EJ, et al. Pneumocystis carinii pneumonia in HIV-negative patients with haematologic disease. *Infection* 1997; 25(2):78–81.

67. Worth LJ, Dooley MJ, Seymour JF, Mileshkin L, Slavin MA, Thursky KA. An analysis of the utilisation of chemoprophylaxis against Pneumocystis jirovecii pneumonia in patients with malignancy receiving corticosteroid therapy at a cancer hospital. *Br J Cancer* 2005;92(5):867–872.

68. Pagano L, Fianchi L, Mele L, et al. Pneumocystis carinii pneumonia in patients with malignant haematological diseases: 10 years' experience of infection in GIMEMA centres. *Br J Haematol* 2002;117(2):379–386.

69. Peters SG, Prakash UB. Pneumocystis carinii pneumonia. Review of 53 cases. *Am J Med* 1987;82(1):73–78.

70. Roblot F, Le Moal G, Godet C, et al. Pneumocystis carinii pneumonia in patients with hematologic malignancies: a descriptive study. *J Infect* 2003; 47(1):19–27.

71. Yale SH, Limper AH. Pneumocystis carinii pneumonia in patients without acquired immunodeficiency syndrome: associated illness and prior corticosteroid therapy. *Mayo Clin Proc* 1996;71(1):5–13.

72. Vickrey E, Allen S, Mehta J, Singhal S. Acyclovir to prevent reactivation of varicella zoster virus (herpes zoster) in multiple myeloma patients receiving bortezomib therapy. *Cancer* 2009;115(1):229–232.

73. Pour L, Adam Z, Buresova L, et al. Varicella-zoster virus prophylaxis with low-dose acyclovir in patients with multiple myeloma treated with bortezomib. *Clin Lymphoma Myeloma* 2009;9(2):151–153.

74. Robertson JD, Nagesh K, Jowitt SN, et al. Immunogenicity of vaccination against influenza, Streptococcus pneumoniae and Haemophilus influenzae type B in patients with multiple myeloma. *Br J Cancer* 2000;82(7):1261–1265.

75. Butler JC, Breiman RF, Campbell JF, Lipman HB, Broome CV, Facklam RR. Pneumococcal polysaccharide vaccine efficacy. An evaluation of current recommendations. *JAMA* 1993;270(15):1826–1831.

76. Shildt RA, Rubin RR, Schiffman G, Giolma P. Polyvalent pneumococcal immunization of patients with plasma cell dyscrasias. *Cancer* 1981;48(6): 1377–1380.

77. Landesman SH, Schiffman G. Assessment of the antibody response to pneumococcal vaccine in high-risk populations. *Rev Infect Dis* 1981;3 suppl:S184–S197.

78. Lazarus HM, Lederman M, Lubin A, et al. Pneumococcal vaccination: the response of patients with multiple myeloma. *Am J Med* 1980;69(3): 419–423.

79. Gordon DS, Hearn EB, Spira TJ, Reimer CB, Phillips DJ, Schable C. Phase I study of intravenous gamma globulin in multiple myeloma. *Am J Med* 1984;76(3A):111–116.

80. Musto P, Brugiatelli M, Carotenuto M. Prophylaxis against infections with intravenous immunoglobulins in multiple myeloma. *Br J Haematol* 1995;89(4):945–946.

81. Raanani P, Gafter-Gvili A, Paul M, Ben-Bassat I, Leibovici L, Shpilberg O. Immunoglobulin prophylaxis in chronic lymphocytic leukemia and multiple myeloma: systematic review and meta-analysis. *Leuk Lymphoma* 2009;50(5):764–772.

82. Chapel HM, Lee M, Hargreaves R, Pamphilon DH, Prentice AG. Randomised trial of intravenous immunoglobulin as prophylaxis against infection in plateau-phase multiple myeloma. The UK Group for Immunoglobulin Replacement Therapy in Multiple Myeloma. *Lancet* 1994;343(8905):1059–1063.

83. Eleutherakis-Papaiakovou V, Bamias A, Gika D, et al.; Greek Myeloma Study Group. Renal failure in multiple myeloma: incidence, correlations, and prognostic significance. *Leuk Lymphoma* 2007;48(2):337–341.

84. Bladé J, Fernández-Llama P, Bosch F, et al. Renal failure in multiple myeloma: presenting features and predictors of outcome in 94 patients from a single institution. *Arch Intern Med* 1998;158(17): 1889–1893.

85. Leung N, Gertz MA, Zeldenrust SR, et al. Improvement of cast nephropathy with plasma exchange depends on the diagnosis and on reduction of serum free light chains. *Kidney Int* 2008;73(11):1282–1288.

86. Knudsen LM, Hjorth M, Hippe E. Renal failure in multiple myeloma: reversibility and impact on the prognosis. Nordic Myeloma Study Group. *Eur J Haematol* 2000;65(3):175–181.

87. Kastritis E, Anagnostopoulos A, Roussou M, et al. Reversibility of renal failure in newly diagnosed multiple myeloma patients treated with high dose dexamethasone-containing regimens and the impact of novel agents. *Haematologica* 2007;92(4):546–549.

88. Elliott GT, McKenzie MW. Treatment of hypercalcemia. *Drug Intell Clin Pharm* 1983;17(1):12–22.

89. Singer FR, Ritch PS, Lad TE, et al. Treatment of hypercalcemia of malignancy with intravenous etidronate. A controlled, multicenter study. The Hypercalcemia Study Group. *Arch Intern Med* 1991;151(3):471–476.

90. Davenport A, Goel S, Mackenzie JC. Treatment of hypercalcaemia with pamidronate in patients with end stage renal failure. *Scand J Urol Nephrol* 1993;27(4):447–451.

91. Machado CE, Flombaum CD. Safety of pamidronate in patients with renal failure and hypercalcemia. *Clin Nephrol* 1996;45(3):175–179.

92. Gucalp R, Theriault R, Gill I, et al. Treatment of cancer-associated hypercalcemia. Double-blind comparison of rapid and slow intravenous infusion regimens of pamidronate disodium and saline alone. *Arch Intern Med* 1994;154(17):1935–1944.

93. Nussbaum SR, Younger J, Vandepol CJ, et al. Single-dose intravenous therapy with pamidronate for the treatment of hypercalcemia of malignancy: comparison of 30-, 60-, and 90-mg dosages. *Am J Med* 1993;95(3):297–304.

94. Major PP, Coleman RE. Zoledronic acid in the treatment of hypercalcemia of malignancy: results of the international clinical development program. *Semin Oncol* 2001;28(2 Suppl 6):17–24.

95. Sekine M, Takami H. Combination of calcitonin and pamidronate for emergency treatment of malignant hypercalcemia. *Oncol Rep* 1998;5(1):197–199.

96. Binstock ML, Mundy GR. Effect of calcitonin and glutocorticoids in combination on the hypercalcemia of malignancy. *Ann Intern Med* 1980; 93(2):269–272.

97. Wisneski LA, Croom WP, Silva OL, Becker KL. Salmon calcitonin in hypercalcemia. *Clin Pharmacol Ther* 1978;24(2):219–222.

98. Clark WF, Stewart AK, Rock GA, et al.; Canadian Apheresis Group. Plasma exchange when myeloma presents as acute renal failure: a randomized, controlled trial. *Ann Intern Med* 2005;143(11):777–784.

99. Johnson WJ, Kyle RA, Pineda AA, O'Brien PC, Holley KE. Treatment of renal failure associated with multiple myeloma. Plasmapheresis, hemodialysis, and chemotherapy. *Arch Intern Med* 1990;150(4):863–869.

100. Zucchelli P, Pasquali S, Cagnoli L, Ferrari G. Controlled plasma exchange trial in acute renal failure due to multiple myeloma. *Kidney Int* 1988;33(6):1175–1180.

101. Rajkumar SV, Rosiñol L, Hussein M, et al. Multicenter, randomized, double-blind, placebo-controlled study of thalidomide plus dexamethasone compared with dexamethasone as initial therapy for newly diagnosed multiple myeloma. *J Clin Oncol* 2008;26(13):2171–2177.

102. Jagannath S, Durie BG, Wolf J, et al. Bortezomib therapy alone and in combination with dexamethasone for previously untreated symptomatic multiple myeloma. *Br J Haematol* 2005;129(6):776–783.

103. Ludwig H, Zojer N. Renal recovery with lenalidomide in a patient with bortezomib-resistant multiple myeloma. *Nat Rev Clin Oncol* 2010;7(5):289–294.

104. Dimopoulos MA, Christoulas D, Roussou M, et al. Lenalidomide and dexamethasone for the treatment of refractory/relapsed multiple myeloma: dosing of lenalidomide according to renal function and effect on renal impairment. *Eur J Haematol* 2010;[Epub ahead of print].

105. Tosi P, Zamagni E, Cellini C, et al. Thalidomide alone or in combination with dexamethasone in patients with advanced, relapsed or refractory multiple myeloma and renal failure. *Eur J Haematol* 2004;73(2):98–103.

106. Roussou M, Kastritis E, Migkou M, et al. Treatment of patients with multiple myeloma complicated by renal failure with bortezomib-based regimens. *Leuk Lymphoma* 2008;49(5):890–895.

107. Carlson K, Hjorth M, Knudsen LM; Nordic Myeloma Study Group. Toxicity in standard melphalan-prednisone therapy among myeloma patients with renal failure–a retrospective analysis and recommendations for dose adjustment. *Br J Haematol* 2005;128(5):631–635.

108. Ludwig H, Drach J, Graf H, Lang A, Meran JG. Reversal of acute renal failure by bortezomib-based chemotherapy in patients with multiple myeloma. *Haematologica* 2007;92(10):1411–1414.

109. Jagannath S, Barlogie B, Berenson JR, et al.; SUMMIT/CREST Investigators. Bortezomib in recurrent and/or refractory multiple myeloma. Initial clinical experience in patients with impared renal function. *Cancer* 2005;103(6):1195–1200.

110. Chanan-Khan AA, Kaufman JL, Mehta J, et al. Activity and safety of bortezomib in multiple myeloma patients with advanced renal failure: a multicenter retrospective study. *Blood* 2007;109(6):2604–2606.

111. Tauro S, Clark FJ, Duncan N, Lipkin G, Richards N, Mahendra P. Recovery of renal function after autologous stem cell transplantation in myeloma patients with end-stage renal failure. *Bone Marrow Transplant* 2002;30(7):471–473.

112. Badros A, Barlogie B, Siegel E, et al. Results of autologous stem cell transplant in multiple myeloma patients with renal failure. *Br J Haematol* 2001;114(4):822–829.

113. Lee CK, Zangari M, Barlogie B, et al. Dialysis-dependent renal failure in patients with myeloma can be reversed by high-dose myeloablative therapy and autotransplant. *Bone Marrow Transplant* 2004;33(8):823–828.

114. Abildgaard N, Glerup H, Rungby J, et al. Biochemical markers of bone metabolism reflect osteoclastic and osteoblastic activity in multiple myeloma. *Eur J Haematol* 2000;64(2):121–129.

115. Merico F, Bergui L, Gregoretti MG, et al. Cytokines involved in the progression of multiple myeloma. *Clin Exp Immunol* 1993;92(1):27–31.

116. Yaneva MP, Goranova-Marinova V, Goranov S. Palliative radiotherapy in patients with multiple myeloma. *J BUON* 2006;11(1):43–48.

117. Adamietz IA, Schöber C, Schulte RW, Peest D, Renner K. Palliative radiotherapy in plasma cell myeloma. *Radiother Oncol* 1991;20(2):111–116.

118. Leigh BR, Kurtts TA, Mack CF, Matzner MB, Shimm DS. Radiation therapy for the palliation of multiple myeloma. *Int J Radiat Oncol Biol Phys* 1993;25(5):801–804.

119. Mill WB, Griffith R. The role of radiation therapy in the management of plasma cell tumors. *Cancer* 1980;45(4):647–652.

120. Saliou G, Kocheida el M, Lehmann P, et al. Percutaneous vertebroplasty for pain management in malignant fractures of the spine with epidural involvement. *Radiology* 2010;254(3):882–890.

121. Lim BS, Chang UK, Youn SM. Clinical outcomes after percutaneous vertebroplasty for pathologic compression fractures in osteolytic metastatic spinal disease. *J Korean Neurosurg Soc* 2009;45(6): 369–374.

122. Bartolozzi B, Nozzoli C, Pandolfo C, et al. Percutaneous vertebroplasty and kyphoplasty in patients with multiple myeloma. *Eur J Haematol* 2006;76(2):180–181.

123. Diamond TH, Hartwell T, Clarke W, Manoharan A. Percutaneous vertebroplasty for acute vertebral body fracture and deformity in multiple myeloma: a short report. *Br J Haematol* 2004;124(4):485–487.

124. Voormolen MH, Mali WP, Lohle PN, et al. Percutaneous vertebroplasty compared with optimal pain medication treatment: short-term clinical outcome of patients with subacute or chronic painful osteoporotic vertebral compression fractures. The VERTOS study. *AJNR Am J Neuroradiol* 2007;28(3):555–560.

125. Wardlaw D, Cummings SR, Van Meirhaeghe J, et al. Efficacy and safety of balloon kyphoplasty compared with non-surgical care for vertebral compression fracture (FREE): a randomised controlled trial. *Lancet* 2009;373(9668):1016–1024.

126. Buchbinder R, Osborne RH, Ebeling PR, et al. A randomized trial of vertebroplasty for painful osteoporotic vertebral fractures. *N Engl J Med* 2009;361(6):557–568.

127. Gray LA, Jarvik JG, Heagerty PJ, et al. INvestigational Vertebroplasty Efficacy and Safety Trial (INVEST): a randomized controlled trial of percutaneous vertebroplasty. *BMC Musculoskelet Disord* 2007;8:126.

128. Berenson JR, Lichtenstein A, Porter L, et al. Efficacy of pamidronate in reducing skeletal events in patients with advanced multiple myeloma. Myeloma Aredia Study Group. *N Engl J Med* 1996;334(8):488–493.

129. Rosen LS, Gordon D, Kaminski M, et al. Zoledronic acid versus pamidronate in the treatment of skeletal metastases in patients with breast cancer or osteolytic lesions of multiple myeloma: a phase III, double-blind, comparative trial. *Cancer J* 2001;7(5):377–387.

130. Kraj M, Poglód R, Maj S, Pawlikowski J, Sokolowska U, Szczepanik J. Comparative evaluation of safety and efficacy of pamidronate and zoledronic acid in multiple myeloma patients (single center experience). *Acta Pol Pharm* 2002;59(6):478–482.

131. Ruggiero SL, Mehrotra B, Rosenberg TJ, Engroff SL. Osteonecrosis of the jaws associated with the use of bisphosphonates: a review of 63 cases. *J Oral Maxillofac Surg* 2004;62(5):527–534.

132. Durie BG, Katz M, Crowley J. Osteonecrosis of the jaw and bisphosphonates. *N Engl J Med* 2005;353(1):99–102; discussion 99.

133. Badros A, Terpos E, Katodritou E, et al. Natural history of osteonecrosis of the jaw in patients with multiple myeloma. *J Clin Oncol* 2008; 26(36):5904–5909.

134. Pozzi S, Marcheselli R, Falorio S, et al.; Gruppo Italiano Studio Linfomi (GISL). Bisphosphonates-associated osteonecrosis of the jaw: A long-term follow-up of a series of 35 cases observed by GISL and evaluation of its frequency over time. *Am J Hematol* 2009;84(12):850–852.

135. Bagán J, Blade J, Cozar JM, et al. Recommendations for the prevention, diagnosis, and treatment of osteonecrosis of the jaw (ONJ) in cancer patients treated with bisphosphonates. *Med Oral Patol Oral Cir Bucal* 2007;12(4):E336–E340.

136. Chu V; American Association of Oral and Maxillofacial Surgeons; American Dental Association.

Management of patients on bisphosphonates and prevention of bisphosphonate-related osteonecrosis of the jaw. *Hawaii Dent J* 2008;39(5):9–12; quiz 17.

137. Landis BN, Richter M, Dojcinovic I, Hugentobler M. Osteonecrosis of the jaw after treatment with bisphosphonates: is irreversible, so the focus must be on prevention. *BMJ* 2006;333(7576):982–983.

138. Montefusco V, Gay F, Spina F, et al. Antibiotic prophylaxis before dental procedures may reduce the incidence of osteonecrosis of the jaw in patients with multiple myeloma treated with bisphosphonates. *Leuk Lymphoma* 2008;49(11):2156–2162.

139. Lacy MQ, Dispenzieri A, Gertz MA, et al. Mayo clinic consensus statement for the use of bisphosphonates in multiple myeloma. *Mayo Clin Proc* 2006;81(8):1047–1053.

140. Odvina CV, Levy S, Rao S, Zerwekh JE, Rao DS. Unusual mid-shaft fractures during long-term bisphosphonate therapy. *Clin Endocrinol (Oxf)* 2010;72(2):161–168.

141. Napoli N, Novack D, Armamento-Villareal R. Bisphosphonate-associated femoral fracture: implications for management in patients with malignancies. *Osteoporos Int* 2010;21(4):705–708.

142. Koh JS, Goh SK, Png MA, Kwek EB, Howe TS. Femoral cortical stress lesions in long-term bisphosphonate therapy: a herald of impending fracture? *J Orthop Trauma* 2010;24(2):75–81.

143. Kelly JJ Jr, Kyle RA, Miles JM, Dyck PJ. Osteosclerotic myeloma and peripheral neuropathy. *Neurology* 1983;33(2):202–210.

144. Dispenzieri A, Kyle RA, Lacy MQ, et al. POEMS syndrome: definitions and long-term outcome. *Blood* 2003;101(7):2496–2506.

145. Wilson JR, Stittsworth JD Jr, Fisher MA. Electrodiagnostic patterns in MGUS neuropathy. *Electromyogr Clin Neurophysiol* 2001;41(7):409–418.

146. Noring L, Osby E, Hast R, Kjellin KG, Knutsson E, Sidén A. Peripheral neuropathy in patients with benign monoclonal gammopathy–a pilot study. *J Neurol* 1982;228(3):185–194.

147. Nobile-Orazio E, Barbieri S, Baldini L, et al. Peripheral neuropathy in monoclonal gammopathy of undetermined significance: prevalence and immunopathogenetic studies. *Acta Neurol Scand* 1992;85(6):383–390.

148. Kelly JJ Jr, Kyle RA, Miles JM, O'Brien PC, Dyck PJ. The spectrum of peripheral neuropathy in myeloma. *Neurology* 1981;31(1):24–31.

149. Richardson PG, Xie W, Mitsiades C, et al. Single-agent bortezomib in previously untreated multiple myeloma: efficacy, characterization of peripheral neuropathy, and molecular correlations with response and neuropathy. *J Clin Oncol* 2009;27(21):3518–3525.

150. Besinger UA, Toyka KV, Anzil AP, Fateh-Mognadam A, Rouscher R, Heininger K. Myeloma neuropathy: passive transfer from man to mouse. *Science* 1981;213(4511):1027–1030.

151. Roelofs RI, Hrushesky W, Rogin J, Rosenberg L. Peripheral sensory neuropathy and cisplatin chemotherapy. *Neurology* 1984;34(7):934–938.

152. van der Hoop RG, van der Burg ME, ten Bokkel Huinink WW, van Houwelingen C, Neijt JP. Incidence of neuropathy in 395 patients with ovarian cancer treated with or without cisplatin. *Cancer* 1990;66(8):1697–1702.

153. Windebank AJ, Grisold W. Chemotherapy-induced neuropathy. *J Peripher Nerv Syst* 2008;13(1):27–46.

154. Mileshkin L, Stark R, Day B, Seymour JF, Zeldis JB, Prince HM. Development of neuropathy in patients with myeloma treated with thalidomide: patterns of occurrence and the role of electrophysiologic monitoring. *J Clin Oncol* 2006;24(27):4507–4514.

155. Plasmati R, Pastorelli F, Cavo M, et al. Neuropathy in multiple myeloma treated with thalidomide: a prospective study. *Neurology* 2007;69(6):573–581.

156. Argyriou AA, Iconomou G, Kalofonos HP. Bortezomib-induced peripheral neuropathy in multiple myeloma: a comprehensive review of the literature. *Blood* 2008;112(5):1593–1599.

157. Dahut WL, Aragon-Ching JB, Woo S, et al. Phase I study of oral lenalidomide in patients with refractory metastatic cancer. *J Clin Pharmacol* 2009;49(6):650–660.

158. Richardson PG, Blood E, Mitsiades CS, et al. A randomized phase 2 study of lenalidomide therapy for patients with relapsed or relapsed and refractory multiple myeloma. *Blood* 2006;108(10):3458–3464.

159. Gay F, Hayman SR, Lacy MQ, et al. Lenalidomide plus dexamethasone versus thalidomide plus dexamethasone in newly diagnosed multiple myeloma: a comparative analysis of 411 patients. *Blood* 2010;115(7):1343–1350.

160. Richardson PG, Briemberg H, Jagannath S, et al. Frequency, characteristics, and reversibility of peripheral neuropathy during treatment of advanced multiple myeloma with bortezomib. *J Clin Oncol* 2006;24(19):3113–3120.

161. Richardson PG, Sonneveld P, Schuster MW, et al. Reversibility of symptomatic peripheral

neuropathy with bortezomib in the phase III APEX trial in relapsed multiple myeloma: impact of a dose-modification guideline. *Br J Haematol* 2009;144(6):895–903.

162. El-Cheikh J, Stoppa AM, Bouabdallah R, et al. Features and risk factors of peripheral neuropathy during treatment with bortezomib for advanced multiple myeloma. *Clin Lymphoma Myeloma* 2008;8(3):146–152.

163. Hainsworth JD, Spigel DR, Barton J, et al. Weekly treatment with bortezomib for patients with recurrent or refractory multiple myeloma: a phase 2 trial of the Minnie Pearl Cancer Research Network. *Cancer* 2008;113(4):765–771.

164. Suvannasankha A, Smith GG, Juliar BE, Abonour R. Weekly bortezomib/methylprednisolone is effective and well tolerated in relapsed multiple myeloma. *Clin Lymphoma Myeloma* 2006;7(2):131–134.

165. Rosenstock J, Tuchman M, LaMoreaux L, Sharma U. Pregabalin for the treatment of painful diabetic peripheral neuropathy: a double-blind, placebo-controlled trial. *Pain* 2004;110(3):628–638.

166. Tölle T, Freynhagen R, Versavel M, Trostmann U, Young JP Jr. Pregabalin for relief of neuropathic pain associated with diabetic neuropathy: a randomized, double-blind study. *Eur J Pain* 2008;12(2):203–213.

167. Vondracek P, Oslejskova H, Kepak T, et al. Efficacy of pregabalin in neuropathic pain in paediatric oncological patients. *Eur J Paediatr Neurol* 2009;13(4):332–336.

168. Sindrup SH, Andersen G, Madsen C, Smith T, Brøsen K, Jensen TS. Tramadol relieves pain and allodynia in polyneuropathy: a randomised, double-blind, controlled trial. *Pain* 1999;83(1):85–90.

169. Nordström M, Lindblad B, Anderson H, Bergqvist D, Kjellström T. Deep venous thrombosis and occult malignancy: an epidemiological study. *BMJ* 1994;308(6933):891–894.

170. Falanga A, Donati MB. Pathogenesis of thrombosis in patients with malignancy. *Int J Hematol* 2001;73(2):137–144.

171. Hettiarachchi RJ, Lok J, Prins MH, Büller HR, Prandoni P. Undiagnosed malignancy in patients with deep vein thrombosis: incidence, risk indicators, and diagnosis. *Cancer* 1998;83(1):180–185.

172. Kristinsson SY, Fears TR, Gridley G, et al. Deep vein thrombosis after monoclonal gammopathy of undetermined significance and multiple myeloma. *Blood* 2008;112(9):3582–3586.

173. Cavo M, Zamagni E, Cellini C, et al. Deep-vein thrombosis in patients with multiple myeloma receiving first-line thalidomide-dexamethasone therapy. *Blood* 2002;100(6):2272–2273.

174. Camba L, Peccatori J, Pescarollo A, Tresoldi M, Corradini P, Bregni M. Thalidomide and thrombosis in patients with multiple myeloma. *Haematologica* 2001;86(10):1108–1109.

175. Menon SP, Rajkumar SV, Lacy M, Falco P, Palumbo A. Thromboembolic events with lenalidomide-based therapy for multiple myeloma. *Cancer* 2008;112(7):1522–1528.

176. Rus C, Bazzan M, Palumbo A, Bringhen S, Boccadoro M. Thalidomide in front line treatment in multiple myeloma: serious risk of venous thromboembolism and evidence for thromboprophylaxis. *J Thromb Haemost* 2004;2(11):2063–2065.

177. Palumbo A, Rajkumar SV, Dimopoulos MA, et al.; International Myeloma Working Group. Prevention of thalidomide- and lenalidomide-associated thrombosis in myeloma. *Leukemia* 2008;22(2):414–423.

178. Miller KC, Padmanabhan S, Dimicelli L, et al. Prospective evaluation of low-dose warfarin for prevention of thalidomide associated venous thromboembolism. *Leuk Lymphoma* 2006;47(11):2339–2343.

179. Zangari M, Barlogie B, Anaissie E, et al. Deep vein thrombosis in patients with multiple myeloma treated with thalidomide and chemotherapy: effects of prophylactic and therapeutic anticoagulation. *Br J Haematol* 2004;126(5):715–721.

180. Baz R, Li L, Kottke-Marchant K, et al. The role of aspirin in the prevention of thrombotic complications of thalidomide and anthracycline-based chemotherapy for multiple myeloma. *Mayo Clin Proc* 2005;80(12):1568–1574.

181. Zonder JA, Barlogie B, Durie BG, McCoy J, Crowley J, Husscin MA. Thrombotic complications in patients with newly diagnosed multiple myeloma treated with lenalidomide and dexamethasone: benefit of aspirin prophylaxis. *Blood* 2006;108(1):403; author reply 404.

182. Minnema MC, Breitkreutz I, Auwerda JJ, et al. Prevention of venous thromboembolism with low molecular-weight heparin in patients with multiple myeloma treated with thalidomide and chemotherapy. *Leukemia* 2004;18(12):2044–2046.

183. Jiménez-Zepeda VH, Domínguez-Martínez VJ. Acquired activated protein C resistance and thrombosis in multiple myeloma patients. *Thromb J* 2006;4:11.

Index

Note: Page numbers followed by "*f*" and "*t*" denote figures and tables, respectively.